D1348935

Diseases of the Lymphatics

Diseases of the Lymphatics

SIR NORMAN BROWSE, MD FRCS FRCP
Professor of Surgery, Emeritus and
Honorary Consulting Surgeon
St Thomas' Hospital, London

KEVIN G BURNAND, MS FRCS
Professor of Surgery
King's College, London and
Consultant Surgeon
Guy's and St Thomas' Trust, London

PETER S MORTIMER, MD FRCP
Professor of Dermatological Medicine and
Consultant Skin Physician
St George's and The Royal Marsden Hospitals
London

with contributions from
Professor Judit Daróczy, Dr Peter Gloviczki,
Professor J Rodney Levick, Professor Noel McHale,
Professor Thomas Mentzel, Dr Thomas O'Donnell,
Professor Hugo Partsch, Professor Terence Ryan and
Mr John Wolfe

A member of the Hodder Headline Group
LONDON

First published in Great Britain in 2003 by
Arnold, a member of the Hodder Headline Group,
338 Euston Road, London NW1 3BH

http://www.arnoldpublishers.com

Distributed in the United States of America by
Oxford University Press Inc.,
198 Madison Avenue, New York, NY10016
Oxford is a registered trademark of Oxford University Press

Whilst the advice and information in this book are believed to be
true and accurate at the date of going to press, neither the authors
nor the publisher can accept any legal responsibility or liability for
any errors or omissions that may be made. In particular (but
without limiting the generality of the preceding disclaimer) every
effort has been made to check drug dosages; however, it is still
possible that errors have been missed. Furthermore, dosage
schedules are constantly being revised and new side-effects
recognized. For these reasons the reader is strongly urged to
consult the drug companies' printed instructions before
administering any of the drugs recommended in this book.

British Library Cataloguing in Publication Data
A catalogue record for this book is available from the British Library

Library of Congress Cataloging-in-Publication Data
A catalog record for this book is available from the Library of
Congress

ISBN 0 340 76203 9

1 2 3 4 5 6 7 8 9 10

Publisher: Georgina Bentliff
Development Editor: Michael Lax
Production Editor: Wendy Rooke
Production Controller: Bryan Eccleshall

Typeset in 10/12 pt Minion by Charon Tec Pvt. Ltd, Chennai, India
Printed and bound in Malta

What do you think about this book? Or any other Arnold title?
Please send your comments to **feedback.arnold@hodder.co.uk**

Dedicated to

John Bernard Kinmonth
(1917–1983)
foremost amongst lymphologists

Contents

Contributors

Sir Norman Browse MD FRCS FRCP
Professor of Surgery, Emeritus
and Honorary Consulting Surgeon
St Thomas' Hospital
London, UK

Kevin G Burnand MS FRCS
Professor of Surgery
King's College, London and
Consultant Surgeon
Guy's and St Thomas' Trust
London, UK

Judit Daróczy MD
Professor of Dermatology and
Head of 2nd Dermatology Unit
St Stephan Hospital
Budapest, Hungary

Peter Gloviczki MD
Professor of Surgery
Mayo Medical School and
Chair Division of Vascular Surgery
Mayo Clinic and Mayo Foundation
Rochester, Minnesota, USA

J Rodney Levick DSc DPhil MA BM BCh Oxon
Professor of Physiology
St George's Hospital Medical School
London, UK

Noel G. McHale BSc PhD MRPharmS
Professor of Physiology
Queen's University
Belfast, UK

Thomas Mentzel MD
Consultant Pathologist
Department of Dermatohistopathology
Friedrichschafen, Germany

Peter S Mortimer MD FRCP
Professor of Dermatological Medicine and
Consultant Skin Physician
St George's and The Royal Marsden Hospitals
London, UK

Thomas O'Donnell MD
Chairman, Department of Surgery
New England Medical Center
Tufts University School of Medicine
Boston, Massachusetts, USA

Hugo Partsch MD
Professor of Dermatology
Department of Medicine
University of Vienna
Austria

Terence J Ryan
Professor of Dermatology
Oxford Centre for Health Care, Research and Development
Oxford Brookes University
Oxford, UK

John Wolfe MS FRCS
Consultant Vascular Surgeon
St Mary's Hospital
London, UK

Preface

Primary abnormalities of the lymphatic system are rare; secondary abnormalities of the lymphatic system are not uncommon, especially those caused by filariasis. Methods for investigating lymphatic abnormalities did not become available until the 1950s, when John Kinmonth introduced his technique of human clinical lymphangiography. In 1972, after 20 years of clinical investigation, Kinmonth wrote his seminal book *The lymphatics*, in which he described the clinical and lymphographic appearances and treatment of many lymphatic diseases and abnormalities. In the 20 years that have passed since the second edition of that book was published in 1982, the year before Kinmonth's untimely death, our methods of investigating and our understanding of lymphatic physiology and pathology have significantly increased and our treatments, both medical and surgical, improved. It therefore seemed that the time had come to write a new book about diseases of the lymphatics rather than produce a third edition of Kinmonth's book, albeit acknowledging that much of the contents would be derived from his original work supplemented by the work that Professor Burnand and I carried out during the investigation and treatment of the many lymphatic problems we saw during our 20 years' work with Kinmonth in the surgical professorial unit at St Thomas' Hospital and the 20 years since 1982 during which we have continued Kinmonth's work.

It is, however, impossible for two surgeons to write a comprehensive, authoritative textbook on a complicated set of diseases with many medical connotations without the help of an expert physician, so we invited Professor Peter Mortimer of St George's Hospital, a dermatologist interested in lymphatic problems who has been working closely with Professor Burnand over the past few years on the genetics of lymphoedema, to join us in this endeavour. We then asked nine friends to contribute sections on lymphatic topics for which they have an international renown. Their contributions are acknowledged in the book's title pages and in the relevant sections. Nevertheless, each of the three principal authors has read and jointly edited the whole text to ensure a common style of presentation.

We have not attempted to quote every reference in the published literature, many of which are single case reports, but have instead quoted all the references that the reader who wishes to explore a particular subject in greater detail might need. We have illustrated the pathology of many conditions with lymphangiographs, even though lymphangiography is used much less nowadays, because lymphographs provide a far better image of the anatomical and pathological abnormalities than do the current, less-invasive methods of diagnostic investigation.

We hope that the book will become a major reference text for all those interested in diseases of the lymphatics. We have divided it into two parts. The first, which discusses the physiology, pathology and investigation of the lymphatic system, and the principles underlying medical and surgical treatment, is intended mainly for the trainee. The second part discusses the management of specific clinical conditions and is presented in a way that will allow consultants who encounter these conditions in their offices to gain guidance and advice quickly. This means that there is a little duplication, but the emphasis in the chapters of the first part is intentionally quite different from that of those in the second.

My co-authors and I hope that this book will be widely read by physicians and surgeons and be a fitting tribute to the work of John Kinmonth, to whom it is dedicated.

Norman Browse
London, 2002

Acknowledgements

The names of the authors on the many papers published by the St Thomas' Department of Surgery indicate the tremendous contributions to our clinical studies and laboratory research made by our consultant colleagues, our surgical registrars, our research assistants and our laboratory technicians; we thank them all. At St George's, Professor Mortimer has been similarly assisted by his registrars and research assistants and especially by Dr Sahar Mansour, consultant clinical geneticist, and Dr A.W.B. Stanton, post-doctoral scientist. We thank our nursing colleagues, our hospitals' photography departments and our secretarial staffs for their loyal and energetic support, and the staff of Arnold Publishers for their invaluable advice and encouragement. As we all have heavy clinical commitments, this book has been written in the evenings and at weekends, an out-of-working-hours activity made possible by the loving support of our wives and families. To them we owe an incalculable debt.

PART 1

General principles

The invisible vessels: who saw them first?

Written evidence that would reveal whether the physicians and anatomists of ancient Greece, Egypt, Rome, India and China knew of the existence of the lymphatics was lost as each of the early civilizations that produced the world's first great philosophers and scientists was destroyed or collapsed. Consequently, our understanding of their knowledge is based mainly upon copies and translations of their works, many of doubtful authenticity.

If the first physicians had seen the peripheral lymphatics, they would have written and spoken about them, and that knowledge would undoubtedly have been passed down through the ages by word of mouth. As there is no convincing oral or written evidence to suggest that they did see peripheral lymphatics, as opposed to lacteals, we must assume that they did not – presumably because lymphatics are small, transparent and, in dead animals including man, usually empty. This is not a criticism of the failure of these astute, highly intelligent men to notice these minute vessels: there are many modern-day surgeons too who have never knowingly seen a peripheral lymphatic.

This chapter summarises, in chronological order, the evidence that has been collected and published over the years by many learned scholars concerning the discovery of the lymphatics and their function.

460–360 BC: GLANDS AND WHITE BLOOD

Hippocrates certainly knew that there were glands in the axilla.[1] According to Thomas Bartholinus's edition of Hippocrates' works, the latter refers to 'white blood being present in the glands'.[2] If this was a reference to the mesenteric glands, he may have seen chyle in the lacteals and the mesenteric glands, but the Hippocratean school did not practise autopsy or vivisection so a more likely explanation is that the 'white blood' he saw was pus exuding from an infected lymph gland in the neck, axilla or groin, perhaps after it had been lanced.

There is little evidence that Hippocrates knew about the lymphatics. He described three types of vessel – arteries, veins and nerves – the nerves being classified as vessels because they were believed to have a hollow centre.

384–322 BC: ANOTHER SIGHTING IN GREECE?

Aristotle is said to have described 'fibres containing colourless fluid between the blood vessels and the nerves'.[3]

Did he see lymphatics? The lacteals certainly lie between the arteries and nerves, but that is not where most peripheral lymphatics are found. Kanter[4] has suggested that the meaning of the word that Thomas Bartholinus translated as fibre (the Greek word *ines*) is uncertain and concludes that Aristotle probably did not see lymphatics.

334–250 BC: A PROBABLE SIGHTING OF THE LACTEALS IN ALEXANDRIA

The great physicians of the Medical School of Alexandria – **Herophilus** (334–280 BC) and **Erasistratus** (310–250 BC)[5,6] – probably saw the lacteals because they made many of their anatomical and physiological observations on living animals and possibly living men,[4,5] but sadly the only knowledge that we have of their studies comes indirectly through the writings of Galen, none of their own original writings being extant.

According to Cruikshank,[7] Galen wrote how Herophilus taught that 'nature has made in the whole of the mesentery, peculiar veins, destined for the nourishment of the intestines, not passing to the liver, for these veins terminate in certain glandular bodies, whilst all the rest [the mesenteric veins] are carried up to the liver'. In addition, Cruickshank describes Galen's quotation of Erasistratus that 'on dividing the epigastrium along with the peritoneum we may clearly see arteries on the mesentery of sucking kids full of milk'. Aselli also quotes this comment by Galen in his book on the lacteals.[8] As Galen studied in Alexandria, it is reasonable to assume that he saw many of the Alexandrian school's manuscripts and quoted them correctly. If so, we can be reasonably certain that the Alexandrians did see the lacteals and had some understanding of their function.

CIRCA AD 50: MESENTERIC LYMPH NODES

Marinus, much quoted by Galen, is said to have described the mesenteric lymph glands.[4]

129–199: LACTEALS DEFINITELY SEEN BUT THEIR FUNCTION MISINTERPRETED

Galen, whose quotations from the works of the Greek and Alexandrian schools kept the knowledge and practices of those great schools alive, and who added much of his own observations to the practice of medicine, certainly saw the lacteals. According to W.I.H. Duckworth's translation of Galen's *On anatomical procedures*,[9] Galen wrote:

> Further you will see in the mesentery, beside these veins which we have mentioned, others [lacteals] each of which ends at a portion of spongy flesh [mesenteric lymph glands] especially associated with itself. And you will see how the final parts, the extreme endings of these veins [lacteals] which lie in the coverings of the intestines, unite and combine themselves with those veins which come from the portal vein, inasmuch as they travel in the mesentery to the intestines.

This observation is based on his dissections of primates rather than man and reveals that he believed the lacteals to connect with the terminal tributaries of the mesenteric veins in the bowel wall. Galen makes no suggestions about their function.

400–1400: THE 'DARK AGES'

These 1000 years are commonly known as Europe's Dark Ages because they were a period of political turmoil. Invasions from the East, the rise and fall of kingdoms and dynasties, and the control of knowledge and thought by the Christian Church all inhibited the development of medicine. Nevertheless, the teachings of Galen were known and followed throughout Europe and the Arab Islamic Empire, which stretched from the Indus to the Atlantic and the Pyrenees, and were developed by many great European and Arabian physicians. It is therefore possible that some of these physicians knew about the lacteals, although we have found no evidence to suggest that they knew about the peripheral lymphatics.

1514–1564: THE 'FATHER OF ANATOMY' DID NOT SEE THEM

The 'Dark Ages' of medicine ended in the sixteenth century with the publication of a series of anatomy textbooks, the most important of which was the book by **Andreas Vesalius** (1513–64) entitled *De humani corporis fabrica*.[10] This great book does not mention the lymphatics; the only explanation of this deficiency must be the fact that lymphatics are almost invisible in preserved cadavers and that this great anatomist and his contemporaries had no reason to think that the body needed a third set of vessels, and therefore no reason to search for them.

1524–1574: THE FIRST RECORDED OBSERVATIONS OF A THORACIC DUCT

Bartholommeo Eustachio (1513–74) (Fig. 1.1) saw the thoracic duct and the cisterna chyli in a horse and described it in his book *Opuscula anatomica*,[11] published in 1564 (and translated here by J. Lloyd, Head of Classics, Marlborough College, Wiltshire, UK), as follows:

> I have believed on other occasions that the vein of the *horse* relates to this foresight of nature, since it is

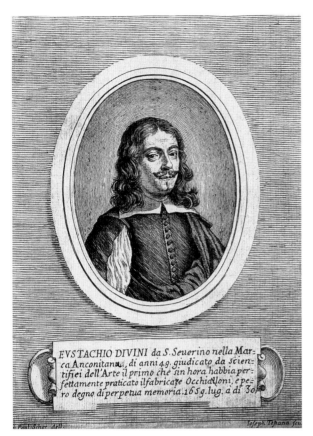

Figure 1.1 *Bartholommeo Eustachio (1513–74): the first physician/anatomist to describe the thoracic duct (albeit in the horse).[11] Reproduced by kind permission of the Wellcome Library, London.*

full of ingenuity and wonder; nor does it lack delight and usefulness. Although it is not at all designed to nourish the thorax, it is worthwhile that it should be explained. And so in these animals from the prominent left branch itself of the jugular vein at the posterior aspect of the root of the internal jugular vein, some sort of big shoot sprouts forth, which apart from the fact that in its origin it has a semicircular ostiola, it is also white and full of white water. And not far from its origin it splits into two parts, shortly afterwards again coming together into one part, near the left of the vertebrae, which has no separate branches. Having gone through the diaphragm, it is then connected to the middle as far as the lumbar region in which place it becomes wider, and occupies a large artery turning in on itself – a very obscure end and one which is still not well understood by me.

Eustachio called this structure the *vena alba thoracis*, which confirms that he appreciated that it was not filled with blood, although he made no suggestions about its function. Eustachio's observation was, however, ignored and forgotten, probably because it appeared to have little to do with the circulation of the blood.

1622: **THE LACTEALS (OF THE DOG) REDISCOVERED**

Gasparo Aselli (1581–1626) (Fig. 1.2a), Professor of Anatomy and Surgery in Milan and Pavia, rediscovered the lacteals while searching the mesentery of a dog for mesenteric glands and, more importantly, appreciated their function. His description of his chance discovery in his book *De lactibus sive lacteis venis, quarto vasorum mesarai corum genere nova invento*,[8] published in 1627 and translated by Foster,[13] was as follows:

On 23rd July, 1622 I had taken a dog in good condition and well fed, for a vivisection at the request of some of my friends who very much wished to see the recurrent nerves. When I had finished this demonstration of the nerves it seemed good to watch the movements of the diaphragm in the same dog, at the same operation. While I was attempting this, and for that purpose had opened the abdomen and was pulling down with my hand the intestines and stomach gathered together in a mass, I suddenly beheld a great number of cords as it were, exceedingly thin and beautifully white, scattered over the whole of the mesentery and the intestine, and starting from almost innumerable beginnings. At first I did not delay, thinking them to be nerves, but presently I saw that I was mistaken in this since I noticed that the nerves belonging to the intestine were distinct from these cords, and wholly unlike them, and, besides, were distributed quite separately from them. Wherefore struck by the novelty of the thing I stood for some time silent while there came into my mind the various disputes, rich in personal quarrels no less than in words, taking place among the anatomists concerning the mesariac veins and their function. And by chance it happened that a few days before I had looked into a little book by Johannes Crostaeus written about this very matter. When I gathered my wits together for the sake of the experiment, having laid hold of a very sharp scalpel, I pricked one of those cords and indeed one of the largest of them. I had hardly touched it when I saw a white liquid like milk or cream forthwith gush out. Seeing this I could hardly restrain my delight, and turning to those who were standing by, to Alexander Tadinus and more particular to Senator Septalius, who was both a member of the great College of the Order of Physicians and while I am writing this, the Medical Officer of Health, *'Eureka'* I exclaimed with Archimedes, and at the same time invited them to see the interesting spectacle of such an unusual phenomenon. And they indeed were much struck with the novelty of the thing.

Aselli's drawings of the lacteals (Fig. 1.2b), which he called *venae lacteae*, are believed to be the first coloured plates of a medical subject ever published.

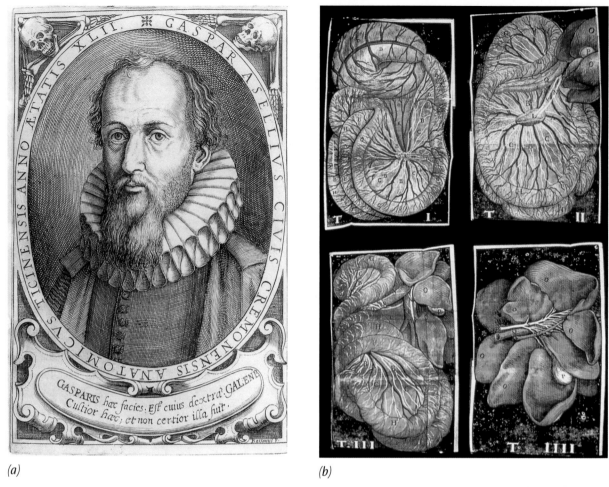

(a)   *(b)*

Figure 1.2 *(a) Gasparo Aselli (1581–1626): the first anatomist to describe the lacteals. (b) Aselli's illustrations of the lacteals.[8] The first coloured plates in a medical publication, probably drawn by Ceare Bassono.[12] Reproduced by kind permission of the Royal College of Surgeons of England.*

Aselli believed that the chyle in the lacteals flowed to the lymph nodes close to the pancreas and then on to the liver, the liver being, according to Galen, the centre of the circulation and the site where blood was produced. Aselli had clearly not heard of Eustachio's discoveries 63 years earlier or he might have realized that the lacteals drained into the strange white vein that Eustachio had seen close to the vertebrae. Although Aselli did not perform human dissections, he assumed that lacteals were also present in man.

1634/47: **HUMAN LACTEALS REDISCOVERED**

Cruikshank, quoting Haller,[7] states that **Johann Veslingius** (1598–1649) (Fig. 1.3a) was the first to see lacteals in *man* and that he published a drawing of them in 1634, 12 years after Aselli. Figure 1.3b, from Veslingius's book *Syntagma anatomicums*,[14] published in 1647, clearly shows the

lacteals, but it is interesting to note that this figure appears in the chapter entitled '*De foetu humano*', which describes other fetal appearances such as the lobulation of the kidneys, and that the lacteals are not shown in the corresponding drawing of the mesenteric vessels in the chapter on the adult abdominal contents. Did Veslingius only see the lacteals in neonates and think they were solely concerned with the absorption of maternal milk or some aspect of fetal life? Whatever the explanation, Veslingius's drawings are almost certainly the first illustrations of human lacteals.

According to Cruikshank, Haller claimed that Veslingius described the human thoracic duct in 1647,[14] 3 years before Pecquet's publication (see below), but whether this latter claim is correct is not certain. There is no drawing of the thoracic duct in Veslingius's 1647 book, so most medical historians give Pecquet the credit for being the first to describe the human thoracic duct.

It is notable that all of Veslingius' manuscripts were left to Thomas Bartholinus (see below), and it is likely this bequest stimulated the latter's interest in the lymphatics.

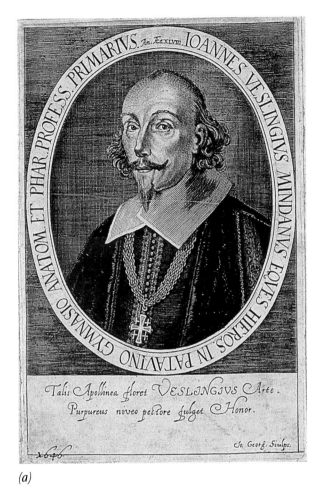

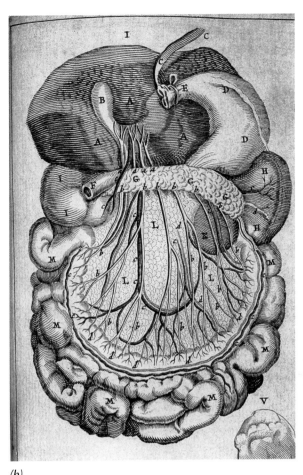

(a)   (b)

Figure 1.3 *(a) Johann Veslingius (1598–1649). Haller is reported, by Cruickshank,[7] to have stated that Veslingius was the first anatomist to see the lacteals and the thoracic duct in man and to have published drawings of them, but we have been unable to find any drawings of the thoracic duct. (b) Veslingius' drawing of the lacteals. From Syntagma anatomicums,[14] Tabula II, Cap. VIII. The legend reads as follows: a.a.a.a. – Venae aliquot lacteae a pancreate ad lecur porrectae, quarum hic pauce, et minores expressae. b.b.b.b. – Venae aliquot lacteae a pancreate ad intestina diffusae, grandiuscule delineate. c.c.c.c. – Rami venea portae meseraicae. d.d.d.d. – Rami arteriarum mesentericarum. Reproduced by kind permission of the Royal College of Surgeons of England.*

1650–1651: RECOGNITION OF THE HUMAN THORACIC DUCT, ITS CONNECTION TO THE LACTEALS AND THEIR JOINT ROLE IN TRANSPORTING CHYLE

In 1651, **Jean Pecquet** (1622–74) (Fig. 1.4a) found and described the thoracic duct in the dog and the connections between it and the lacteals (Fig. 1.4b).[15] He showed quite clearly that chyle drained from the intestines, through the lacteals and mesenteric lymph glands into the receptaculum chyli and then up the thoracic duct into the great veins of the neck. With this observation, he destroyed the belief that had been held since Galen's time that nourishment absorbed in the intestines flowed to the liver.

Pecquet described his discoveries as follows after pointing out the errors of his forebears:

none of them knew that the Chyle was not derived to the liver, nor to the Vena Porta, nor to the Vena Cava near the Emulgenis, as the received error held forth but, which in dissection may be seen to any man more clear than the light, from the Guts to a RECEPTACLE of that bigness which will fill up the interstitium between the lumbar muscles, at least in Beasts.

Now this receptacle above the Vertebers of the loins receives the liquor of the milky veins spread in the mesentery, and rendreth it again by those milky veins, which being hid within the breast, in a continued passage run to the Subclavial venal branches, till within the ascending stem of the Vena Cava about the External Jugulars, being mixed with blood and running into one and the same Channel *it throws itself headlong into the whirlpool of the heart.* (Emphasis added.)

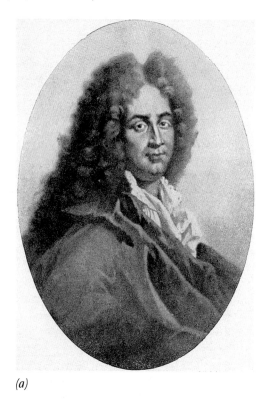

(a)

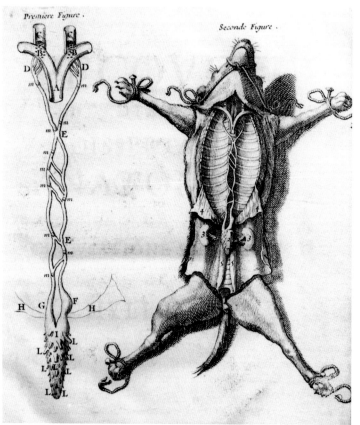

(b)

In 1651, Pecquet conducted a serious of autopsies on executed criminals, confirming that the situation in man was similar to that which he had observed in the dog.

In 1628, 6 years after Aselli's description of the lacteals and 22 years before Pecquet's discoveries, **William Harvey** published his description of the circulation of the blood entitled *Exercitatio anatomica de motu cordis et sanguini in animalibus*,[16] having first presented these discoveries in a Lumlean lecture at the College of Physicians of London on 17 April 1616. It was therefore not too difficult for Pecquet to contradict Galen's teaching that the liver was the seat of the circulation and affirm that the chyle that was necessary for the formation of blood and the body's nutrition was carried via the thoracic duct to the bloodstream. He clearly accepted Harvey's description of the circulation.

Surprisingly, Harvey was dismissive of the work of both Aselli and Pecquet. In a letter to a Dr Morrison of Paris,[17] written in April 1650 soon after hearing of Pecquet's discoveries, Harvey wrote:

> With regard to the lacteal veins discovered by Aselli and by the further diligence of Pecquet, who discovered the receptacle or reservoir of the chyle (digested contents of the intestine) and traced the canals thence to the subclavian veins, I shall tell you freely, since you ask me what I think of them. I had already in the course of my dissections, I venture to say even

Figure 1.4 *(a) Jean Pecquet (1622–74) described the thoracic duct in the dog and its connection with the lacteals in 1651, thus contradicting Galen's teaching that all nourishment absorbed from the intestine flowed to the liver. (b) Pecquet's drawing of the cisterna chyli and thoracic duct of the dog. Reproduced by kind permission of the Royal College of Surgeons of England.*

before Aselli had published his book, observed these white canals but for various reasons and led by several experiments I could never be brought to believe that the milky fluid was chyle conducted hither from the intestines, and distributed to all parts of the body for their nourishment; but that it was rather met with occasionally and by accident, and proceeded from too ample a supply of nourishment and the peculiar vigour of concoction.

Harvey also stated: 'All Pecquet's assertions constitute a novelty that I shall perhaps be ready to believe when they have been satisfactorily proved, and when they introduce something useful and convenient *in morborum curatione, quo excepto*, I will have nothing to do with them.'[18]

It is clear that if Harvey thought that the sole function of the lacteals and the thoracic duct was to convey the nutrition occasionally provided by excess eating to the circulation, it was of little relevance to his own great discovery – the way in which the blood circulated. It was another 100 years before the role of the lymphatics in assisting interstitial fluid clearance, and therefore in maintaining blood volume, was recognized, so perhaps Harvey's intransigence can be excused; it is, however, always comforting to we lesser mortals to discover that the greatest of scientific investigators may occasionally have feet of clay.

1652

In 1652, **Johannes Van Horne** (1621–64), Professor of Anatomy in Leyden, independently found and described the human thoracic duct and its connection with the lacteals,[19] although precedence for this must go to Pecquet.

1652: 'A FOURTH SET OF VESSELS'

Although Aselli and Pecquet described the lacteals and thoracic duct, they did not see the peripheral lymphatics. In 1653, according to William Harvey, Francis Glisson (see below) and Robert Boyle, as quoted by Cruikshank,[7] **George Jolyffe** (1618–58) saw and gave a lecture at the College of Physicians on 'a fourth set of vessels'. As Harvey recorded: 'Jolyffe made some discoveries of that fourth sort of vessels, plainly differing from veins, arteries and nerves now called lymphatics.' Boyle said, 'by accident too, as himself have told me did our industrious anatomist Dr Jolyffe first light upon these yet freshly detected vessels, which afterwards the ingenious Bartholinus, without being informed of them, or seeking for them, hath met with and acquainted the world with under the name of "vasa lymphatica"'. Glisson, Jolyffe's teacher, states as an aside, in his book *Anatomia hepatis*,[20] that Jolyffe had, at the beginning of June 1652, asserted, as a result of his dissections, that a fourth kind of vessel existed in the body, one entirely distinct from veins, arteries and nerves, which conducted an aqueous humour.

Similar quotations from different sources but with different years of attribution make it difficult to know which date is correct, but the evidence suggests that Jolyffe discovered the peripheral lymphatics some years before Rudbeck (see below) and Bartholinus. Had his lectures or his thesis been published or preserved, we might have been able to accord Jolyffe the accolade of being the discoverer of the peripheral lymphatics.

1652: **THE LYMPHATICS ARE DEMONSTRATED TO A QUEEN AND THE WORLD**

Queen Christina of Sweden was fascinated by the developments of science and anatomy that were appearing all round her and invited **Olaf Rudbeck** (1630–1702) (Fig. 1.5a), the 22-year-old Professor of Anatomy in Uppsala, to demonstrate to her the new vessels that he had found, which he called the vasa serosa.[21] The demonstration took place in Uppsala in April 1652.

Rudbeck had noticed some years earlier, while dissecting a calf, a milky-white fluid near the supraclavicular notch. This led him to dissect more than 300 animals and to his discovery of the thoracic duct, the lymphatics of the colon and rectum, and their drainage route into the cisterna chyli. He also looked for and found lymphatics all over the body and appreciated that together they formed a system separate from the blood-carrying vessels.

At the time of his demonstration, Rudbeck did not know about Pecquet's discovery of the thoracic duct 2 years earlier, so it must have been most embarrassing when a member of the audience (perhaps one of the Court physicians – Palmcron, Bromsius or Wullen) told him, in front of the Queen, of Pecquet's find. Nevertheless, Rudbeck's observations on the peripheral lymphatics were original and of great importance. He defended his thesis in May 1652 and published his book entitled *Nova exercitatio anatomica exhibens ductus hepaticos aquosos et vasa glandularum serosa, nunc primum in venta, aeneisque figuris delineata*[22] in the autumn of 1653 (Fig. 1.5b).

Not far from Uppsala, **Thomas Bartholinus** (1616–80) (Fig. 1.6a), Professor of Anatomy in Copenhagen, had also become interested in the lymphatics, perhaps through the legacy of Veslingius's papers, perhaps after hearing of Pecquet's work or perhaps from a colleague who was at Rudbeck's demonstration. Whatever the stimulus, Bartholinus also looked for and found the thoracic duct and the peripheral lymphatics. He published his findings on the thoracic duct in May 1652[23] but did not report his findings on the peripheral lymphatics until May 1653 (Fig. 1.6b). This latter publication, entitled *Vasa lymphatica nuper Hafniae in animalibus inventa, et hepatis exsequiace*[24] gave the lymphatics their modern name.

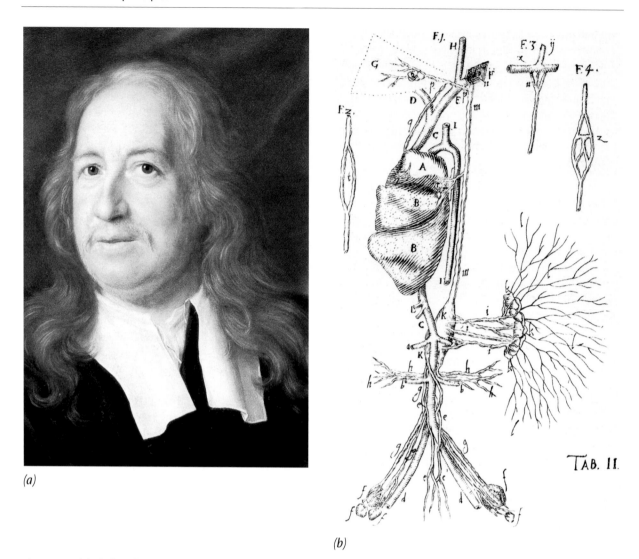

(a)

(b)

Figure 1.5 *(a) Olaf Rudbeck (1630–1702) was the first to give a full demonstration of the peripheral lymphatics, lacteals and thoracic duct in man. (b) Rudbeck's drawing of the lymphatic system, published in 1653.*

There then followed a prolonged dispute between Bartholinus and Rudbeck, both claiming priority for the discovery of the lymphatics, as opposed to the lacteals. Neither knew of the work of Jolyffe, which may have pre-dated them by 10–15 years. The following timetable of events clearly favours Rudbeck's precedence, as does the quality and detail of his work and illustrations:

- Pre-1650: some years of extensive animal dissections by Rudbeck.
- c.1650–51: Bartholinus was stimulated by Pecquet's discoveries.
- April 1652: Rudbeck's public demonstration of the lymphatics (the modern equivalent of a publication in a scientific journal).
- May 1652: Rudbeck defended his thesis.
- May 1652: Bartholinus published his book on the thoracic duct.
- May 1653: Bartholinus published his book on the lymphatics.

- Winter 1653: Rudbeck published his book on the lymphatics.

To be fair to both men, one must conclude that both made independent original observations. Rudbeck was the first to establish that the lymphatics, lacteals and thoracic duct formed a comprehensive system separate from the blood vessels; Bartholinus confirmed this and gave them their name. If there was written evidence rather than hearsay, both would, however, have to yield to Jolyffe, just as Pecquet should probably yield to Veslingius over the thoracic duct and Aselli to the Alexandrians over the lacteals.

1665: THE VALVES

The first clear drawings and descriptions of the valves in the lymphatics were published by **Frederick Ruysch** (1638–1731) (Fig. 1.7) in 1712,[25] but it seems most unlikely

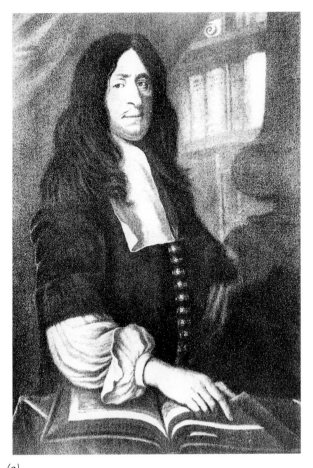

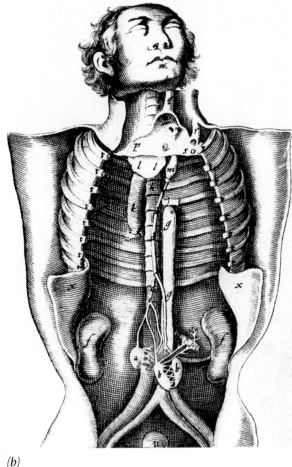

(a)   *(b)*

Figure 1.6 *(a) Thomas Bartholinus (1616–80), who described the human thoracic duct in a publication in 1652 and the peripheral lymphatics in 1653. Evidence suggests that Rudbeck made his discoveries just before those of Bartholinus (see text). Bartholinus did, however, give these vessels their modern name – lymphatics. (b) Bartholinus' drawing of the thoracic duct and the lymphatics of some of the abdominal viscera.*

that men as observant as Rudbeck and Bartholinus failed to see them. Rudbeck's drawings of the lymphatics (Fig. 1.5b) clearly show them to have a beaded appearance. This is caused by the dilatation of the vessel at the level of the valve sinus. Perhaps because it was known that all veins had valves, these scientists considered that the presence of valves in lymphatics was not unexpected or worthy of note.

1654: **THE FUNCTION OF THE LYMPHATICS**

The recognition of the absorbent function of the lymphatics is usually attributed to William Hunter (see below), but in 1654 **Francis Glisson** (1597–1677) (Fig. 1.8) wrote, in his book *Anatomia hepatis*,[20] 'the lymphatics carry back to the blood vessels the lymph which has lubricated the cavities of the body, and their function is to absorb, in contrast to those who thought that they were merely continued from small arteries'.

Although he is referring primarily to the lymphatics draining the liver, Glisson clearly considers them to be

quite separate from the small arteries and to have an absorbent function. He describes the method of production of fluid from smaller arteries as 'effusion' and assigns to the lymphatics the role of collecting this effused fluid and returning it to the bloodstream via the thoracic duct.

1746–1783: **THE ABSORBING VESSELS**

William Hunter (1718–83) (Fig. 1.9), in his series of anatomy lectures, which he started in 1746,[26] was the first to describe how the lymphatic system absorbed tissue fluid and returned it to the blood. He believed that he had discovered this function and wrote thus:

I think I have proved that the lymphatic vessels are the absorbing vessels, all over the body; that they are the same as the lacteals; and that these altogether, together with the thoracic duct, constitute one great and general system, dispersed through the whole body for absorption; that this system only does

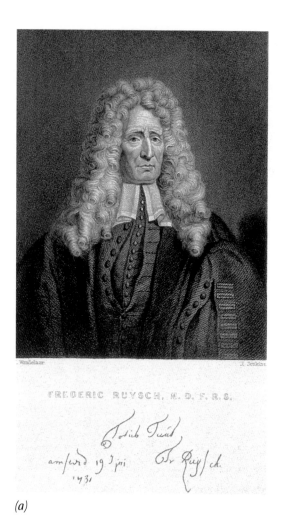

(a)

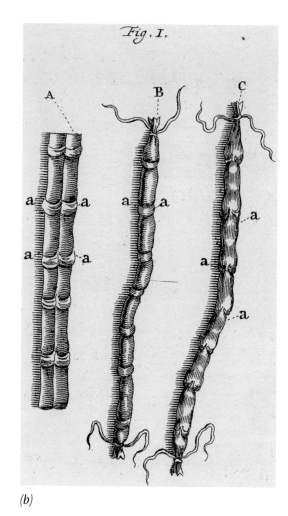

(b)

(c)

Figure 1.7 *(a) Frederick Ruysch (1638–1731) was the first to publish detailed drawing of the lymphatics' many valves. (b) An example of Ruysch's demonstration of the valves of a peripheral lymphatic, with the vessel collapsed (A), distended (B) and opened longitudinally (C). (c) Ruysch's drawing of the valves in the lacteals and the efferent lymphatics of the mesenteric lymph glands. (a) Reproduced by kind permission of the Wellcome Library, London; (b, c) reproduced by kind permission of the Royal College of Surgeons of England.*

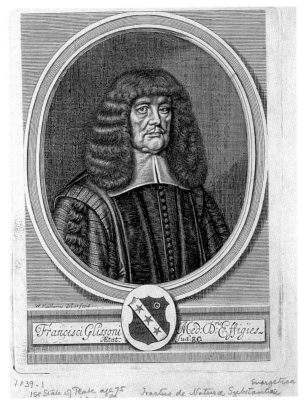

Figure 1.8 *Francis Glisson (1597–1677), the first physician to state that the lymphatics had an absorbent function. Reproduced by kind permission of the Wellcome Library, London.*

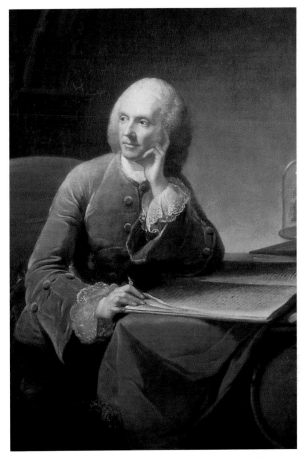

Figure 1.9 *William Hunter (1718–83), who thought he was the first to describe the absorbent function of the lymphatics but later acknowledged Glisson's precedence. A portrait by Robert Edge Pine, reproduced by kind permission of the Royal College of Surgeons of England.*

absorb, and not the veins; that it serves to take up, and convey, whatever is to make, or to be mixed with the blood, from the skin, from the intestinal canal, and from all the internal cavities or surfaces whatever. This discovery gains credit daily, both at home and abroad, to such a degree, that I believe we may now say that it is almost universally adopted; and if we mistake not, in a proper time, it will be allowed to be the greatest discovery, both in physiology and in pathology, that anatomy has suggested, since the discovery of the circulation.

To his great credit, Hunter, when he later learnt of Glisson's description of the role of the lymphatics[27] 100 years earlier, generously acknowledged Glisson's precedence:

I have several times met with my own observations in books after having long believed them peculiar to myself. It must be the case with every man who is more entertained with nature than with books. The present dispute [with Monro] has given me a fresh instance of it. Glisson having been quoted, I considered what he had advanced on this subject and had the pleasure and mortification to find that he gave exactly the same account for transudation and of absorption; so that I can no longer call it, what I really believed it to be a *new opinion*, but Glisson's *revived and confirmed*, for in him it was a mere

opinion and accordingly was overlooked or rejected by his successors, as happened to the doctrine of the circulation in the writings of Servetus and Caesalpinus. (Emphasis added.)

This acknowledgement made the 'present dispute' that he was having with **Alexander Monro secundus** (1733–1817), Professor of Anatomy in Edinburgh, almost superfluous.

Monro, when injecting mercury into the vas deferens, noticed that if he injected too forcibly, the seminiferous tubules burst and mercury appeared in the lymphatics. In his thesis, published in 1755,[28] he stated: 'Valvular lymphatic vessels, in all parts of the body are absorbent veins, they do not emanate from arterial twigs as is generally believed.' On the basis of this statement, he claimed that he had described the lymphatics as absorbing vessels before Hunter. An acrimonius argument followed, but Hunter was able to show that he had ascribed an absorbent function to the lymphatics in his lectures ever since 1746, long before Monro wrote his thesis in 1755.

Monro must have been deeply concerned about his status in the academic world, for a few years later, in 1768

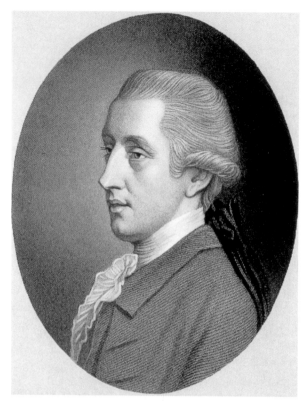

Figure 1.10 *William Hewson (1739–74) described the lymphatic systems of birds, fish and reptiles as well as that of many mammals while working in close collaboration with John Hunter and William Cruickshank. Reproduced by kind permission of the Royal College of Surgeons of England.*

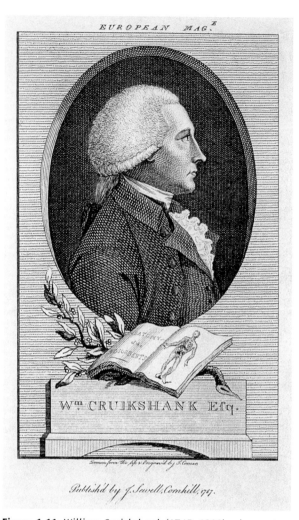

Figure 1.11 *William Cruickshank (1745–1800), who wrote the first comprehensive description of the anatomy of the human lymphatics,[7] including important references to the history of their discovery. Reproduced by kind permission of the Wellcome Library, London.*

and 1769, he published two papers[29,30] strongly criticizing **William Hewson's** (1739–74) (Fig. 1.10) claim to be the first to have described the lymphatics of birds, fishes and other animals, to which Hewson replied in detail.[31] All the evidence points to Hewson's precedence for these discoveries rather than Monro's. In addition to his work on the comparative anatomy of the lymphatics, Hewson also subdivided lymphatics into deep and superficial, and suggested that they played a part in the spread of poison and infection.

1786: A COMPREHENSIVE TEXTBOOK ON THE LYMPHATICS

Contemporary with William Hunter and William Hewson, and a colleague of both, lived **William Cruikshank** (1745–1800) (Fig. 1.11). It was Cruikshank who, in 1784, published one of the first all-embracing books on the lymphatics – *The anatomy of the absorbing vessels of the human body*[7] – which described the history of their discovery, their anatomy and their physiology.

Cruikshank described in some of detail the contributions of his contemporaries, including those of John Hunter, William's brother, who made many injection studies of the lymphatics and was the first to describe lymphatics in the crocodile and goose. Among Cruikshank's own original observations were those of the presence of autonomic nerve fibres running to the thoracic duct and a belief that the lymphatics played a role in the defence of the body against infection and in the production of oedema.

1650–1800: DISSECTION, INJECTION, CORROSIVE CASTS AND MICROANATOMY

The syringe was invented by Ktesibios in Alexandria in the third century BC but was not used for the display of anatomical features until the seventeenth and eighteenth centuries AD. Rudbeck and Bartholinus injected lymphatics with coloured water, milk and air to help to identify them during dissection. **Jan Swammerdam** (1637–80) injected lymphatics with a mixture of suet and wax.[32]

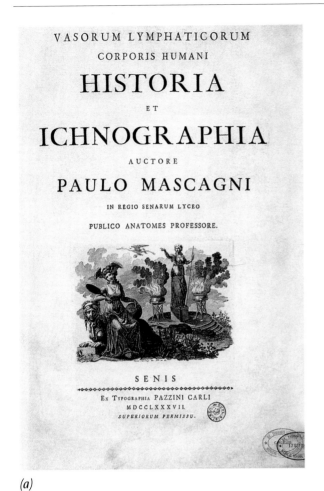
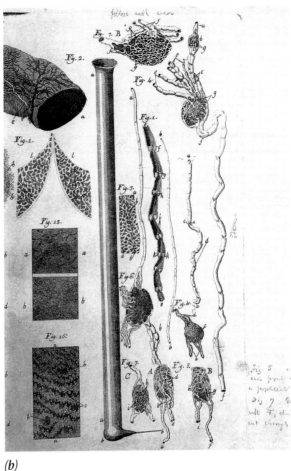

(a)   *(b)*

Figure 1.12 *(a) The title page of the atlas of the lymphatic system prepared by Mascagni,[35] whose illustrations have never been bettered. (b) Mascagni's illustration of peripheral lymphatics, lymph glands, valves and the pipette used for lymphatic injection.*

Anton Nuck (1650–92) is believed to be the first person to use mercury, in 1692, having combined it with other substances such as lead and zinc to make an amalgam.[33] Unfortunately, his prescription is lost. By using an amalgam of mercury that set hard, he was able to dissolve the tissues around the lymphatics and so produce corrosion casts. Modern methods using a variety of plastics can now produce beautiful casts of the smallest vessels.

In 1690, **Marcello Malpighi** (1628–94) wrote a letter to the Royal Society[34] pointing out that lymphatics entered and left the 'conglobate' glands, as they were called, and that these glands were not just fibrous swellings.

Ruysch used injection techniques to display the valves.[25]

1787: AN ANATOMICAL ATLAS OF THE LYMPHATICS

In 1787, **Paolo Mascagni** (1755–1815) published an atlas of the anatomy of the lymphatics[35] that was of incredible beauty and detail (Fig. 1.12). We have used some of Mascagni's plates to illustrate the chapter on anatomy for they have never have been bettered.

Mascagni also said that lymph from any organ passes through at least 8–10 glands on its way to the thoracic duct or a large vein; this became known as Mascagni's Rule.

THE NINETEENTH AND TWENTIETH CENTURIES: **MICROANATOMY**

As the quality of microscopes, microdissection and corrosion casting developed, many researchers studied the anatomy of the small lymphatics.

In 1745, **Johann Lieberkühn** (1711–56) showed that the lacteals reached to the very tips of the intestinal villi.[36] **Johannes Meckel**[37] and later **Vincenz Fohmann**[38] found lymphovenous communications. **Gustav Weirich**[39] described nerve endings in the walls of very small lymphatics, whereas **Albert Koelliker**[40] demonstrated the terminal buds of the lymphatic capillaries. **Friedrich von Recklinghausen**[41] claimed to have found clefts in the tissues between the arterial capillaries and the lymphatics through which lymph was filtered, but these were later shown to be artefacts. **Philibert Sappey**[42] produced a detailed atlas of the lymphatics and counted their valves.

He found between 60 and 80 valves in the lymphatics that ran the length of the arm, one valve occurring approximately every centimetre. All this work greatly increased our knowledge of the anatomical features of the lymphatics but did not help to elucidate their physiological role.

LYMPH PROPULSION

In 1833, **Johannes Müller** described the lymph 'hearts' of amphibians.[43] It was clear that these pulsating sacs on the sides of the lymphatics helped to propel the lymph onwards, but no lymph hearts were found in humans. In 1861, **Wilhelm Weiss** showed that the negative intrathoracic pressure produced by ventilation in fact sucked the lymph forwards.[44]

Arnold Heller, in 1896, noticed spontaneous contractions in a lymphangioma,[45] so, knowing that there was a muscle coat in the larger lymphatics, postulated that spontaneous rhythmical contractions of the lymphatic wall assisted lymph movement, a hypothesis that was not confirmed until recent years.

Karl Generisch[46] and **Wilhelm Paschutin**,[47] in 1871 and 1872 respectively, showed that both passive and active movements of a limb increased lymph flow.

LYMPH FORMATION

The anatomical and lymphodynamic discoveries described above unfortunately made little contribution to the vital question everyone was asking – how is lymph produced? For 40 years, many theories on this were proposed and then destroyed.

In 1858, **Carl Ludwig** (1816–95) postulated that lymph was produced by the process of *filtration*, the interstitial fluid that became lymph being forced through the capillary wall by the intracapillary blood pressure.[48] It was, however, soon shown that lymph production was not solely dependent upon intracapillary blood pressure, and so **Rudolf Heidenhain** postulated, in 1891, that lymph production was an active process – the *secretion* of fluid by the cells of the capillary wall.[49] In 1895, **W. Cohnstein** combined the idea of the processes of filtration and effusion, and called lymph a *transudation* from the capillaries.[50]

The arguments continued until, in 1909, **Ernest Starling** (1866–1927) (Fig. 1.13) showed that the production of interstitial fluid depended upon the balance between the hydrodynamic pressures inside and outside the capillaries and the oncotic pressure of the plasma and interstitial fluid, the balance being set in such a way that fluid left the capillaries at their arterial end and returned to them at their venous end, the fluid that did not return to the venules being taken up by the lymphatics and

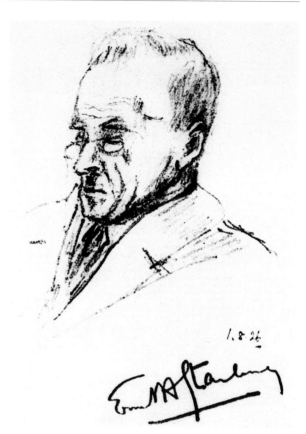

Figure 1.13 *Ernest Starling (1866–1927), who was the first to define the forces that determined the production and reabsorption of interstitial fluid, from and back into the blood vessels, thus defining the need for a special system of excess fluid and protein absorption – the lymphatics. A sketch believed to have been drawn at a committee meeting by Professor Henry Barcroft FRS.*

returned to the circulation via the thoracic duct.[51] Starling's hypothesis gained support as methods for measuring capillary, interstitial and hydrodynamic pressure, and plasma and interstitial fluid oncotic pressure, developed.[52–60]

The mechanism by which interstitial fluid enters the lymphatics is still not clear. When **W.G. MacCallum** showed that the terminal (or original) buds of the lymphatics were closed and completely lined with epithelium,[61] it became apparent that the movement of interstitial fluid into the lymphatics could not be purely a passive process. Chapter 3 analyses the current views on this problem, the study of the capillary circulation, interstitium, interstitial fluid and lymph formation now being a highly sophisticated and specialized branch of physiology.

LYMPHATICS IN THE LIVING

It became clear over successive centuries that there were many clinical conditions and diseases caused by

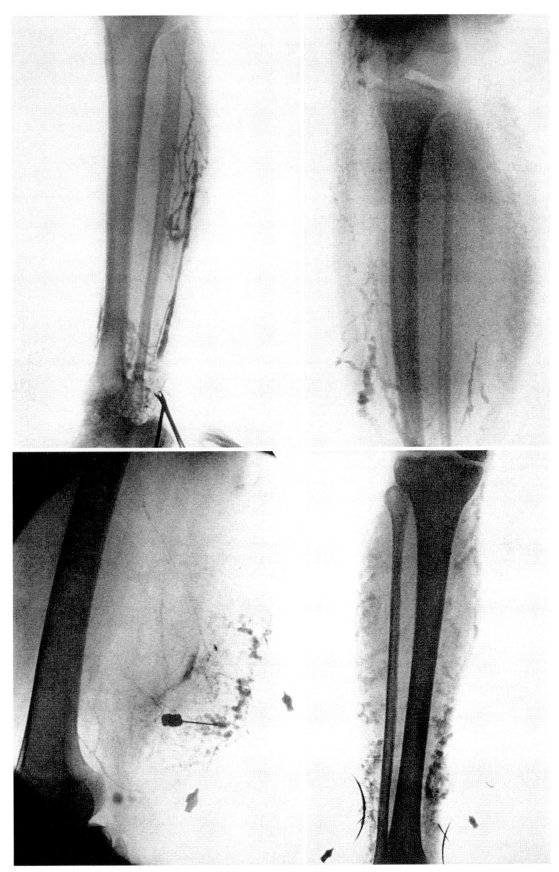

Figure 1.14 *Abnormal incompetent lymphatics displayed on 22 November 1945 by Servelle and Deysson during a reducing operation on the thigh by injecting thorium dioxide into a grossly enlarged lymphatic exposed in the thigh.*[64] *Although these radiographs were not published until 1951, they are almost certainly the first radiographs of human (abnormal) lymphatics. Reproduced from the* Annals of Surgery *1951;* **133:** *234, by kind permission of the publishers.*

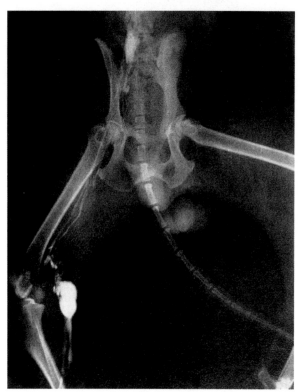

Figure 1.15 *A normal canine lymphangiograph obtained by Glenn[65] by injecting pyelographin into a lymphatic on the paw previously visualized and exposed by the interstitial injection of a vital dye. Although these radiographs were not published until 1981, they were obtained in 1948 and are almost certainly the first radiographs of normal mammalian lymphatics. Reproduced from the* Archives of Surgery *1981;* **116:** *992. Copyrighted (1981), American Medical Association.*

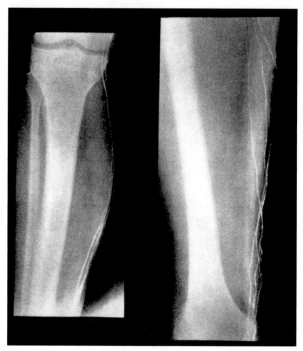

Figure 1.16 *The first normal human lymphangiographs, obtained in 1952 by Professor J.B. Kinmonth, by injecting Diodone into an exposed lymphatic on the dorsum of the foot, previously identified by injecting Patent Blue Violet into the web spaces.*

abnormalities of the lymphatics. Radiological methods for opacifying and visualizing the arteries and veins during life became available through the work of **Moniz** in 1927,[62] but the small hidden lymphatics seemed to be beyond our reach.

Physiologists had known since the 1750s that it was possible to show up the lymphatics of animals by injecting coloured dyes into the interstitial space, but most of these dyes were made up of small molecules and quickly diffused out of the lymphatics. When a dye with a larger molecular size, such as Patent Blue Violet, became available, **Hudack** and **McMaster** took the very brave step of injecting themselves intradermally to see whether the dye entered their dermal lymphatics.[63] In the paper they published in 1933, these authors showed, with serial photographs, how quickly the dye spread through their dermal lymphatics after the injection.

Once the small peripheral lymphatics could be visualized, the next step was to cannulate and inject them. This was first achieved in November 1945 by **Servelle** and **Deysson** who, during a reducing operation on a patient with severe lymphoedema caused by incompetent

lymphatics, injected the grossly dilated incompetent lymphatics *retrogradely* with thorium dioxide (Thorotrast) and took a series of X-rays, which they published 6 years later (Fig. 1.14).[64] The first lymphographs of *normal* mammalian lymphatics were probably those of a dog obtained in 1948 by **Glenn** using pyelographin, although these were not published until 1981 (Fig. 1.15).[65]

The first human lymphangiographs were produced by **John Kinmonth** (1916–83) in 1952 (Fig. 1.16).[66] He used Patent Blue Violet to detect a suitable lymphatic on the dorsum of the foot and then, using a specially made fine needle and an infusion pump, slowly injected the contrast medium Diodone. The X-ray images he obtained showed the lymphatics from the foot to the groin but gradually faded as the water-soluble contrast medium diffused out of the lymphatics into the interstitial space. This problem was solved when a safe non-diffusible oily medium of poppy seed oil and iodine (Lipiodol) was introduced by **Brunn** and **Engeset**.[67,68] The way was then open for the study of every conceivable condition involving the lymphatics – the lifetime work of J.B. Kinmonth – to whom this book is dedicated.

The only technique developed since the 1950s that has helped to simplify clinical diagnosis and management is isotope lymphography (*see* Chapter 6). Other new techniques such as fluorescence microlymphography and indirect lymphography are not employed clinically but are useful research tools.

REFERENCES

1. Majno G. *The healing hand*. Cambridge, MA: Harvard University Press, 1977.
2. Seger. Epistol ad Th. Bartholinus de editione Hippocrates nova. Lymphaticorum vestigia ex Hippocrate, Ejusdem locus correctus. In Th. Bartholinus Epist.
3. Bartels P. *Das Lymphgefasssystemen*. Jena Fischer, 1909.
4. Kanter MA. The lymphatic system: a historical perspective. *Plastic and Reconstructive Surgery* 1987; **79:** 131–9.
5. Perrott JW. Advances in the anatomical investigation in the lymphatic system with special reference to some pathological applications. *Edinburgh Medical Journal* 1954; **61:** 50.
6. Allbutt TC. *Greek medicine in Rome*. London: Macmillan, 1901.
7. Cruikshank WC. *The anatomy of the absorbing vessels of the human body*. London: G Nicol, 1786.
8. Aselli G. *De lactibus sive lacteis venis, quarto vasorum mesarai corum genere nova invento*. Milan: JB Biddelli, 1627.
9. Galen. *On anatomical procedures*. Lyons MC, Towers B eds (trans. Duckworth WIH). Cambridge: Cambridge University Press, 1962.
10. Vesalius A. *De humani corporis fabrica*. Basle: J Oporinns, 1543.
11. Eustachio B. *Opuscula anatomica*. Venetiis: V Luchinus, 1564.
12. Arvy L. Some errors about Asellius and the chyliferous vessels. *Lymphology* 1972; **5:** 49–51.
13. Foster M. *Lectures on the history of physiology*. Cambridge: Cambridge University Press, 1901.
14. Veslingius J. *Syntagma anatomicums*. Patavii: Frambotti, 1647.
15. Pecquet J. *Experimenta nova anatomica quibus incognitum chyli receptaculum, et ab eo per thoracem in ramos uque subclavis vasa lactea defergunter*. Paris: S & G Carmoisy, 1651.
16. Harvey W. *Exercitatio anatomica de motu cordis et sanguini in animalibus*. Frankfurt: W Fitzer, 1628.
17. Wyall H. *William Harvey*. London: Parsons, 1924.
18. Chauvois L. *William Harvey*. London: Hutchinson, 1957.
19. Van Horne J. *Novus ductus chyliferus, nun primum delineatus descriptus et eruditorum examini expositus*. Leydon: Hack, 1652.
20. Glisson F. *Anatomia hepatis*. London: DuGardionis, 1654.
21. Skandalakis JE. I wish I had been there: highlights in the history of lymphatics. *American Surgeon* 1995; **61:** 799–808.
22. Rudbeck O. *Nova exercitatio anatomica, exhibens ductus hepaticos aquosos et vasa glandularum serosa, nunc primum in venta, aeneisque figuris delineata*. Vesteras: E Lauringer, 1653.
23. Bartholinus T. *De lacteis thoracicis in homine brutisque nuperrime observatis*. Copenhagen, 1652.
24. Bartholinus T. *Vasa lymphatica nuper Hafniae in animalibus inventa, et hepatis exsequiae*. Hafniae. P Hakins, 1653.
25. Ruysch F. *Dilucidatio valvularum in vasis lymphaticis et lacteis. Mangeti bibl. anat.* II 1712, p. 712.
26. Hunter W. *Hunter's lectures of anatomy*. London: Elsevier, 1972.
27. Hunter W. *Medical commentaries*. No. 26. London: 1762.
28. Monro A II. *De testibus et de semine in variis animalibus*. MD thesis, University of Edinburgh, 1755.
29. Monro A II. *A State of facts concerning the discovery of the lymphatics valvular absorbent system of vessels in oviparous animals*. Edinburgh, 1770.
30. Monro A II. *The structure and physiology of fishes*. Edinburgh, 1785.
31. Hewson W. *Experimental enquiries. Appendix relating to the discovery of the lymphatic system in birds, fish and the animals called amphibians*. London, 1774.
32. Swammerdam J. *Bibia naturae*. Leyden: 1737; Boerhaave ed. Leipzig: 1752.
33. Nuck A. *Adenographia curiosa et uteri foeminei anatome nova*. Lugd. Batav. 1692.
34. Malpighi M. *De structura glandularum conglobatorum crusimiliumque partium epistota*. Leyden: 1690.
35. Mascagni P. *Vasorum lymphaticorum corporis humani descriptio et iconographia*. Sienna: P Carli, 1787.
36. Lieberkühn JN. *Dissertatio de fabrica et actione villorum intestinorum tennium*. Leyden: 1745.
37. Meckel JF. Dissertatio epistolaris de vasis lymphaticus glandulisque conglobat. In Haller, Berolini. 1772.
38. Fohmann V. *Memoires sur les vaisseaux lymphatiques avec les veines et sur les vaisseaux absorbant du placenta et du cordon ombilical*. Liège: J Desoer, 1832.
39. Weirich G. *The morphology of the walls of the thoracic duct and of other lymph vessels*. Yurev: Tartu, 1851.
40. Koelliker A. *Handbuch der Gewebelehre*, 4. Leipzig: Aufl, 1863.
41. von Recklinghausen F. Zur Fettresorption. *Virchows Archivs* 1863; **26:** 172.
42. Sappey P. *Anatomie, physiologie, pathologie des vaisseaux lymphatiques considérés chez l'homme et les vertèbres*. Paris: A Delahaye & E Lecroisnier, 1874/1885.
43. Müller J. On the existence of four distinct hearts having regular pulsations connected with the lymphatic system in certain amphibious animals. *Philosophical Transactions of the Royal Society of London* 1833; **123:** 89–94.
44. Weiss W. Experimentale Untersuchungen über den Lymphstrom. *Archiv der Pathologie, Anatomie, Physiologie und klinische Medizin* 1861; **22:** 525.

45. Heller A. Ueber Selbstandige rhythmische Contractionen der Lymphgefasse bei Saugethieren. *Centralblatt Medizine Wissenschaft* 1896; **7**: 545.

46. Generisch K. Die Aufnanhme der Lymphe durch die Sehnen und Fascien der Skelettmuskeln. *Arb. Physiol. Aust. Leipzig* 1871; **5**: 53.

47. Paschutin WW. Ueber die Absonderung der Lymphe in Arme des Hundes. *Arb. Physiol. Aust. Leipzig* 1872; **7**: 197.

48. Ludwig C. *Lehrbuch der Physiologie des Menschen.* Leipzig: CF Winter, 1856–61.

49. Heidenhain R. Versuche und Fragen zur Lehre de Lymphbildung. *Pflugers Archivs* 1891; **49**: 209.

50. Cohnstein W. Weitere Beitrage zur Lehre von der Transudation und zur Theorie der Lymphbildung. *Pflügers Archivs* 1895; **59**: 350.

51. Starling EH. *The fluids of the body: the Herter lectures.* Chicago: WT Keener, 1909.

52. Carrier EB, Rehberg PB. Capillary and venous pressure in man. *Scandinavian Archives of Physiology* 1923; **44**: 20.

53. Govaerts P. Recherches clinique sur le rôle de la progression osmotique des proteines du sang dans la pathogenie des oedemes et de l'hypertension artérielle. *Bulletin d'Academie Royal de Médecin Belgique* 1942; **161**.

54. Rusznyak I. Untersuchungen über die Entstehung des Odems bei nieren Krankern. *Zeitschrift Experimentale Medizin* 1924; **41**: 532.

55. Landis EM. The capillary pressure in frog mesentery as determined by micro-injection methods. *American Journal of Physiology* 1925; **75**: 548.

56. Landis EM. Capillary pressure and capillary permeability. *Physiology Review* 1934; **14**: 404.

57. Drinker CK. *The lymphatic system. Its part in regulating composition and volume of tissue fluid.* Stanford, CA: Stanford University Press, 1942.

58. Pappenheimer JR, Renkin REM, Borrero LM. Filtration, diffusion and molecular seiving through peripheral capillary membranes: contribution to pore theory of capillary permeability. *American Journal of Physiology* 1951; **137**: 13.

59. Pappenheimer JR. Passage of molecules through capillary walls. *Physiology Review* 1953; **33**: 387.

60. Guyton AC. A concept of negative interstitial pressure based on pressures in implanted perforated capsules. *Circulation Research* 1963; **12**: 399.

61. MacCallum WG. On the mechanism of absorption of granular material from the peritoneum. *Bulletin of the Johns Hopkins Hospital* 1903; **14**: 105.

62. Moniz E. L'encephalographie artérielle son importance dans la localisation des tumeurs cérébrales. *Reviews of Neurology* 1927; **2**: 72.

63. Hudack SS, McMaster PD. The lymphatic participation in human cutaneous phenomena. *Journal of Experimental Medicine* 1933; **57**: 751.

64. Servelle M, Deysson M. Reflux of intestinal chyle in the lymphatics of the leg. *Annals of Surgery* 1951; **133**: 234–39.

65. Glenn WLW. The lymphatic system. *Archives of Surgery* 1981; **116**: 909–95 .

66. Kinmonth JB. Lymphangiography in man. *Clinical Science* 1952; **11**: 13–20.

67. Brunn S, Engeset A. Lymphadenography. A new method for the visualisation of enlarged nodes and vessels. *Acta Radiologica* 1951; **45**: 389–95.

68. Guiney EJ, Gough MH, Kinmonth JB. Lymphography with fat-soluble contrast media. *Journal of Cardiovascular Surgery* 1964; **5**: 346–54.

2

Anatomy

The lymphatics begin as minute, blind-ended, endothelial-lined sacs in the intercellular spaces of all tissues. In the limbs, they are found mainly in the skin and subpapillary dermal plexus, whereas in the solid organs of the abdomen and thorax, they are closely related to the capillaries and small blood vessels. The minute end-sacs join together to form a delicate plexus of small vessels within the interstitial spaces and then continue to join together in the tissues around the arterioles and venules. These are the minute vessels that can be seen when a small volume of Patent Blue Violet is injected into a solid organ or the skin (visual lymphangiography) (Fig. 2.1). These very small vessels then progressively unite to form large collecting vessels that lie in the subcutaneous, perivascular, retroperitoneal and retromediastinal tissues. These are the vessels that, having been identified by an interstitial injection of Patent Blue Violet, are large enough to be injected with Lipiodol (X-ray lymphangiography).[1]

This chapter gives a brief description of the normal anatomy of the lymphatics and lymph nodes of the lower and upper limbs, the abdomen, the chest, the head and neck, and the organs of the abdomen and thorax . Each section is subdivided into the cadaver anatomy and the anatomy displayed by X-ray lymphography, the lymphographic anatomy.

The descriptions of the cadaveric anatomy are short because the accompanying engravings by Mascagni,[2] which were based upon careful cadaver dissections, often after injecting the lymphatics with an amalgam of mercury, show clearly and instantly what it would take hundreds of words to describe, and because detailed descriptions may be found in many textbooks of anatomy.[3–6] Although the normal lymphangiographic anatomy has also been described in many publications, it is repeated and illustrated

here because it is important to know the normal lymphangiographic appearances when investigating patients suspected of having lymphatic disease. All our normal lymphangiograms come from studies made on patients suspected of having some lymphatic or lymph gland disease who were eventually proved to be disease free.

LYMPHATICS OF THE LOWER LIMB

Cadaver anatomy

Most of the collecting vessels of the lower limb begin on the dorsum of the foot and around the ankle and run up the medial side of the leg, quite close to the long saphenous vein, to end in the inguinal lymph nodes (Fig. 2.2a and b). A second smaller group that begins on the heel and lateral side of the foot runs up the back of the calf to enter the popliteal lymph gland. The efferents of this gland join the deep lymphatics (Fig. 2.3a). A valve is found every 2 or 3 mm (Fig. 2.3b).

In addition to the lymphatics on the medial and posterolateral aspects of the lower leg, there are others that run upwards and medially across the leg's anterior and posterior surface to join the medial group and, higher up, vessels that run across the back of the thigh, the buttock and the perineum to reach the inguinal region. Lymphatics that run obliquely upwards and *laterally* are invariably abnormal. Surprisingly, the lymphatics do not increase much in diameter (1–2 mm) as they run proximally, presumably because each lymphatic carries a relatively fixed amount of lymph and is not joined by multiple tributaries.

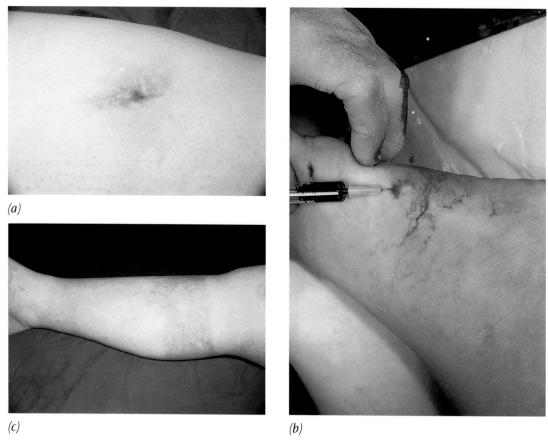

(a)

(c)

(b)

Figure 2.1 *The small intradermal lymphatics that are revealed by the intradermal injection of Patent Blue Violet. In a normal limb, the dye spreads only 1–2 cm (a). If there is any degree of lymphatic obstruction, the intradermal vessels dilate (b), and the dye may spread over the whole limb (c).*

There are many fewer deep lymphatics. One or two small lymphatics usually run alongside the anterior and posterior tibial and peroneal arteries on the deep surface of the interosseous membrane. In the popliteal fossa, they become larger and are closely related to the surface of the popliteal vessels. In the upper part of the popliteal fossa, they are joined by the efferent vessels of the popliteal gland (Fig. 2.4a). After traversing the subsartorial canal, they drain into the small medial inguinal glands that lie on the medial side of the femoral vein.

Lymphographic anatomy

The injection of Patent Blue Violet between the toes usually shows up four or five collecting trunks on the dorsum of the foot suitable for injection. When Lipiodol is injected into one of these lymphatics, it invariably enters the lymphatics that run up the medial side of the limb (*see* Fig. 2.2c). Only between two and five lymphatics are filled at the level of the knee, but between five and 15 lymphatics fill in the upper thigh (*see* Fig. 2.2d and e). In fact, the lymphatics divide into more vessels as they progress up the limb, resembling the delta of a river, rather

than reducing in number by being joined by other vessels from other parts of the limb. Consequently, the number of vessels filled is significantly affected by the rate, pressure and volume of Lipiodol injected. In spite of this variability of filling, we consider that the opacification of fewer than five or more than 15 lymphatics in the upper thigh is abnormal, usually an indication of hypoplasia/ obliteration and hyperplasia respectively. The efferent vessels of the inguinal glands are much larger than the afferent vessels (*see* Fig. 2.2f).

The lateral group of lymphatics is not filled by an injection on the dorsum of the foot. If it is necessary to opacify these vessels, an injection must be made into a lymphatic behind the lateral malleolus.

There is occasionally a lymphatic accompanying a small vein that runs from the short saphenous vein, just before it passes through the deep fascia, upwards and medially around the back of the thigh to join the medial cutaneous vein of the thigh. This lymphatic carries lymph that has come up from the lateral side of the heel with those which normally pierce the popliteal fascia. Thus, lymph from the lateral side of the foot may enter the medial collecting trunks of the thigh and pass into the medial and/or deep inguinal glands (Fig. 2.4b).

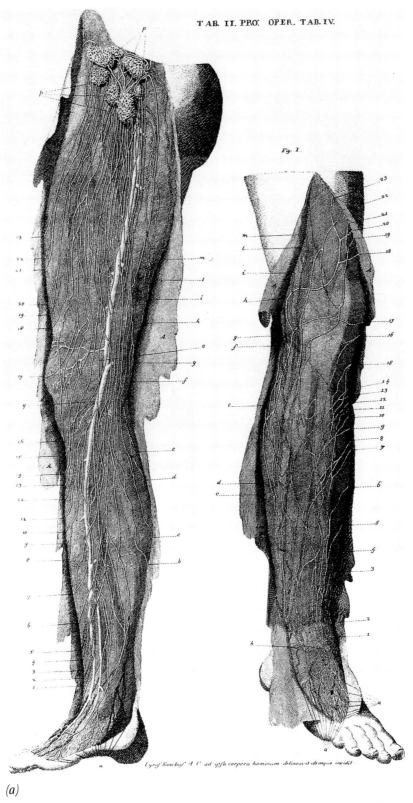

Fig. I.

(a)

Figure 2.2 (Continued on pp. 24–5) *(a, b) The normal lymphatics of the lower limb and groin as dissected and illustrated by Mascagni. (c–f) The normal lymphatics of the lower limb as revealed by X-ray lymphangiography. Because only one lymphatic on the dorsum of the foot is injected, only a few vessels are filled below the knee (c), but in the upper thigh lymphangiography usually fills 5–15 vessels (d, e). The efferent lymphatics of the inguinal glands are invariably larger and more tortuous than the glands' afferent vessels (f).*

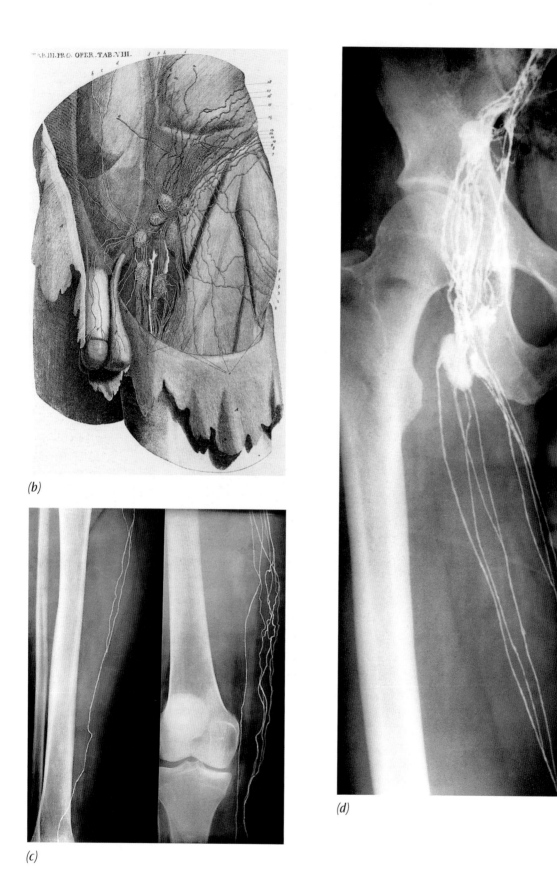

(b)

(c)

(d)

Figure 2.2b,c,d Continued.

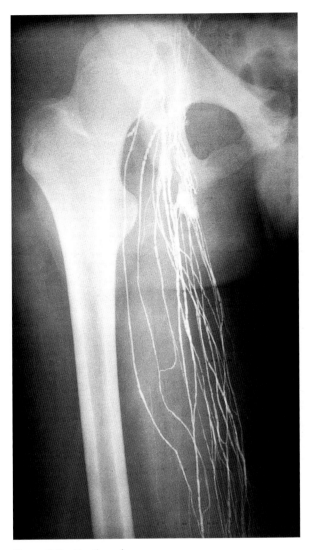

Figure 2.2e Continued.

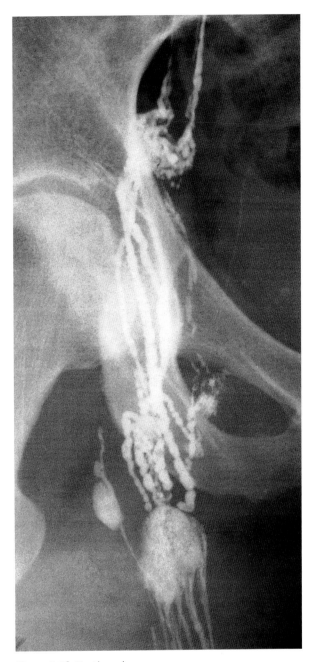

Figure 2.2f Continued.

The deep lymphatics are not usually seen when a superficial foot lymphatic is injected unless it happens to run into the popliteal lymph gland, which drains into the lymphatics that accompany the popliteal and femoral vein (Fig. 2.4a).

The deep lymphatics can be displayed by injecting a lymphatic adjacent to the vascular bundles in one of the deep compartments of the leg just above the ankle.

LYMPH GLANDS OF THE LOWER LIMB

Cadaver anatomy

There are a number of lymph glands in the lower limb below the groin. Small tibial lymph glands have been described along the surface of the anterior and posterior interosseous membrane associated with the deep lymphatics. There is usually also a small single gland or cluster of glands in the fat of the popliteal fossa, close to the end of the short saphenous vein, which receives the vessels that accompany the short saphenous vein. The efferent lymphatics from these glands join the deep lymphatics alongside the femoral neurovascular bundle. Ectopic glands are sometimes seen on the medial aspect of the thigh.

The inguinal lymph glands receive all the lymphatics of the lower limb, perineum, external genitalia, lower quadrant of the anterior abdominal wall and buttock (Fig. 2.5). They occupy an elongated triangle whose base corresponds to the line of the inguinal ligament and whose apex is at the junction of the middle and upper thirds of the thigh. They vary in size and number (*see* Figs 2.2b, d

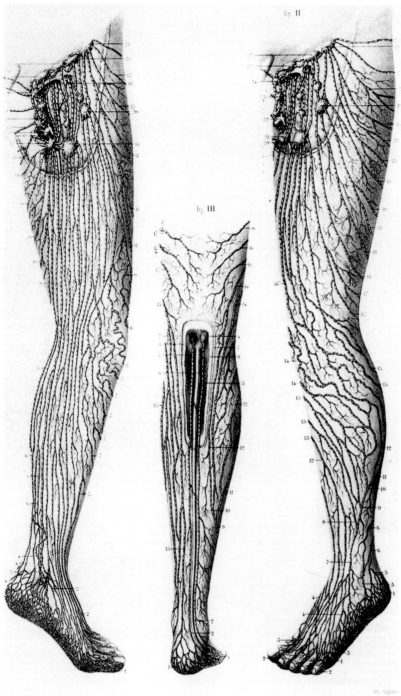

VAISSEAUX LYMPHATIQUES SUPERFICIELS OU CUTANÉS DU MEMBRE INFÉRIEUR.

Figure 2.3a *Sappey's drawing showing the many valves (one per centimetre) in all the lymphatics, and the group of lymphatics that begin on the lateral side of the heel and end in the popliteal lymph node. Reproduced by kind permission of the Royal College of Surgeons of England.*

and 2.6). They are subdivided into superficial and deep, the former being further divided into superior, inferior, medial and lateral. None of these anatomical groupings has any great physiological or pathological significance; of greater significance are the areas they drain.

Figure 2.5 shows, diagrammatically, the tissues that drain into the inguinal lymph glands. There is a reasonable chance that, draining in such a radial fashion, lymph from any particular area will first enter the gland nearest to that area, often called that area's 'sentinal node', but

this route of drainage cannot be guaranteed as some lymphatics bypass the nearest gland and enter others of the group.

Lymphographic anatomy

It is difficult, on a lymphadenograph, to separate the inguinal from the external iliac glands. In such cases, the inguinal lymph glands are classified as those glands which lie below a line drawn from the anterior superior iliac

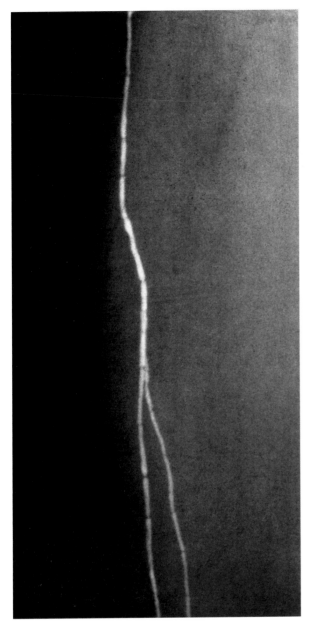

Figure 2.3b *An enlarged lymphograph showing many valves and distended valve sinuses.*

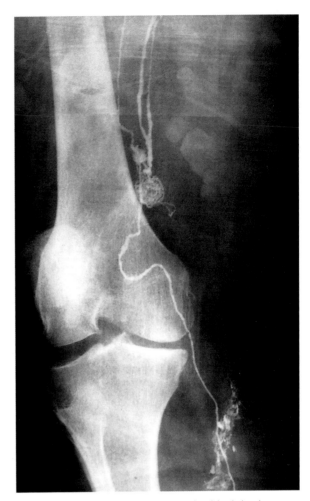

Figure 2.4a *A lymphangiograph obtained by injecting a lymphatic on the lateral side of the ankle. The vessels from this area run up to the popliteal node, the efferent vessels of the popliteal node usually joining the deep lymphatics accompanying the femoral vein.*

spine to the pubic tubercle on an X-ray taken in the supine position.

There are usually 10–20 inguinal glands (Fig. 2.6a). The proximal glands are usually small and circular, the lower ones larger and oval. The glands are usually discrete; it is not common to see the fused chains of glands that are seen in the pelvis (Fig. 2.6b). The deep inguinal glands are usually small, approximately 1 cm in diameter, and can be identified by their proximity to the medial end of the superior ramus of the pubis just below the femoral canal.

The typical pattern of a lymph gland full of Lipiodol on an X-ray lymphadenograph can be seen in many of

the illustrations in this chapter, being best described as a diffuse, fine, punctate or reticular pattern. As the lower limbs are frequently the site of chronic infection, cellular hyperplasia may make the glands larger and lead to a coarser X-ray pattern. There may also be small filling defects caused by fibrosis or fatty deposits, although fatty deposits are not as common in the inguinal glands as they are in the glands of the axilla.

The efferent vessels from the distal inguinal lymph glands run to the proximal glands, whose efferents continue on into the external iliac glands. Sometimes, however, the lymphatics of the thigh bypass the lower inguinal glands, and similarly some of the efferent vessels of the lower inguinal glands may bypass the upper inguinal glands and run straight up into the external iliac glands (Fig. 2.7). The efferent lymphatics of each gland are larger than its afferent lymphatics and often follow a torturous, corkscrew course.

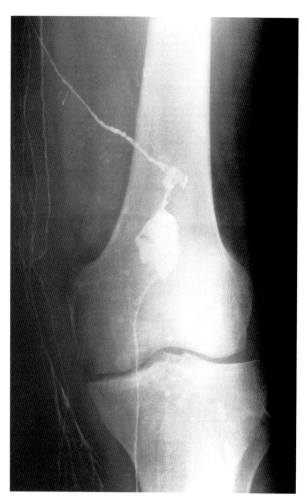

Figure 2.4b *The efferent vessels of the popliteal node sometimes pass superficially to join the medial thigh lymphatics.*

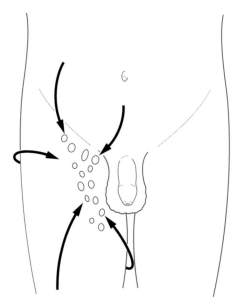

Figure 2.5 *The tissues that drain to the inguinal lymph glands.*

ILIAC LYMPHATICS AND LYMPH GLANDS

Cadaver and lymphographic anatomy

The iliac lymphatics collect together into three sets of vessels, one on either side of the external iliac artery and a third on the medial side of the external iliac vein. (Fig. 2.8).[7–9] Many interconnections exist between the vessels of each chain and between the three chains, forming an extensive plexus of lymphatics around both blood vessels.

Associated with these three sets of vessels are lateral, intermediate and medial chains of lymph glands. The medial chain of glands is joined by lymphatics coming up from the pelvis alongside the internal iliac vessels. These vessels also have associated lymph glands on the side wall of the pelvis. The glands of the medial chain are usually thin, elongated and often fused together. The lowest gland of the medial chain is often called the obturator gland. The lymph glands on the lateral aspect of the external iliac artery are usually larger. The lowermost gland of the lateral chain, which lies just above the inguinal ligament, close to the origin of the inferior epigastric artery, is semilunar in shape and sometimes called the lateral external iliac or semilunar gland (Fig. 2.9). The glands between the artery and vein tend to be small and sparse. The medial iliac lymph glands will normally receive lymph from the medial inguinal glands and hence from the perineum and genitalia, but, because of the many interconnections between the vessels, lymph from the lateral inguinal lymph glands may reach the medial iliac glands.

At the bifurcation of the common iliac artery and vein, the intermediate and lateral external lymphatics unite to form a single set of vessels on the lateral side of the common iliac artery. The medial group continue on the medial side of the common iliac artery, and a few new vessels from the rectum and the floor of the pelvis run up alongside the medial side of the common iliac vein. There are thus still three chains of lymphatics and a number of glands related to the common iliac vessels, although the medial chain is small. The efferent vessels from the uppermost common iliac glands continue upwards to become the para-aortic lymph chain.

There are many small glands alongside the common iliac vessels, but there is frequently a gap in the chain on the lateral side of the right common iliac artery where it crosses the right common iliac vein. The number of nodes is extremely variable but, with the exception just mentioned, they form an almost continuous chain from the inguinal ligament to the sacral promontory. To identify the exact position and appearance of these glands, it is essential to take oblique X-rays as the nodes are often superimposed in anteroposterior films.

The internal iliac glands are not opacified by pedal injections. They can only be displayed by injecting the lymphatics draining the pelvic organs.

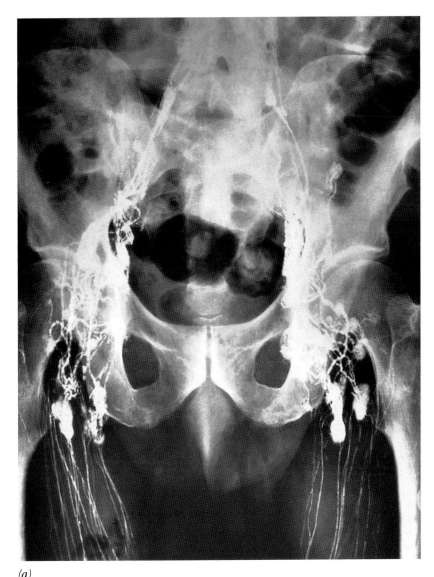

(a)

Figure 2.6 *Normal inguinal lymphadenographs. (a) Early filling of the inguinal glands 1.5 hours after commencing the pedal injection of ultrafluid Lipiodol.*

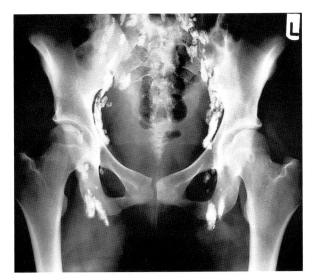

Figure 2.6b *A 24 hour post-injection inguinal/iliac lymphadenograph. The inguinal glands are separate, whereas some of the iliac glands are fused and elongated.*

LUMBAR LYMPHATICS AND LYMPH GLANDS

Cadaver anatomy

The lumbar lymphatics, which are the continuation of the common iliac lymphatics, ascend on either side of the aorta as two main trunks, the right and left lumbar lymph trunks. They are in reality not single vessels but a plexus of vessels that freely connect with each other via lymphatics lying in front and behind the aorta (Fig. 2.10a). The pre-aortic (intestinal) lymphatics, above the origin of the inferior mesenteric artery, receive lymph from the large and small bowel, duodenum, pancreas, stomach and liver.

The lumbar lymph glands form four groups named according to their relationship to the aorta:

1 the *pre-aortic* glands, which drain all the derivatives of the alimentary canal;

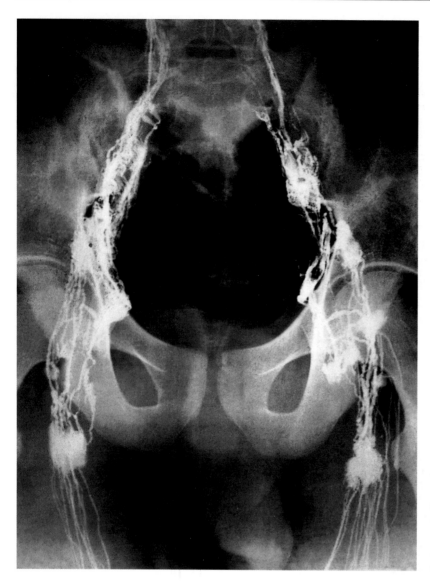

Figure 2.7 *An example of the variable pattern of the inguinal lymphatics. On the patient's left-hand side, three lymphatics bypass the lowermost inguinal glands to enter the upper glands. On the right, the lateral efferent lymphatics of the lower glands bypass the upper glands and enter the external iliac glands. The 'sentinel node' concept cannot be applied to the lymph drainage of the lower limb.*

2   the *left para-aortic* glands, which receive lymph from the left kidney, pelvic viscera and lateral abdominal wall;

3   the *right para-aortic* glands, which receive lymph from the right kidney, pelvic viscera and lateral abdominal wall and are further subdivided according to their relationship to the inferior vena cava;

4   the *retro-aortic* glands, which often unite with the nodes on either side of the aorta.

Lymphographic anatomy

The lymphographic appearance of the lumbar lymphatics[10] is similar to their cadaveric appearance, with two or three sets of vessels either side of the aorta and vena cava (Fig. 2.10b) and many functioning connections between them. This has been confirmed by an analysis of unilateral lymphangiograms,[11] which showed that lymph crossed over from the right to the left chain in 55 per cent of patients and from the left to the right in 32 per cent.

There are many glands of various sizes in the four lumbar chains (Fig. 2.11). They often coalesce, but as a rule there are eight (range 2–26) in the right para-aortic chain, five (range 2–16) in the pre-aortic chain and 12 (range 6–28) in the left chain.[10] In an anteroposterior lymphadenograph of a normal subject, the lymph glands never extend laterally beyond the tips of the transverse processes.

The left-hand chain of glands reaches up to the level of L1 in 50 per cent of patients. In contrast, the right and middle chains reach this level in only about 30 per cent of patients. This is of practical importance because the absence of filling of the upper parts of the right chain must not be interpreted as being caused by replacement with metastatic tumour. In 25 per cent of lymphadenographs, the right chain reaches up to the level of L3, whereas 95 per cent of left-side chains reach up to L2.

The chain of lymph glands on the left side is usually continuous, although 45 per cent of right-side chains show a gap at the level of the L3/4 vertebra, an interesting

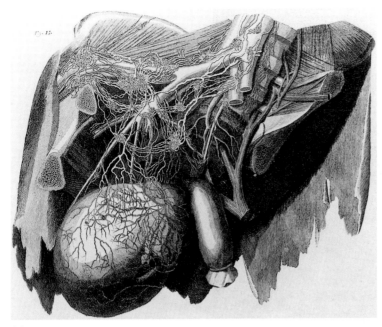

(a)

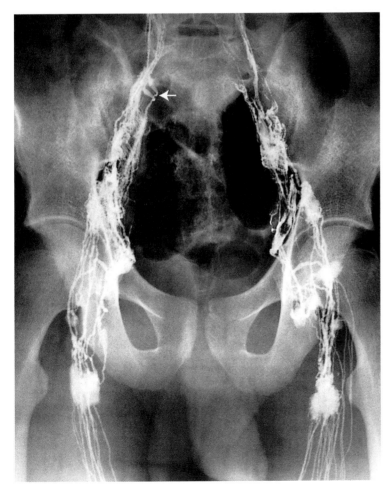

(b)

Figure 2.8 *(a) Mascagni's illustration of the lymphatics around the external, internal and common iliac vessels. (b) Lymphangiograph of the iliac lymphatics. The position of the common and external iliac artery is clearly visible. The vessels of the medial chain are obscured by those of the intermediate chain. These vessels may have large ampullae above their valves (arrowed), which is not abnomal.*

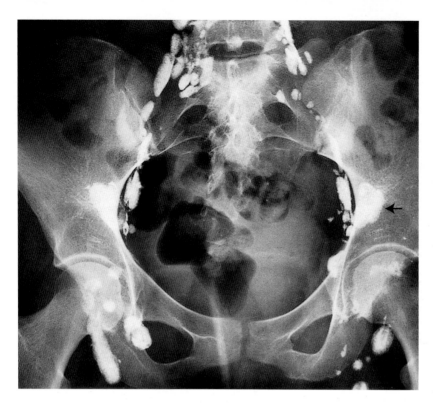

Figure 2.9 *An example of a patient with a relatively small number of large glands. The large lateral external iliac 'semilunar' nodes are particularly noticeable (arrowed).*

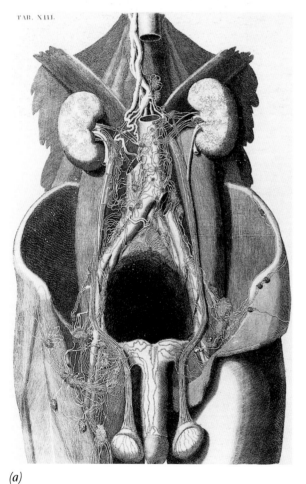

(a)

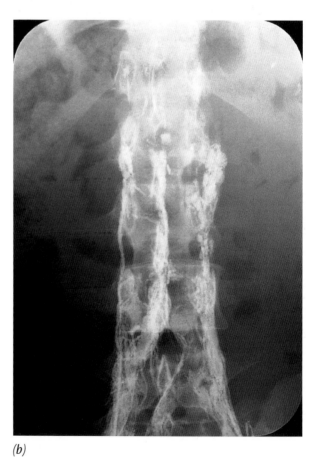

(b)

Figure 2.10 *(a) Mascagni's illustration of the extensive pre- and para-aortic plexus of lymphatics. (b) Lymphangiograph showing three chains of vessels between and either side of the aorta and vena cava. There appear to be only a few vessels connecting the central and right-hand chains, and none between the central and left chains, but in reality the three chains have many interconnections.*

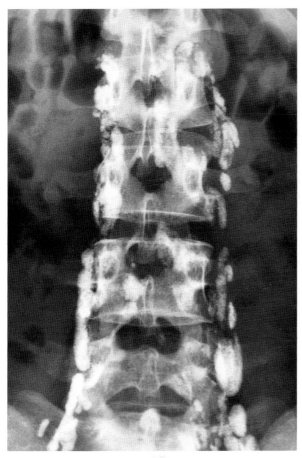

Figure 2.11 *A normal lumbar lymphadenograph. The three chains of glands are clearly visible.*

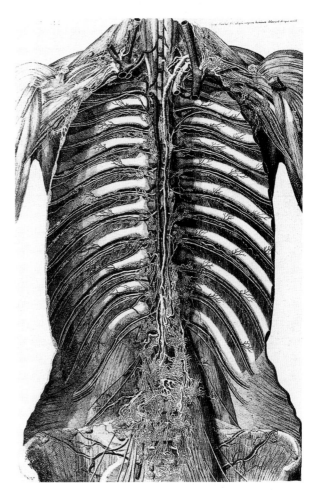

Figure 2.12a *Mascagni's illustration of the cisterna chyli and thoracic duct.*

feature that was also noted by Mascagni. The reason for this is unknown. About 25 per cent of normal lymphadenographs show a large clump of glands in the upper part of the left chain at the level of L1/2. This left upper lumbar clump must not be misinterpreted as reactive hyperplasia or infltration by tumour.

CISTERNA CHYLI

Cadaver anatomy

The cisterna chyli lies to the right of the aorta in front of the first and second lumbar vertebrae and partly behind the right crus of the diaphragm. It is formed by the junction of the right and left lumbar lymph trunks, the pre-aortic (intestinal) lymph trunk and other small lymphatics arising from retroperitoneal structures. Thus, this single sac, which is the dilated start of the thoracic duct, receives all the lymph from the lower half of the body and the abdominal contents. It is usually 1–2 cm wide and up to 5 cm long. It narrows to 5 mm in width as it passes into the thorax to become the thoracic duct (Fig. 2.12a).

Lymphographic anatomy

The cisterna chyli is only opacified during bipedal lymphography if at least 5 mL Lipiodol is injected into each leg and serial films are taken to monitor the progress of the Lipiodol to catch the moment at which it reaches the cisterna as the Lipiodol quickly moves on into the thoracic duct. The opacified cisterna is seen as a single sac at the level of L1/T12 that is usually 1 cm wide and 2 cm long; it is rarely seen to be as large as the typical anatomy textbook description (Fig. 2.12b).

THORACIC DUCT

Cadaver anatomy

The thoracic duct begins as the continuation of the cisterna chyli. It enters and ascends through the thorax on the right side of the aorta, between the aorta and the azygos vein, on the anterior surface of the bodies of the vertebrae until, at the level of the fifth thoracic vertebra, it bends to the left behind the arch of the aorta, to continue

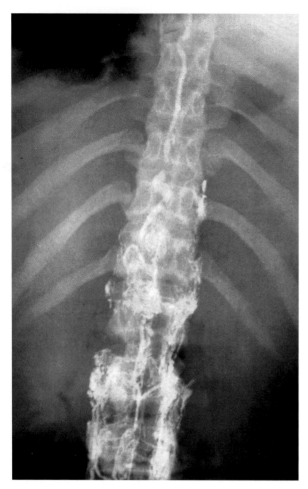

Figure 2.12b *A lymphangiograph showing a 2 cm long, rather tortuous cisterna and the lower portion of the thoracic duct.*

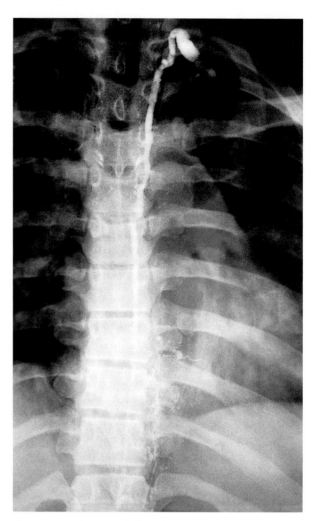

Figure 2.13 *The normal thoracic duct, which can be opacified if 7 mL ultrafluid Lipiodol are injected into each limb and the patient is tipped head down and screened intermittently for 2–3 hours until the oil fills the duct. The valves in the upper portion of the duct are clearly visible, as is the ampullary dilation of the duct just before it joins the subclavian vein.*

upwards on the left side of the oesophagus behind the left subclavian artery. In the root of the neck, it swings forwards to join and empty into the junction of the left subclavian and internal jugular veins (Fig. 2.12a). The thoracic duct is sometimes double.

Throughout the thorax it is joined by many intercostal lymphatics. In the neck, it receives the left jugular lymph trunk, carrying lymph from the left side of the head and neck, and the left subclavian trunk, carrying lymph from the left upper arm. The right side of the head and neck, and the right arm, are drained by a short vessel called the right lymphatic duct, which joins the venous system at the junction of the right internal jugular and subclavian veins.

The intercostal lymphatics on the right side sometimes form a right thoracic duct, above the level of the azygos vein, which stays on the right side of the oesophagus and, when it reaches the neck, replaces the right lymphatic duct and receives lymph from the neck and right arm. There is always a valve in the thoracic duct (and the right duct if present) just before it joins the vein, which prevents blood refluxing into and down the duct.

Lymphographic anatomy

The thoracic duct, when opacified with Lipiodol, appears as a relatively straight, 4–5 mm wide, slightly beaded structure following the course described above, with a definite widening of its terminal centimetre, sometimes called the ampulla (Fig. 2.13).[12] Lipiodol injected into the dorsum of the foot takes 2–3 hours to reach and fill the whole duct.

Although the tributaries of the duct in the thorax and neck are valved, the last few centimetres of some are filled in 50 per cent of lymphographs. When Lipiodol does reflux into a tributary, it may reach one or two small adjacent lymph glands.[13] Figure 2.14 shows the number of glands seen in the chest and neck close to the course of the thoracic duct in the lymphographs of 92 normal patients. The presence of Lipiodol in the duct for more than 2 hours suggests obstruction or malfunction.

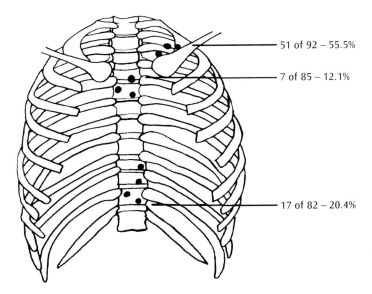

51 of 92 – 55.5%

7 of 85 – 12.1%

17 of 82 – 20.4%

Figure 2.14 *The cervical and mediastinal lymph glands filled during the bipedal lymphangiograms of 92 patients with a normal lymphatic system. Redrawn from reference 13.*

LYMPHATICS OF THE UPPER LIMBS

Cadaver anatomy

The general pattern of the lymphatics of the arm is similar to that of the leg, with long collecting vessels running the whole length of the limb and ending in the axillary lymph glands (Fig. 2.15a). Those on the medial side follow the course of the basilic vein in the forearm but then, at the elbow, pierce the deep fascia to join the deep lymphatics around the brachial artery. Others, after passing through the epitrochlear lymph gland, continue up the medial side of the upper arm to the axilla. The lymphatics on the lateral side of the limb follow the cephalic vein and then either continue up the lateral side of the arm to pierce the clavi-pectoral fascia just below the middle third of the clavicle to join the apical axillary glands, or cross the anterior aspect of the forearm to join the medial group. The efferent lymphatics from the apical axillary glands join with other lymphatics around the subclavian artery to become the left subclavian lymph trunk.

Lymphographic anatomy

When Patent Blue Violet is injected in the web spaces at the base of the fingers, it fills many collecting vessels on the back of the hand. Lipiodol that is injected into one of these lymphatics usually runs into the medial group of lymphatics but may enter the lateral group. It then follows one of the courses described above (Fig. 2.15b). The lymphatics of the arm bifurcate and occasionally join together in a seemingly random way similar to those of the leg. About 10 cm below the head of the humerus, the lymphatics leave the line of the humerus and pass obliquely towards the chest wall (Figs 2.15c and 2.16).

LYMPH GLANDS OF THE UPPER LIMB

Cadaver anatomy

Anatomy textbooks describe the axillary glands as forming a three-sided pyramid with a chain of glands along each edge: the lateral (brachial), anterior (pectoral) and posterior (subscapular) groups (Fig. 2.17). This description is based upon cadaver dissections with the arm abducted, but lymphadenographs rarely show this pattern because they are taken in an anteroposterior projection with the arm often only slightly abducted.

Lymphographic anatomy

The lymphadenogram suggests that the axillary lymph glands have the configuration of an arrow lying flat against the chest between the upper end of the humerus and the ribs (Fig. 2.18). The collecting glands for the arm are positioned at the base of the stem of the arrow. Two smaller groups of glands, the pectoral and subscapular groups, which collect lymph from the breast and anterior chest wall, and the subscapular region and posterior chest wall respectively, lie higher up and drain into one or more collecting glands along the stem of the arrow. The apical glands lie at the tip of the arrow.

The large collecting glands at the base of the arrow are usually easy to see, but the three groups are indistinguishable higher up. All that can be seen is a multitude of glands filling the space between the neck of the scapula, and the clavicle. Although lymph from the arm or breast normally flows to the first gland of the group draining its area, it may, once in the axilla, move in any direction (Fig. 2.19).

There may be as many as 40 axillary lymph glands. The uppermost apical glands lie just behind the middle of the clavicle. Filling defects caused by fatty deposits are quite common in the axillary glands.

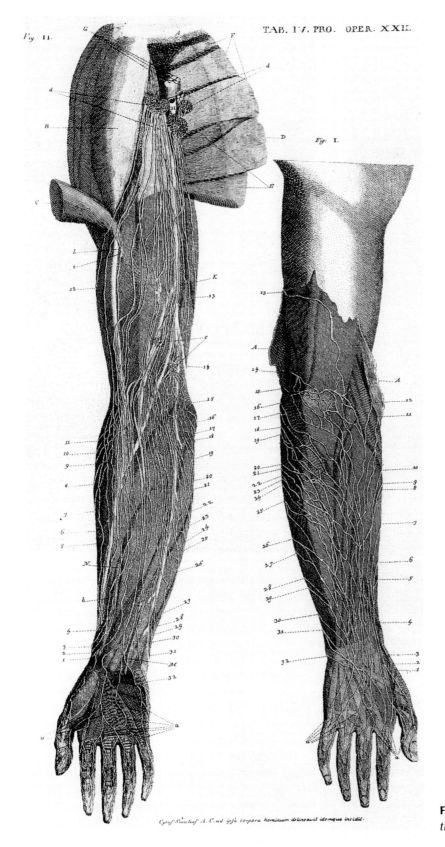

TAB. IV. PRO. OPER. XXII.

Figure 2.15a *Mascagni's dissection of the lymphatics of the upper limb.*

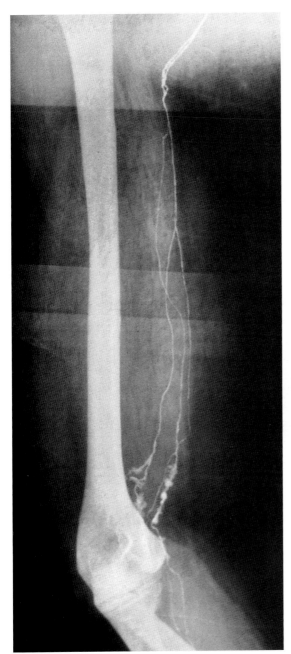

Figure 2.15b *The lymphatics of the arm.*

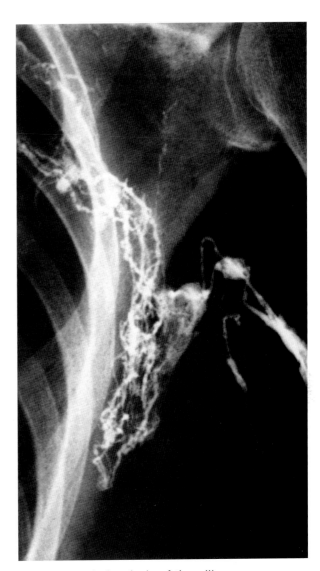

Figure 2.15c *The lymphatics of the axilla.*

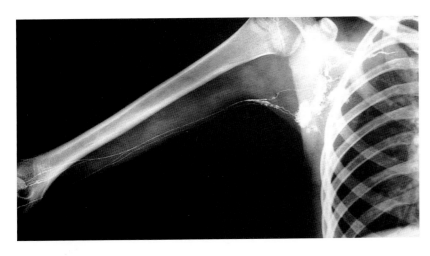

Figure 2.16 *The central lymph glands of the axilla.*

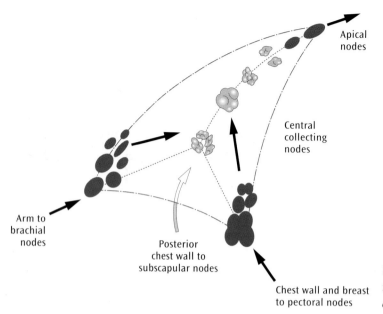

Figure 2.17 *A diagramatic representation of the position of the axillary lymph glands as described in anatomy textbooks.*

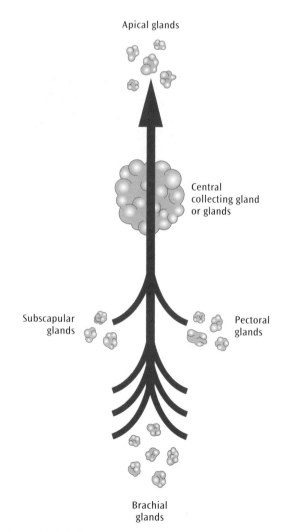

Figure 2.18 *A diagramatic representation of the position of the axillary lymph glands as seen on a lateral lymphadenograph. In the anteroposterior view, they appear to be a curved string of glands against the chest wall.*

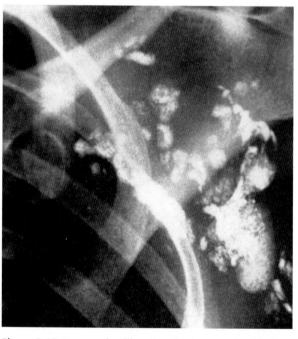

Figure 2.19 *A normal axillary lymphadenograph with the arm slightly abducted, showing the large arm collecting gland and many small glands, which receive lymph from the pectoral and subscapular regions. The apical glands lie high up between the clavicle and the first rib.*

LYMPHATICS AND LYMPH GLANDS OF THE HEAD AND NECK

Cadaver anatomy

The lymphatics of the head and neck are described in detail in many anatomy textbooks and were well illustrated by Mascagni (Fig. 2.20).[2]

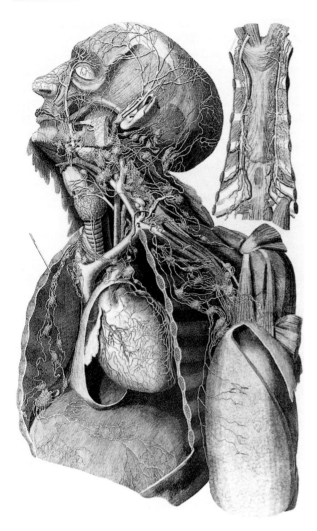

Figure 2.20 *Mascagni's[2] detailed dissection of the normal lymphatics of the head, neck and axilla.*

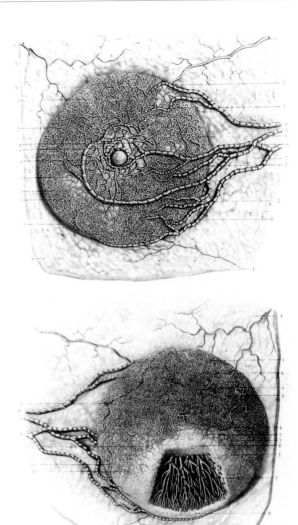

Figure 2.21 *Sappey's[6] dissection of the normal superficial and deep lymphatics of the breast. Reproduced by kind permission of the Royal College of Surgeons of England.*

There are many lymphatics in the subcutaneous tissues of the head that drain to small groups of lymph glands in the occipital, mastoid, parotid and facial regions. The superficial lymphatics of the neck similarly drain to small collections of lymph glands in the submandibular, submental, anterior cervical and superficial cervical areas. All drain to the deep cervical glands, superior and inferior, which lie close to the internal jugular vein, beneath the sternomastoid muscle.

Lymphographic anatomy

Apart from in a few rare cases of facial oedema, we have had little cause to perform lymphograms on the head or neck.

The injection of Patent Blue Violet just behind the mastoid process or in the temporal region usually reveals a lymphatic large enough to inject just in front of, or below, the ear. The resulting lymphograph shows vessels and glands similar in position, size and appearance to those seen in a cadaver dissection.

LYMPHATICS OF THE BREAST

Cadaver anatomy

The anatomy of the lymphatics of the breast was described in detail and illustrated by Sappey in 1874.[6] Figure 2.21 shows the subareolar plexus, which receives lymphatics from the interlobular spaces and the peri-areolar skin and then drains to the pectoral group of axillary lymph glands. Some lymphatics from the deeper part of the breast drain to the lymphatics on the fascia of pectoralis major and then to the axilla.

Patent Blue Violet injected subcutaneously into the lateral half of the breast drains, in 85–90 per cent of patients, to a single pectoral lymph node. This 'sentinel gland' is nowadays used by many surgeons as a sampling site when searching for micrometastases of breast carcinoma.

Unusually, and often associated with obstruction of the lateral lymphatic pathways, lymph from the medial half of the breast may drain through the pectoralis major muscle alongside the anterior intercostal vessels to the internal mammary lymph glands, or sometimes across the midline to the other breast.

Lymphographic anatomy

Apart from an unpublished lymphographic study of the state of the axillary lymph nodes in patients with carcinoma of the breast, obtained by injecting collecting vessels found in the subcutaneous tissues over the upper outer quadrant of the breast, we have not performed lymphograms of the breast. This study was difficult because the lymphatics at this site are very small and, even when successfully injected, failed to provide information of clinical value.

LYMPHATICS AND LYMPH GLANDS OF THE GASTROINTESTINAL TRACT

Cadaver anatomy

Lymphatics are present in all layers of the wall of the gastrointestinal tract. Those of the submucosal and periglandular tissues of the stomach are small and difficult to see, whereas the lymphatics in the centre of the

intestinal villi are large and, when filled with milky chyle, sometimes visible to the naked eye.

The stomach and small and large bowel walls contain an extensive network of lymphatics beneath their mucosal lining whose afferent vessels pierce the muscularis mucosa and join together to form an uninterrupted submucous plexus. As the vessels from this plexus pass through the inner layer of circular muscle, they join with the lymphatics of the muscle to form a plexus between its inner circular and outer longitudinal layers. The efferents from this plexus then pass through the outer longitudinal muscle layer to form a plexus of larger vessels in the subserosa before coalescing into large collecting vessels that run alongside the mesenteric blood vessels to the lymph glands (Fig. 2.22).

The lymph glands of the stomach, small bowel and large intestines are divided into three categories: those close to the wall of the bowel, those in the mesentery close to the divisions and branches of the supplying arteries and those close to the origin of the principal arteries of supply, the coeliac, superior mesenteric and inferior mesenteric.

Lymphographic anatomy

A lymphangiogram of the lymphatics of the small bowel is sometimes necessary as part of the investigation of protein-losing enteropathy. Patent Blue Violet injected beneath the serosa of the bowel rapidly fills the subserosal and collecting lymphatics in the mesentery (Fig. 2.23a).

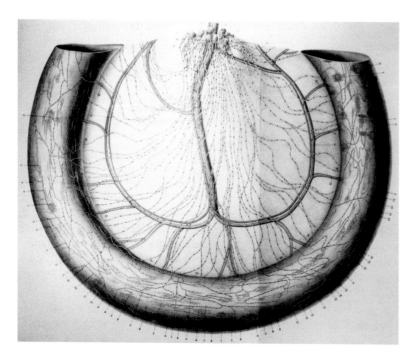

Figure 2.22 *Sappey's[6] dissection of the lymphatics of the small bowel, clearly showing their straight, direct course between the bowel wall and the lymph glands at the base of the mesentery, in contrast to the arcades formed by the arteries and veins. Reproduced by kind permission of the Royal College of Surgeons of England.*

Figure 2.23b is an intestinal lymphangiograph demonstrating how the small bowel lymphatics run a straight course from the bowel wall to the glands at the root of the mesentery. Unlike the arteries and veins, mesenteric lymphatics do not form arcades, so if the lymphatic drainage of a segment of bowel is to be preserved, the mesenteric pedicle must be kept as wide as the segment of bowel (*see* Chapter 16). If the injection of Lipiodol is followed by serial X-rays, good images can be obtained of the pre-aortic lymph glands, cisterna chyli and thoracic duct.

LYMPHATICS AND LYMPH GLANDS OF THE SOLID ORGANS

Liver and gallbladder

The lymphatics of the liver appear to start in the perilobular tissue (Glisson's capsule) rather than in the potential spaces between the columns of cells that form each lobule, (the spaces of Disse). They collect together into ascending trunks that accompany the hepatic veins to join the lymph glands around the end of the inferior vena cava just below the diaphragm, or into descending trunks that run alongside the portal veins to the porta hepatis to join the superior pancreatic and pre-aortic glands.

There is also a superficial subserous plexus over the whole surface of the liver whose efferent vessels, depending on their site of origin, drain to the glands around the termination of the vena cava or porta hepatis. The deep lymphatics between the lobules and the superficial capsular lymphatics are not widely interconnected.

The gallbladder has lymphatic plexuses in its subserous, muscular and submucosal layers. The networks join together to form collecting ducts at the level of the cystic duct. These vessels drain into the hepatic and superior pancreatico-splenic lymph glands.

Spleen

The spleen has a network of periarterial lymphatics running throughout its parenchyma. These collect together to drain into the pancreatico-splenic lymph glands.

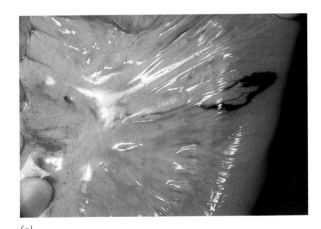

(a)

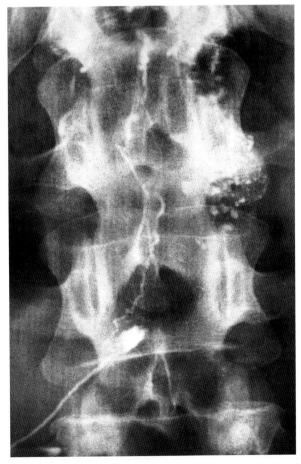

(b)

Figure 2.23 *(a) Normal small bowel lymphatics visualized by injecting Patent Blue Violet into the subserosal layer of the bowel. (b) Normal small bowel lymphangiograph. The injected lacteal (bottom left) ran directly to a mesenteric gland without dividing or joining any other lacteals. The Lipiodol then flowed on to the cisterna chyli (centre top). The Lipiodol in the gland anterior to the left side of the L1 vertebra is the residue of a previous pedal lymphangiogram.*

Kidney

The lymphatics of the kidney begin in three plexuses. One is situated deep in the parenchyma with its end-sacs between the tubules but not in the glomeruli, whereas the other two are superficial, one lying immediately beneath the capsule, the other within the extracapsular perirenal tissues. The deeper lymphatics accompany the arteries and veins to the hilum, the two superficial plexuses intercommunicate freely and drain towards the renal vein as it leaves the hilum. These all then combine into a number of collecting vessels that accompany the renal vein and drain into the para-aortic lymph glands.

Testis and ovary

The testis has two lymphatic plexuses, one within the substance of the testis, the other under the tunica vaginalis. These join to form 4–8 collecting trunks, which run upwards alongside the testicular artery to drain into the para- and pre-aortic lymph glands.

The collecting vessels of the vas deferens drain into the external iliac lymph glands.

The lymphatics of the ovary follow a pattern and course similar to those of the testis.

Uterus

The lymphatics from the plexus beneath the endometrium and those from the subserosa of the uterus and fallopian tubes drain to the pre- and para-aortic lymph glands. The lymphatics of the cervix drain to the external iliac, internal iliac and sacral lymph glands.

Heart

The lymphatic capillaries of the heart form plexuses in the subendocardium, myocardium and subepicardium. The efferent vessels from these plexuses join to form right and left collecting trunks in the subepicardial layer. Then, following retrogradely the branches of the coronary arteries, the left trunks drain to the inferior tracheobronchial lymph glands, and the right trunks to the innominate glands in the superior mediastinum.

Lungs and pleura

The lymphatics of the lung, whose end-sacs are close to the capillaries and bronchioles of the lung substance, but probably not around the alveoli, drain alongside the pulmonary blood vessels to the hilum and then into the bronchopulmonary lymph glands. The large bronchi also have a lymphatic plexus beneath their mucosa as well as one in the peribronchial tissue. The efferent vessels from the parenchyma and the peribronchial tissues drain to the bronchopulmonary lymph glands.

The lungs also have an extensive superficial network of lymphatics situated just beneath the pleura. These lymphatics do not normally communicate with the deep parenchymal lymphatics until they reach the hilum of the lung, where they continue on with the deep lymphatics to the bronchopulmonary lymph glands. There are, however, some connections between the two systems, which may open up if one or the other is obstructed.

The lymphatics of the parietal pleura drain to the intercostal, internal mammary, diaphragmatic or mediastinal lymph glands according to the anatomical position of the area of pleura from which they originate.

Brain

There are no lymphatics in the substance of the central nervous system or the meninges,[14,15] but there are lymphatics on the outer surface of the spinal dura mater and lymphatics within the epineural tissues of major nerves and among the nerve fibres.[16]

REFERENCES

1. Kinmonth JB. Lymphangiography in man. *Clinical Science* 1952; **11:** 13–20.
2. Mascagni P. *Vasorum lymphaticorum corporis humani descriptio et ichnographia.* Sienna: P Carli, 1787.
3. Bartels P. Das Lymphgefasssystem. In: Bardeleben KV ed. *Handbuch der Anatomie des Menschen.* Jena: Fischer, 1909.
4. Poirier P, Cuneo B, Delamere G. *The lymphatics* (transl. Leaf CH). London: Constable, 1903.
5. Rouviere H. *Anatomy of the human lymphatic system* (transl. Tobias). Ann Arbor, MI: MJ Edwards, 1938.
6. Sappey P. *Anatomie, physiologie, pathologie des vaisseaux lymphatiques considérés chez l'homme et les vertèbres.* Paris: A Delahaye, 1874.
7. Wirth W. Zur Röntgenanatomie des Lymphsystems der Inguinalen, Pelvinen und Aortalen Region. *Fortschrift Röntgenstr.* 1966; **105:** 441–52.
8. Gregl A, Eydt M, Fernandez-Redo E, Krack V, Keinle J, Yu D. Die lymphographische Anatomie des Retroperitonealraumes. *Fortschrift Röntgenstr.* 1968; **109:** 547–56.
9. Fuchs WA. *Lymphography in cancer.* London: Heinemann, 1969.
10. Jackson BT, Kinmonth JB. The normal lymphographic appearances of the lumbar lymphatics. *Clinical Radiology* 1974; **25:** 175–86.
11. Jackson BT, Kinmonth JB. Lumbar lymphatic crossover. *Clinical Radiology* 1974; **25:** 187–93.

12. Cox SJ, Kinmonth JB. Lymphography of the thoracic duct. *Journal of Cardiovascular Surgery* 1975; **16:** 120–2.
13. Negus D, Edwards JM, Kinmonth JB. Filling of cervical and mediastinal nodes from the thoracic duct and the physiology of Virchow's node. *British Journal of Surgery* 1970; **57:** 267–71.
14. Pigalew I. Methoden zur Trennung des Subarachnoidalraumes bei Hunden in chronischen Experiment. *Zeitschrifte Ges. Experimentale Medizin* 1928; **61:** 1–15.
15. Magnus R. Über die Enstetehung der Hautodeme bei experimenteller hydramischer Plethora. *Archives of Experimental Medicine* 1899; **42:** 250–62.
16. Zhdanov DA. *General anatomy and physiology of the lymphatic system.* Leningrad: Medgiz, 1952.

3

The physiology of lymph production and propulsion

J RODNEY LEVICK AND NOEL McHALE

The principal roles of the lymphatic system are: (1) the prevention of oedema, achieved by returning capillary filtrate and plasma proteins to the circulation; (2) immunosurveillance and the circulation of lymphocytes; and (3) the transport of particulate matter such as chylomicra. This chapter focuses chiefly on the first of these functions and emphasizes recent advances in understanding the lymphatic pump and the formation of interstitial fluid, the precursor of lymph. For reviews on interstitial fluid formation, the reader is referred to Aukland and Reed (1993),[1] Michel (1997)[2] and Levick (2003);[3] and for reviews of lymphatic function to Yoffey and Courtice (1970),[4] Nicoll and Taylor (1977),[5] Olszewski (1985),[6] Schmid-Schönbein (1990)[7] and McHale (1995).[8]

THE TURNOVER OF EXTRACELLULAR FLUID

Water, small solutes and small amounts of plasma protein pass continuously from the microcirculation into the interstitial spaces to form interstitial fluid. At the same time, interstitial fluid is removed by a network of initial lymphatic vessels, thereby preventing the accumulation of fluid. The ionic and protein composition of prenodal lymph indicates that it is essentially interstitial fluid that has drained into the initial lymphatic network.[9–11] The initial lymphatic plexus drains via 'collectors' into afferent lymph trunks, which possess smooth muscle and actively pump the lymph to the regional lymph nodes. Here some fluid is absorbed, antigens are processed and lymphocytes are added. The modified, efferent lymph is actively pumped back into the circulation, chiefly via the thoracic duct, which drains into the subclavian vein in the neck. Smaller cervical trunks return lymph from the head to the neck veins. There is also evidence for lympatico-venous communications at more peripheral locations,[12] but the amount of fluid returned by these pathways is probably small (less than 2 per cent) under normal conditions. The brain and eye lack a lymphatic system but have other specialized fluid drainage systems.

Magnitude of net lymph flow and concentration of lymph in lymph nodes

Fistulae of the human thoracic duct pour out 1–3 L lymph per day. From this it has been estimated that an adult produces up to approximately 4 L efferent lymph per day, inclusive of cervical lymph.[4] This flow of efferent lymph was traditionally taken as a measure of the rate of formation of afferent lymph and hence the net microvascular filtration rate. It now appears, however, that afferent lymph flow may be up to double the efferent lymph flow,

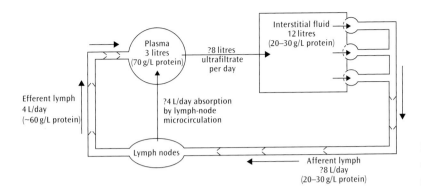

Figure 3.1 *Estimate of extravascular circulation of fluid and plasma protein in a 65 kg human. Adapted from reference 3.*

Table 3.1 *Regional variation in efferent lymph flow and composition in different tissues in man*

	Flow (% of total thoracic duct flow)	L/P ratio (concentration of plasma protein in lymph relative to plasma)
Thoracic duct	1–3 litres per day	0.66–0.69
Liver	30–49%	0.66–0.89
Gastrointestinal tract	~37%	0.50–0.62
Kidneys	6–11%	0.47
Lungs	3–15%	0.66–0.69
Limbs and cervical trunks	<10%	0.23–0.58

Adapted from reference 4.

i.e. up to 8 L per day (Fig. 3.1).[13] This upward revision arose from the discovery that as much as half of the water in lymph can be absorbed directly into the bloodstream as the lymph passes through the regional lymph nodes.[14–16] The lymph proteins are not absorbed at the same time so the protein concentration in efferent lymph is up to twice that in afferent lymph. The proteins are chiefly plasma proteins that have leaked from the microcirculation into the interstitial compartment.

Turnover times

The human circulation contains approximately 3 L plasma. Since afferent lymph production is of the order of 4–8 L per day, the entire plasma water mass must circulate through the interstitial compartment (in the region of 12 L) and lymphatic system in 9–18 hours. In other words, the extravascular circulation of fluid is relatively rapid. Because of this, the lymphatic system has a major impact on interstitial and plasma volumes. This is demonstrated clinically by the rapid formation of lymphoedema following lymphatic obstruction. Conversely, pharmacological arrest of the dorsal lymph 'hearts' in amphibia causes a rapid fall in plasma volume.[17]

Regional differences in lymph flow and composition

Roughly 30–50 per cent of human thoracic duct lymph is derived from the liver. Hepatic lymph contributes disproportionately to the plasma protein content of thoracic duct

lymph because hepatic capillaries are discontinuous (sinusoidal) and therefore unusually permeable to protein. Table 3.1 summarises the lymph flow and composition from various tissues. The marked regional differences in lymph protein content arise from differences in local capillary permeability and filtration rate.

As well as plasma-derived solutes such as electrolytes, urea and glucose, lymph contains a low concentration of hyaluronan that has leached out of the interstitial matrix. The hyaluronan is avidly taken up and cleared in lymph nodes by highly specific receptors, probably the recently discovered receptor LYVE-1.[18,19]

FORMATION OF MICROVASCULAR FILTRATE: LYMPHATIC 'LOAD'

In the steady state, i.e. when a tissue is neither swelling nor shrinking, the volume of fluid drained by the afferent lymphatic system must equal that produced by microvascular filtration. The filtration rate is thus the ultimate determinant of lymph flow in the steady state. Advances in understanding capillary filtration have so far passed largely unreported in standard textbooks, and are reviewed below.

Starling principle of capillary filtration

In his seminal paper of 1896, Starling[20] pointed out that microvascular endothelium forms a semipermeable membrane, albeit a slightly leaky one, between plasma and interstitial fluid.[2,21] Consequently, the rate and direction of fluid exchange in capillaries and venules depends in principle on four pressures. Filtration is driven by capillary blood pressure, P_c, minus the opposing pressure of interstitial fluid, P_i. Absorption of fluid, when it occurs (see below), is driven by the colloid osmotic pressure of plasma (π_p), minus π_i. π_i is defined here as the colloid osmotic pressure of fluid at the abluminal surface of the semipermeable pores. π_i has traditionally been assumed to be the same as interstitial fluid colloid osmotic pressure, which is quite large as a consequence of the leaked plasma proteins, but recent evidence of pore exit microgradients has raised doubts about this assumption, as discussed below.

The crucially important Landis–Starling equation tells us that the microvascular filtration rate J_v, and hence lymph flow in the steady state, is determined by the algebraic sum of the four pressures multiplied by the hydraulic conductance of the wall (hydraulic permeability, L_p) and the wall area (A). Thus:

$$J_v = L_p A\{[P_c - P_i] - \sigma[\pi_p - \pi_i]\}$$

The sum of all the L_pA values in 100 g tissue is called the tissue's capillary filtration capacity (CFC). The term σ is the reflection coefficient, which is a measure of the osmotic 'effectiveness' of the membrane. For a perfect semipermeable membrane, the reflection coefficient is 1 (100 per cent reflection of the plasma proteins), whereas for a totally leaky membrane it is zero. Most estimates of σ for healthy capillaries lie in the range 0.80–0.95.

Effects of microvascular pressure and inflammation

Figure 3.2 shows how filtration into the interstitial compartment depends on microvascular pressure and plasma colloid osmotic pressure, and how the relationship is altered during acute inflammation. The control results in the lower panel show that filtration rate increases linearly with microvessel blood pressure above a certain value but is zero at a certain, relatively high pressure. The positive pressure intercept shows that there must be a pressure opposing filtration, namely the plasma colloid osmotic pressure.

The slope of the relation represents the endothelial hydraulic permeability L_p. The hydraulic permeability is increased many fold by inflammatory agonists such as serotonin, histamine and bradykinin because of the formation of μm-wide gaps through and between the endothelial cells.[23] In addition, the pressure intercept shifts to the left during inflammation, indicating that the effective osmotic pressure across the wall is reduced. This is caused by a fall in the reflection coefficient σ as gaps form in the endothelial layer. As a consequence of these changes, fluid with a high protein content pours rapidly into inflamed tissue, causing local oedema and increased lymph flow. The exudate and lymph are particularly enriched in the larger plasma proteins such as fibrinogen, which can lead to adhesions in certain clinical situations.

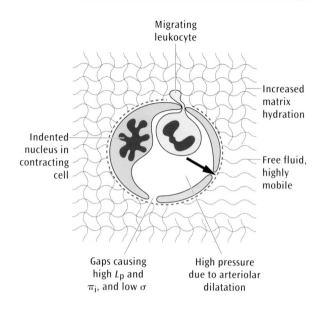

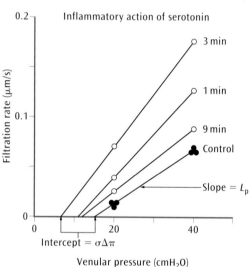

Figure 3.2 *(Top) Effect of inflammation on filtration into interstitial compartment. The large inflammatory gaps are not present in normal vessels. (Bottom) Transient effect of an inflammatory mediator (serotonin, applied continuously) on filtration rate, hydraulic conductance and osmotic reflection coefficient in a single rat venule. See text for details. Data from reference 22.*

Pathways across microvascular endothelium

Recent experimental and theoretical work indicates that the microstructure of the transendothelial pathway is likely to be an important factor slowing the formation of interstitial fluid and lymph (see below). In the continuous capillaries of the skin, muscle, connective tissue and lung, the water and small hydrophilic solutes (glucose, salts, etc.) pass through a long, narrow paracellular pathway consisting of clefts approximately 20 nm wide between adjacent endothelial cells – the intercellular junctions.[24]

In the fenestrated capillaries of the synovium, intestinal mucosa, kidney and all endocrine and exocrine glands, water and small solutes also pass through circular, ultra-thin windows in the cell body called fenestrae. The entrances to the intercellular clefts and fenestrae are covered by the glycocalyx, a layer of fibrous molecules. There is evidence that the glycocalyx is so dense (effective pore radius in the region of 4 nm) that it reflects the plasma proteins. The glycocalyx has therefore been proposed as the anatomical site of the 'small-pore system' that confers the property of semipermeability.[23]

A separate pathway is responsible for the slow transfer of plasma proteins across the endothelium into the interstitial fluid and lymph; this is called the 'large-pore system'.[24,25] The physical identity of the 'large pores' is controversial because pores as such are rarely seen. There is considerable evidence for the transcytosis of proteins by endothelial vesicles approximately 60 nm in diameter, but other structures, such as rare transendothelial pores, may also contribute.[23,25]

HYPOTHESES OF LYMPH FORMATION, OLD AND NEW

We have adopted above the simple view that capillary *filtration* generates the fluid that enters the lymphatic system, but there is a tenaciously held, albeit poorly substantiated, alternative hypothesis of lymph formation. This is the traditional view that most of the filtrate produced by the arterial capillaries, where pressure is high, is continuously *reabsorbed* by the downstream, venous microvessels, where pressure is low, leaving behind a small, concentrated fraction of the original filtrate to drain away as lymph.

There is now considerable evidence against the concept of continuous downstream reabsorption in most tissues, as described below.

Adding up the four Starling pressures in venous microvessels

The first issue is whether the four traditional Starling forces actually add up to a net absorptive force in venous microvessels. Figure 3.3 shows on the left the conventional schema for lymph formation in human skin at heart level, based on micropuncture measurements of human skin capillary pressure.[24] Blood pressure falls along the capillary because of the resistance to flow. By the time the blood reaches the venous capillaries, its pressure is less than the plasma colloid osmotic pressure so a sustained downstream reabsorption has been assumed. This would only be true, however, if the interstitial hydraulic and colloid osmotic pressure were negligibly small or cancelled each other out, and modern measurements of the interstitial forces show that neither is the case.[2,13,27,28]

The right side of Fig. 3.3 incorporates interstitial forces measured directly in the human arm.[26] Interstitial pressure measured by a subcutaneous wick-in-needle is *negative* relative to atmospheric pressure (-2 mmHg), in keeping with the seminal studies on dogs by Guyton *et al.*[29] Interstitial colloid osmotic pressure measured on samples obtained by a soaked subcutaneous wick is far from negligible, namely 15.7 mmHg. The combined interstitial term $P_i - \sigma_i$ tips the conventional sum of the Starling pressures in the venous skin capillary towards a slight net filtration pressure (Fig. 3.3, rightside).

The example in Fig. 3.3 is just one of many data sets obtained from a variety of tissues and species in which

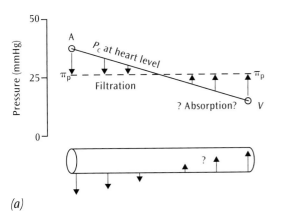

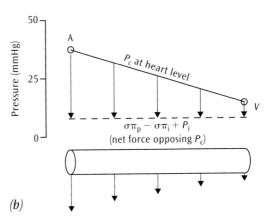

(a)   (b)

Figure 3.3 *Traditional (left) and recent (right) hypotheses of interstitial fluid formation in the human arm at heart level. See text for symbols. (Left) Capillary blood pressures measured by micropuncture of nailfold capillaries. The two interstitial Starling pressures were thought to be roughly equal and opposite, and thus had little overall effect on exchange. Lymph formation is viewed as being a slight imbalance between upstream filtration and downstream reabsorption. Based on reference 24. (Right) Net filtration force along the microvascular axis when measurements of subcutaneous interstitial pressure (−2.1 mmHg, wick-in-needle) and interstitial colloid osmotic pressure (15.7 mmHg, soaked wick method) are taken into account. Same capillary pressure and plasma colloid osmotic pressure as on left. A, arterial end of capillary; V, venous end of capillary. Data from reference 26.*

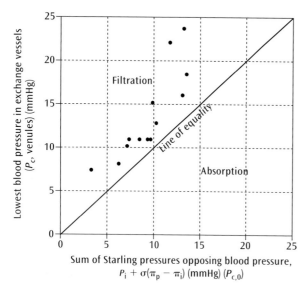

Figure 3.4 *Lowest pressure in the downstream exchange vessels (venules) versus the sum of the other three Starling pressures in the same tissue (net absorption term,* $P_{c0} = P_i + \sigma\pi_p - \sigma\pi_i$*): dog lung (lowest point), human arm, rat tail, rabbit knee, rabbit subcutis, rabbit elbow and shoulder joints, fasting rat mucosa, human chest, dog muscle, rabbit omentum, rabbit mesentery and cat mesentery (highest point). Data as reviewed in reference 28.*

summation of the conventional four Starling pressures reveals no net absorptive force in venous capillaries and venules.[28] Figure 3.4 compares the blood pressure in the venules with the sum of the other three conventional Starling pressures for 13 sets of data. Without exception, the data refute the traditional hypothesis of lymph formation through upstream filtration and sustained downstream reabsorption. Instead, the balances indicate that, in most tissues, lymph is produced by a net filtration force that dwindles along the microvascular axis (Fig. 3.3, rightside). The magnitude of the net filtration force is, however, probably less than the values calculated above using conventional Starling pressures because of the microgradients at the small pore exits (see below).

Direct observations of the direction of fluid exchange at low capillary pressures

An important test of the filtration–reabsorption hypothesis was conducted by Michel and Phillips[30] (Fig. 3.5). These authors measured fluid exchange at controlled pressures in individual mesenteric capillaries by observing the motion of red cells after stopping the blood flow. At pressures typical of arterial capillaries, filtration was observed, as expected. When the pressure was reduced to venous levels well below the plasma colloid osmotic pressure, the direction of fluid exchange altered with time.

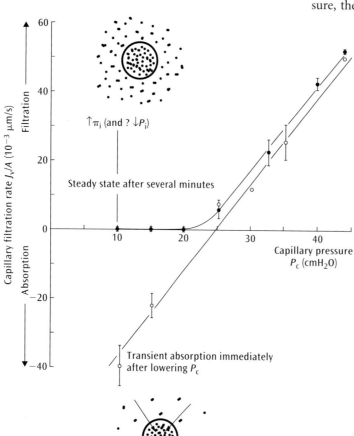

Figure 3.5 *Effect of reducing pressure to venular levels upon fluid exchange across single capillaries in the saline-superfused frog mesentery. Absorption occurred transiently at capillary pressures below the plasma colloid osmotic pressure (approximately 30 cmH$_2$O) (open circles). When the pressure was held at venular levels for several minutes to establish a steady state, absorption no longer occurred (filled circles). This was attributed chiefly to a rise in pericapillary π_i in response to the change in transendothelial flow (inset sketches: thin arrows, water flow; thick arrow and dots, protein). Data from reference 30.*

Immediately after the pressure reduction, a transient absorption of interstitial fluid was observed, in accordance with the Starling principle. (Transient absorption is medically important during hypotensive episodes such as haemorrhagic shock because it contributes to an 'internal fluid transfusion' that boosts the depleted plasma volume.) When the capillary was perfused at the same, low pressure for several minutes, however, *the process of absorption dwindled and ceased*, even though fluid was freely available for absorption, since the mesentery was superfused with saline. Sustained absorption could not be produced no matter how much the microvascular pressure was reduced.

Abluminal colloid osmotic pressure: why downstream absorption is not sustained

The reason that downstream absorption cannot in general be sustained is that the colloid osmotic pressure on the

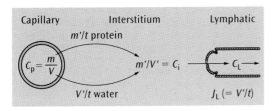

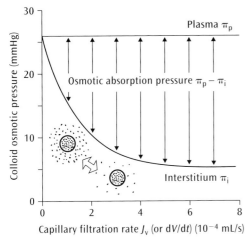

Figure 3.6 *Effect of capillary filtration on interstitial colloid osmotic pressure. (Top) The mass of protein entering the interstitium over a given time (m'/t) is diluted by the volume of filtrate over the same time (V'/t) to form interstitial fluid of concentration C_i and colloid osmotic pressure π_i. This drains away as lymph. (Bottom) Relation between filtration rate (measured as lymph flow) and bulk interstitial colloid osmotic pressure (calculated from the lymph protein concentrations) in dog paw during graded venous congestion. Data from reference 13. The conventional absorption force $\pi_p - \pi_{i\ bulk}$ falls when the filtration rate decreases and would be zero at zero filtration because of protein equilibration across the slightly permeable endothelial barrier.*

abluminal side of the capillary pores is not a fixed quantity but a variable whose magnitude depends on the capillary filtration rate (Fig. 3.6). This is well established on the macroscopic scale; that is to say, bulk interstitial protein concentration varies inversely with microvascular filtration rate,[13,27] which is in accordance with the predictions of the molecular sieving theory.[30] The greater the filtration rate, the greater the dilution of the interstitial proteins (and π_i), as explained in the upper panel of Fig. 3.6. Conversely, the lower the filtration rate, the higher the interstitial protein concentration and π_i (see insets to lower panel, Fig. 3.6). At zero filtration rate, the plasma and interstitial concentrations will eventually equilibrate if the capillary permeability to protein is finite (Fig. 3.6, lower panel). If fluid is reabsorbed, π_i will rise even more quickly because reflected interstitial protein begins to accumulate around the capillary (see insets to Fig. 3.5) and also inside the paracellular pathway (see below). Thus, the absorption term $\pi_p - \pi_i$ falls when filtration is reduced or reversed, until a net absorption force no longer exists. Therefore, unless the tissue has certain structural specializations (see the following section), fluid absorption is a self-cancelling process, contrary to the filtration–reabsorption hypothesis of lymph formation.[2,28,31]

This new perspective on fluid exchange, namely a state of dwindling filtration along the microvascular axis, reinforces the importance of lymphatic function because lymphatic drainage emerges as the only effective means of removing capillary filtrate from most tissues in the steady state.

Exceptions to the rule: microvessels that can sustain fluid absorption

In contrast to the microcirculations in Figs 3.3–3.5, the fenestrated renal peritubular capillaries and gut mucosa capillaries (after water ingestion) absorb fluid for long periods, this being an inherent part of the normal function of these tissues. Sustained absorption is made possible by breaking the coupling between the interstitial colloid osmotic pressure and the capillary filtration rate so that the relation in Fig. 3.6 no longer applies. The coupling is broken by a second source of water input into the interstitial compartment. Interstitial colloid osmotic pressure is prevented from rising during fluid absorption because the interstitial space is continuously *flushed by an independent stream of fluid*. The independent stream comprises water pumped through the interstitial compartment by epithelium in the kidney and mucosa, and the afferent lymph stream pumped through lymph nodes.

A second factor that helps to sustain the absorptive process in the above tissues is the presence of fenestrations. Interstitial plasma proteins that are reflected during the reverse ultrafiltration (fluid absorption) across the fenestrations can readily diffuse away from the unconfined fenestrations into the interstitium. This is very different from the situation deep inside the long, narrow intercellular clefts of non-fenestrated capillaries, as described in the next section.

Paradox of low lymph flow and insights into pore exit microgradients

As noted earlier, the production of afferent lymph may be as much as double the earlier estimates (*see* Fig. 3.1), a finding that is in keeping with the absence of sustained, downstream reabsorption in most tissues. The rate of afferent lymph production is nevertheless so small that its explanation presents a serious challenge. Overnight lymph production by the human foot, for example, is only 0.22 mL/100 g per hour.[32] Calculations of the expected microvascular filtration rate, based on the relation $J_v = $ CFC × (sum of Starling pressures), give values that are an order of magnitude bigger than the observed lymph flows. This can be called the 'low lymph flow paradox'. Several factors may contribute to this paradox.[31]

Arteriovenous gradient of permeability

The magnitude of CFC is usually determined by a venous congestion experiment and may be unduly weighted by venular permeability. The latter is up to seven times greater than capillary permeability. In arterial capillaries, where the filtration pressure is highest, the wall permeability is low. Thus, filtration calculations using a global CFC and averaged Starling pressures may overestimate the net filtration rate.

Arteriolar vasomotion

Vasomotion may influence fluid balance in certain tissues. Intermittent contraction of the arterioles at 2–3 cycles per minute repeatedly stops the blood flow through the capillaries in some muscle. During this cessation of flow, the capillary pressure will inevitably fall towards venular levels. This could cause short but repeated periods of transient fluid absorption.[33] If this idea proves correct, the traditional view of spatial (axial) filtration–reabsorption near-balance would be replaced by one of temporal (intermittent) filtration–reabsorption near-balance. The intermittency of capillary flow is, however, much less marked in most tissues than it is in skeletal muscle. In the skin of supine adults, for example, blood flow in individual capillaries stops for only 4 per cent of the time, rising to 35 per cent in the skin of the foot during orthostasis.[34]

Pore exit microgradients

A step towards resolving the low lymph flow paradox came with advances in understanding the protein concentration gradients at fenestral exits[35] and within the paracellular clefts of continuous capillaries.[2] Colloid osmotic pressure is generated across small pores of radius approximately 4 nm (see above). Since the pore exit is probably the underside of the glycocalyx, which overlies both the long, deep intercellular cleft and the very shallow fenestration, the relevant liquid osmotically is not the bulk interstitial fluid per se but the fluid at the pore exit, which, in the case of continuous capillaries, means the fluid deep inside the 750 nm-long intercellular cleft (Fig. 3.7). To reach this point, interstitial protein has to diffuse up the cleft against a continuous stream of filtrate. Because of the continuous washout of proteins, the protein concentration and osmotic pressure within the cleft at the pore exit, during filtration across vessels of high hydraulic permeability, is up to an order of magnitude smaller than in the interstitial fluid.[36] The effective osmotic pressure across the pore is then closer to plasma colloid osmotic pressure, i.e. $\pi_p - 0$, than to the conventional Starling term π_p − bulk interstitial colloid osmotic pressure. The true filtration rate is consequently lower than that predicted by the Landis–Starling equation, and lymph production is much reduced. Analogous reasoning also applies, albeit to a less extreme degree, to the exit

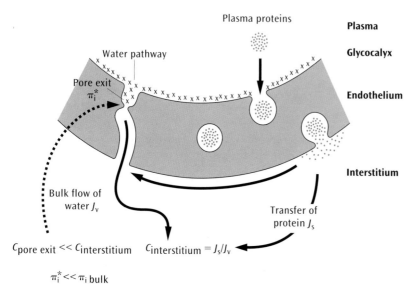

Figure 3.7 *Sketch of the endothelial cell junction (cleft on the left). The small-pore exit on the underside of the glycocalyx 'sees' intracleft fluid of lower protein concentration ($C_{pore\ exit}$) and osmotic pressure (π_i^*) than bulk interstitial fluid ($C_{interstitium}$, $\pi_{i\ bulk}$); see text for details. Plasma proteins reach the interstitial fluid chiefly via the 'large-pore' system (probably vesicles). The true force opposing filtration, $\pi_p - \pi_i^*$, is larger than $\pi_p - \pi_{i\ bulk}$. This may contribute to the low rate of lymph formation rate. Adapted from references 2 and 36.*

region around the fenestrations[35] and to capillaries of lower hydraulic permeability such as muscle capillaries.

If the above reasoning is correct, it follows that bulk interstitial colloid osmotic pressure should have less effect on filtration rate than does π_p. This inference is supported by experimental evidence. Changes in bulk interstitial colloid osmotic pressure have less effect on fluid exchange than do changes in π_p in synovial joints, where the capillaries are fenestrated.[37] In an elegant and dramatic test of the glycocalyx/junctional strand model, Hu *et al.*[38] showed that raising the bulk interstitial colloid osmotic pressure caused almost *no* change in filtration rate across continuous mesenteric capillaries, in agreement with the pore exit microgradient model.

If the above 'pore-in-cleft' model is correct, the traditional filtration–reabsorption hypothesis becomes increasingly untenable for such capillaries. Interstitial plasma protein will be washed *into* the cleft during the early, transient stage of fluid absorption. Reflection at the interface between pore and cleft raises the local protein concentration and osmotic pressure in the confined space. This gradually reduces the osmotic pressure difference that is driving the absorption process.[38] Whether an equally extreme process would occur in continuous capillaries of lower hydraulic permeability, such as those in skeletal muscle, awaits investigation.

PHYSIOLOGICAL AND PATHOLOGICAL FACTORS AFFECTING LYMPHATIC LOAD

Tissues with a high capillary density (large endothelial area) and high hydraulic permeability (fenestrated and discontinuous capillaries), such as liver, gut and kidneys, generate more lymph than those with a low density of continuous capillaries, such as skin, fat and connective tissue.

Inflammation

Inflammation greatly increases local microvascular filtration (*see* Fig. 3.2).[3] As a result, the local lymph flow is increased. In the case of snake or spider envenomation, the increase in lymph flow caused by the bite is highly dangerous. Lymph flow from the bitten limb can be greatly reduced by proximal compression of the lymphatic trunks using a cuff or bandage, although a compression pressure of 40–70 mmHg is required to overcome the contractile power of the lymphatics.[39]

Hypoproteinaemia

Hypoproteinaemia raises lymph flow because plasma colloid osmotic pressure is the only force that acts to retain water within the plasma compartment. Experimental reductions in plasma protein concentration cause marked increases in lymph formation.[13,40,41] The severe hypoproteinaemias associated with the nephrotic syndrome, hepatic failure and malnutrition cause the capillary filtration rate to exceed the maximum lymphatic drainage rate, leading to clinical oedema.

Increased capillary pressure

Raised capillary pressure is a common cause of increased microvascular filtration and thus lymph flow. Capillary pressure is increased by exercise, gravity (posture) and many pathological conditions, as follows.

Exercise causes arteriolar dilatation, which raises the local capillary pressure. This leads to marked increases in lymph flow from exercising human legs[42–44] and a 3–6-fold increase in the clearance of labelled interstitial colloid.[45]

Pathological conditions that raise microvascular pressure chronically and lead to oedema include cardiac failure, deep venous thrombosis, portal hypertension and over-transfusion. The enhancing effect of venous congestion on lymph flow has been demonstrated many times since the seminal work of Heidenhain in 1891,[46] for example by Olszewski *et al.*,[42] Aarli *et al.*[41] and Renkin *et al.*[47]

Leg lymph flow alters during *orthostasis*. Gravity raises the filtration pressure in the microvessels below heart level, which form the majority of vessels in man. The weight of the vertical column of blood raises the local arterial and venous pressures in proportion to the vertical distance. Micropuncture studies on human toe capillaries show that capillary pressure increases with distance below heart level but does not rise by as much as the arterial and venous pressures.[48] This is because an active, precapillary vasoconstriction (postural vasoconstriction) helps to protect the capillaries from the increased arterial pressure. Postural vasoconstriction shifts the capillary pressure towards its lowest limit, which is the current venous pressure. Even so, P_c reaches around 120 cmH$_2$O (95 mmHg) in the human foot during standing. This increases the lymph formation rate[42] and raises the initial lymphatic pressure 2.5-fold.[49] The lymph protein concentration falls because of the ultrafiltration mechanism illustrated in Fig. 3.6.

The dermal lymphatic plexus in the human leg appears to be more highly developed than in the forearm,[50] which implies that the lymphatic system has adapted anatomically to cope with a high lymph load in the human leg. If the lymphatic system fails to remove the interstitial fluid as fast as it forms, oedema of the leg develops. This increases further the local interstitial fluid pressure[51] and raises the initial lymphatic pressure in the leg.[52,53]

Safety factors that limit lymphatic load

Several factors help to protect tissues against excessive capillary filtration and oedema.[27,54] *Postural cutaneous vasoconstriction* has been mentioned above. The resulting sluggish blood flow allows a substantial local *haemoconcentration* to develop during plasma transit through the capillary. This raises the colloid osmotic pressure of the plasma entering the distal microcirculation, reducing the venular filtration rate.

Another important protective mechanism in the legs is the *calf muscle pump*, in which movement lowers the venous pressure (and with it capillary pressure) to around 30 mmHg during walking.[3] The pump fails if the venous valves become incompetent, resulting in chronic ambulatory venous hypertension and oedema. Reduction of the *interstitial colloid osmotic pressure* by dilution has to date been seen as an important factor opposing filtration (*see* Fig. 3.6). Whereas this view may still be true for some tissues, the issue may require re-evaluation for other tissues in view of the dramatic findings of Hu *et al.*,[38] described earlier. Finally, a rise in *interstitial fluid pressure* by 1 mmHg or so opposes filtration.[27,55] Despite the above protective mechanisms, however, some increase in local filtration is inevitable in response to venous congestion, orthostasis, etc.

We next consider how the microvascular filtrate crosses the interstitial compartment to reach and enter the lymphatic system.

INTERSTITIAL COMPARTMENT: PRESSURE, VOLUME, FLOW AND EXCLUSION

Interstitial compliance curve (pressure–volume relation)

Interstitial fluid pressure, P_i, affects both capillary filtration and drainage into the lymph vessels. Interstitial fluid pressure is a function of interstitial fluid volume. A plot of pressure P_i as a function of volume is highly non-linear in a loose connective tissue such as the subcutis.[29] The relation is steep at normal tissue hydration, small changes in fluid volume causing marked changes in the subatmospheric P_i. This 'buffers' the fluid exchange across the microcirculation. At the increased volumes typical of overhydration and oedema, however, the value of P_i is just above atmospheric pressure and the compliance curve is very flat, so that large volumes of fluid can accumulate with little increase in P_i to oppose filtration.[27,29] Interstitial pressure is typically around -2 mmHg in normally hydrated human subcutis (a common site for oedema) and between $+1$ and $+2$ mmHg in oedematous subcutis.[1,26,51]

Interstitial resistance to flow, effective 'pore' size and pitting

Although water accounts for two thirds or more of the interstitium, it cannot normally be easily displaced because the interstitial matrix has a low hydraulic conductivity. This arises from the hydraulic drag exerted by long chains of glycosaminoglycan and other interstitial biopolymers. The polymer chains subdivide the μm-wide spaces between the cells into submicroscopic, interconnected voids. The average size of these irregular spaces can be characterized by the ratio of the fractional

water content (void volume) to the surface area of the polymer chains. This ratio is called the 'mean hydraulic radius' of the matrix and ranges from 3 nm in articular cartilage to approximately 300 nm in vitreous humor.[56] Because the mean hydraulic radius is so small in most tissues, the interstitial hydraulic conductivity is likewise small, namely $10^{-10}-10^{-13}$ cm^4/s per dyne. This is nevertheless sufficient to allow the capillary filtrate to percolate slowly through the matrix to the lymphatic plexus under a small pressure gradient, which can be as little as 0.004 cmH$_2$O/μm.[57] The low interstitial conductivity, however, prevents the rapid displacement of the fluid when an external force is applied. Consequently, normal tissue does not 'pit' in response to brief (1 minute) applications of external pressure.

Protein transport and exclusion in the interstitium

Escaped plasma proteins and water are transported through the interstitial matrix towards the draining lymphatic system by convective transport or 'wash-along'. The characteristic transport distance is determined by the width of a unit ring in the 'chicken wire' network of initial lymphatic capillaries, namely in the region of 500–1000 μm in human skin.[50,58,59] Small solutes such as fluorescein (379 Da) diffuse quickly across this space, passing from the plasma to the initial lymphatic in 2–3 minutes in rat mesentery.[60] Macromolecules take much longer; labelled intravascular albumin, for example, takes 2–3 days to reach a steady-state concentration in the interstitium and lymph of the rabbit leg.[61] Such macromolecules can experience considerable restriction to movement through the interstitium because of the narrowness of the voids between the matrix polymer chains.[62]

The narrowness of the interchain voids not only restricts the diffusional velocity of macromolecules, but also excludes macromolecules from some of the interstitial water space.[1,62,63] Albumin, for example, is excluded from 20–50 per cent of the interstitial water space in subcutis and muscle. As a result, the effective interstitial protein concentration, and with it the interstitial colloid osmotic pressure, is greater than the apparent concentration calculated as protein mass/total water volume. The greater the matrix glycosaminoglycan concentration, the smaller the average void size and the greater the degree of macromolecular exclusion. Conversely, when glycosaminoglycan concentration falls as a consequence of oedema formation, the exclusion effect is reduced. An increased fraction of the water space is then available to the proteins so the fall in effective protein concentration is 'amplified', i.e. the dilution is greater than expected from the increase in tissue water seen. This causes an amplified fall in interstitial colloid osmotic pressure, which may help to attenuate the filtration rate in some tissues.[55,64]

It has been suggested that, rather than fluid percolating diffusely through the interstitial matrix, flow might be carried preferentially by definable prelymphatic, trans-interstitial pathways.[65,66] The structural evidence for such pathways has, however, been challenged.[67] In addition, the magnitude of interstitial conductivity provides no grounds for postulating such a pathway.[56] The observation that large proteins pass across the interstitial compartment into the lymphatic system in a shorter time than small proteins is sometimes cited as indirect evidence of preferential flow channels, but the difference in transit time may simply be related to the greater distribution volume that is available to the smaller solute.[63] In support of this, solute transit time is found to be size dependent even in a homogeneous glycosaminoglycan solution in vitro.[68]

FILLING OF LYMPHATIC CAPILLARIES

Having followed the capillary ultrafiltrate through the interstitial compartment, we consider next how it enters the lymphatic system. It needs to be stated plainly at the outset that, although plausible inferences can be drawn concerning how lymphatics fill, the supporting evidence is often sketchy.

Openings in the vessel wall

The initial lymphatic network is usually a blind-ending system of anastomosing lymphatic capillaries approximately 50–200 μm in diameter (e.g. skin), or sometimes a system of closed end-bulbs (e.g. bat wing).[49,50,58,69,70] A notable exception is provided by the open-ended lymphatic stomata of parietal pleura, especially over the diaphragm. These drain away the pleural fluid.[71–73] The wall of a lymphatic capillary consists of a thin layer of endothelium and an incomplete basal lamina, with no smooth muscle investment in most tissues.[74] Crucially, some of the endothelial intercellular junctions are 14 nm or more wide.[69] This renders the wall highly permeable to water, interstitial plasma proteins and even fine particulate matter. Human skin microlymphatic vessels are freely permeable to small solutes[75] and 40 kDa dextran, but less so to dextrans of 150 kDa or more.[76]

Endothelial flap valves and tethering filaments

The endothelial cell junctions run very obliquely in lymphatic capillaries, as a result of which the margins of adjacent cells overlap. It is thought that this enables the junctions to act as flap valves. When the interstitial pressure exceeds the intraluminal pressure, the flap on the luminal side is pushed open, and interstitial fluid flows into the lymphatic lumen. Conversely, when the lymph pressure rises above the interstitial fluid pressure, the luminal flap is pressed onto the abluminal flap, preventing a reflux of lymph into the tissue.[7,70,77]

The outer surface of the lymphatic capillary is tethered to the surrounding tissue by radiating fibrils

called anchoring filaments.[74] These probably act to prevent lymphatic collapse when the interstitial pressure is high, as in oedema.[70]

Fluid velocity in lymph vessels

Fluid velocity in lymphatic capillaries is 5–500 μm/s in human skin[58] and mouse tail.[78] The initial network drains into collecting vessels, where semilunar valves first appear, directing the flow centrally. The larger vessels acquire a contractile coat of smooth muscle and have fluid velocities of around 33–50 μm/s (2–3 cm/min) in human and dog limbs.[12,39]

What force fills the lymphatic capillary? Initial lymphatic pressures

The answer to the above question is poorly resolved in most tissues. The interstitial fluid is probably driven through the lymphatic intercellular gaps by a very small, intermittent, hydraulic pressure gradient (1 cmH$_2$O or less), such as that illustrated in Fig. 3.8. Supporting evidence has been found in bat wing[79] and rabbit pleura.[72] The lymphatic end-bulbs in the bat wing are, however, actively contractile,[80] unlike most lymphatic capillaries. In the rabbit pleural space, the normal liquid pressure is around −3.9 mmHg, and the diaphragmatic lymphatics can suck in fluid down to −(8–9) mmHg.[72] Their capacity to pump fluid out of the pleural cavity may be powered by the contraction of the diaphragm.

In contrast, in the exposed rat mesentery, which has neither contractile initial lymphatics nor contiguous

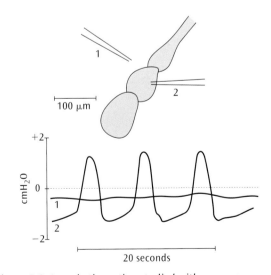

Figure 3.8 *Lymphatic suction studied with pressure-recording micropipettes in the interstitium and contractile lymphatic end-bulb of the bat wing. The interstitial pressure (micropipette 1) exceeded the lymphatic pressure (micropipette 2) during intervals of lymphatic relaxation, which constituted 43 per cent of the period. Adapted from reference 57.*

skeletal muscle, the pressure gradient does not appear to favour filling; the measured lymphatic pressures of 0–4 mmHg are slightly higher than the interstitial fluid pressure.[81] Occasional, transient dips of mesenteric initial lymphatic pressure to −1 cmH$_2$O have been noted, which might induce intermittent filling.[82] In human skin, the interstitial fluid pressure is between −2 mmHg (chest and arm) and +1 mmHg (foot). Although the mean pressure in fluorescein-filled dermal lymphatic capillaries is higher than this (2.6 ± 2.8 mmHg[53]), pressure oscillations with transient dips as low as −7 mmHg have been observed.[76,83] Some of the difficulty experienced in demonstrating a gradient in favour of fluid uptake may arise from the high conductance of the initial lymphatic wall; because of the high wall conductance, the required pressure difference may be as little as 0.12 cmH$_2$O.[7]

The mechanisms proposed for the intermittent generation of a favourable pressure gradient across the walls of non-contractile lymphatic capillaries are as follows:

1 The vessel may fill intermittently by a recoil process akin to the filling of a rubber teat. An external squeeze resulting from tissue movement first empties the lymphatic capillary proximally. Then elastic recoil, aided by the special tethering filaments, creates a transient, low luminal pressure that establishes a filling gradient.[57,79,84]

2 An intermittent, subatmospheric pressure might be created in contractile, proximal vessels as they relax and recoil. Flow into the relaxing segment from the periphery might then reduce the pressure in the feeding lymphatic plexus. Set against this, however, is the observation that pulsating pressures in the contractile lymphatics of exposed mesentery are supra- rather than subatmospheric, and increase by approximately 2 cmH$_2$O (1.5 mmHg) as lymph progresses centrally from one intervalve segment to the next.[82]

3 Many small lymphatic vessels, including initial lymphatics in muscle, lie alongside pulsating arterial vessels. Transmitted pulsations may help to pump fluid along non-contractile lymph vessels.[33,85,86]

4 A complex uptake mechanism based on translymphatic osmosis was proposed by Casley-Smith,[87] but this currently lacks experimental support.[10,11]

COUPLING BETWEEN LYMPH FLOW AND CAPILLARY FILTRATION RATE

A fixed rate of lymph drainage cannot guarantee tissue volume homeostasis. To achieve this, the lymph flow has to be coupled (linked) to the net microvascular filtration rate. In other words, the lymphatic system needs, somehow, to be responsive to the microvascular filtration rate. Coupling is an important property because it enables a change in filtration rate to be matched in a relatively short time by a change in lymphatic drainage rate. Coupling has been demonstrated in studies of

thoracic duct lymph flow,[88] canine hindlimb,[64] lung,[54,89] diaphragm,[72,90] bat wing,[80] mesentery[91] and rat tail.[41] In all these cases, an increase in fluid load on the interstitium, caused by increased filtration, is followed by an increase in lymph flow from the tissue.

What mechanism produces this coupling? Interstitial fluid pressure is one possible coupling factor because it is affected by microvascular filtration rate and is itself the 'uphill' end of the pressure gradient into the lymphatic capillary. The increase in local lymph flow in response to increased fluid pressure in the pleural cavity is shown in the upper panel of Fig. 3.9. The lower panel of Fig. 3.9

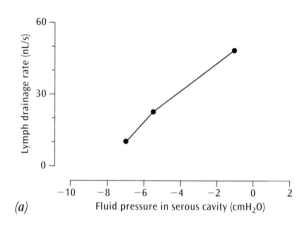

(a)

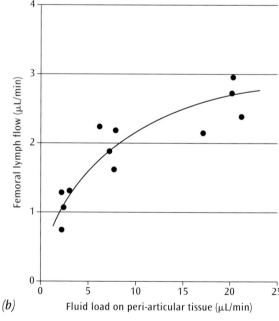

(b)

Figure 3.9 *(a) Effect of subatmospheric fluid pressures on lymph drainage from the pleural and peritoneal cavities in rabbits. Based on reference 72. (b) Femoral lymph flow during progressive experimental oedema of the tissue around a rabbit knee. Fluid was driven from the joint cavity into the peri-articular tissue at increasing intra-articular pressure over several hours. Unpublished data, S. Sabaratnam and J.R. Levick.*

shows that, when flow into an interstitial compartment is increased to the point of oedema, the lymphatic drainage rate responds non-linearly and tails off at high fluid loads. This presumably underlies oedema formation since oedema develops only when the lymphatic drainage rate is slower than the input of fluid to the interstitial compartment.

Several groups have argued that interstitial *volume* rather than pressure is the coupling factor, at least in oedematous tissue.[41,64,80] Interstitial fluid volume and pressure are themselves interlinked through the compliance curve described earlier. As a result of the non-linearity of the compliance curve, there is little change in pressure in response to large increases in volume in an oedematous tissue, so pressure would be a poor coupling mechanism in oedema. Increased interstitial fluid volume may pull open the intercellular junctions by increasing the tension in the anchoring filaments,[70] thus facilitating lymphatic filling.

Because the lymphatic system comprises differing elements plumbed in series (non-contractile initial lymphatics and contractile trunk segments), it is vital that some form of coupling should also exist between the initial lymphatic plexus and the contractile draining vessels, as well as between one segment of contractile vessels and the next. This aspect of coupling involves an active 'distension–pumping' relation, and is described next.

ROLES OF PASSIVE AND ACTIVE TRANSPORT IN INITIAL LYMPHATIC PLEXUS VERSUS CONTRACTILE LYMPH TRUNKS

Three mechanisms have been proposed to explain lymph propulsion in mammals: (1) '*vis a tergo*' (force from behind), i.e. lymph might flow from a region of higher pressure in the periphery to one of lower pressure in the central veins, (2) extrinsic pumping and (3) intrinsic pumping.

Vis a tergo

This mechanism seems unlikely for at least two reasons. First, even at the relatively low flow encountered in the lymphatic system, a pressure gradient as high as 30 mmHg between lymphatic capillaries and central veins could be required to overcome the resistance to flow. This is unrealistic under normal conditions. Second, this mechanism implies that lymph pressure should drop as one moves from the lymphatic capillaries to the thoracic duct. Where direct measurements have been made, such as those of Zweifach and Prather,[82] the opposite has been found to be true. These authors found that pressure rose from 0.6 mmHg in ducts near the terminals to more than 40 mmHg in the larger collecting ducts. Such measurements are consistent with a pump rather than a *vis a tergo*. The next question is therefore whether the pump is an extrinsic or an intrinsic one.

Extrinsic pumping

The idea that the massaging effects of muscular contractions and arterial pulsation are primarily responsible for lymph propulsion is so intuitively appealing that it has been widely, if uncritically, accepted as the main mechanism of lymph flow. Thus, Generisch observed in 1871[92] that very little lymph flowed from resting limbs, whereas Heidenhain found, in 1891,[46] a threefold increase in thoracic duct flow in response to passive movement of a dog's hind limb. Many other studies have confirmed the role of muscular contraction or passive limb movement in promoting lymph flow.[93–95] These results are usually cited as evidence that the role of movement is to enhance propulsion by a 'muscle pump' action similar to that found in veins, and it was on this basis that early reviews, such as those of Drinker and Yoffey[96] and Courtice and Simmonds,[97] argued that lymph transport was essentially passive. An alternative interpretation of the above evidence is, however, that passive movement enhances the entry of interstitial fluid into the lymphatic terminals, lymph propulsion thereafter depending on the intrinsic pumping of the larger lymph ducts.

Intrinsic pumping

Many observations have been made of spontaneous contractility in lymphatic vessels.[98–100] Smith[101] argued convincingly, on the strength of experiments conducted on mice, rats and guinea-pigs, that spontaneous contractions are an important means by which lymph is propelled. He suggested that even if lymph were propelled from the extremities by passive movement, it would remain pooled in the proximal, freely distensible lymph vessels of the leg and thigh in the absence of an intrinsic propulsive mechanism.

Studies with anaesthetized and conscious sheep strongly support this argument.[102] Intermittent compression of the hoof region significantly increased lymph flow from a cannulated metatarsal vessel, but when the intermittent compression was applied over the lymphatic itself, there was no significant increase in flow. This was taken to mean that the lymph duct's intrinsic contractions were keeping it fairly empty so that there was little fluid upon which the external compressive forces could act. When the metatarsal duct was cannulated at both ends and the inflow connected to a constant pressure reservoir of saline, intermittent compression over the (now filled) lymphatic vessel was very effective in promoting flow. These results indicate that external compression is likely to be more effective when the intrinsic pump fails than when it is functioning normally. It is interesting to note, however, that when these animals were allowed to recover, there was no correlation between walking movements and fluid propulsion. This indicates that normal walking movements in sheep do not assist pumping in the meta-tarsal lymphatics, even when these are filled with fluid.

PUMP ACTIVITY OF LYMPHATIC SEGMENTS

The pump cycle

It is now generally agreed that, in normal healthy tissue, passive movements are important only in the initial or pre-contractile lymphatic vessels. Once the fluid has entered the muscular collecting ducts, it is propelled mainly by the intrinsic contractions of the smooth muscle in their walls. The pumping cycle has interesting similarities to that of the heart (Fig. 3.10). A given segment first enters a diastolic filling phase during which the peripheral inflow valves are open and the proximal outflow valves are closed. As contraction begins, a small rise in pressure closes the peripheral inflow valves and isovolumetric contraction quickly raises the pressure until this forces open the proximal outflow valves. This is followed by the ejection phase, which delivers a 'stroke volume' into the upstream segment. As relaxation supervenes, closure of the outflow valve marks a brief isovolumetric relaxation phase, during which the pressure quickly falls. The inflow valves then open, and diastolic filling recommences.

How are the force (stroke volume) and frequency (rate) of intrinsic pumping controlled? How is the rate of fluid delivery from the initial vessels (which may be to a large extent determined by random extrinsic movements) coupled to the pumping rate of the contractile vessels? The main mechanism appears to be an autoregulatory one, although this can be modulated by extrinsic regulatory factors such as autonomic nerve impulses and circulating vasoactive substances.

Autoregulation

Lymphatic vessels respond to increased distension by increasing the force and frequency of their spontaneous contractions. The elevation in transmural pressure can be caused by either an increased preload (an increase in the rate of lymph production) or an increased afterload (an increase in the upstream resistance to flow). There is an optimum value for distending pressure beyond which flow decreases as a result of a drop in stroke volume (Fig. 3.10), which is reminiscent of the decompensation phase of the cardiac Starling curve. Flow falls even though frequency continues to increase.

Figure 3.11 shows the effect of changing the transmural pressure from 0 to 21 cmH_2O in an isolated, doubly cannulated bovine mesenteric lymphatic. Flow increased with increasing transmural pressure up to a maximum at 8 cmH_2O as a result of an increase in both frequency of contraction and stroke volume. A further increase in transmural pressure above 10 cmH_2O caused flow to decline because the stroke volume decreased, despite a continued increase in frequency of contraction. These results have been confirmed in the conscious sheep,[104] except that considerably higher pressures could be tolerated before the pump began to fail. Human leg lymph vessels can pump to at least 40–50 mmHg,[43] and an external pressure of 40–70 mmHg is required to prevent the transmission of snake venom up the human limb lymphatic system.[39]

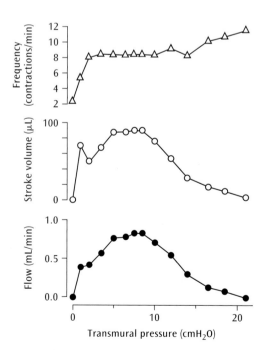

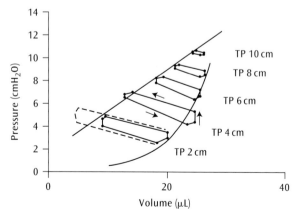

Figure 3.10 *Pressure–volume cycles in sheep mesenteric lymph vessel at increasing diastolic distensions. TP, transmural pressure. The dashed loop shows increased contractility and ejection fraction after a haemorrhage. Adapted from reference 103.*

Figure 3.11 *Flow, stroke volume and frequency of contraction in a spontaneously pumping isolated bovine mesenteric lymphatic during an experiment in which transmural pressure was increased from 0 to 21 cmH_2O. Data of N. McHale.*

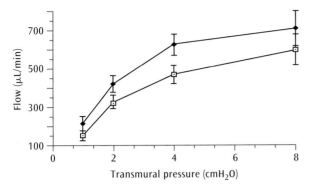

Figure 3.12 *The effect of changing the transmural pressure from 1 to 8 cmH₂O on fluid propulsion in control conditions (open squares) and during field stimulation of the local nerve fibres at 4 Hz (closed diamonds). Data from reference 112.*

Nerves and circulating vasoactive substances

It has been known, at least from the eighteenth century, that lymph vessels are innervated, but the significance of this is not yet fully understood. Lymphatic trunk vessels are known to have noradrenergic, purinergic, cholinergic and peptidergic nerves.[105–109] The first two of these are known to be excitatory, whereas the role of the last two is unclear.

Stimulation of the sympathetic nerves, both in isolated lymphatic vessels and in the intact animal, increases the frequency of spontaneous contractions and hence lymph flow. This occurs even when blood flow is depressed,[110] indicating that sympathetic stimulation can enhance pumping even when input to the initial lymphatic plexus is reduced. A direct effect of nerve stimulation on lymphatic pumping can be confirmed by using a preparation of the sheep main mesenteric lymphatic in situ, in which fluid input pressure is held constant. Under these conditions, stimulation of the splanchnic nerve causes a significant increase in frequency and fluid propulsion, confirming a direct neural effect on lymphatic smooth muscle.[104,111] Similar results were obtained using isolated bovine vessels, in which field stimulation shifted the pressure–flow curve to the left.[112] Figure 3.12 shows the effect of pressure on flow under control conditions and during field stimulation at 4 Hz. Flow was significantly increased at each distending pressure by the positive chronotropic effect of sympathetic stimulation. In contrast to the heart, however, there is no positive inotropic effect of sympathetic nerves on the lymph pump. It therefore seems that stimulation of the excitatory nerves renders the autoregulatory mechanism more sensitive to stretch.

These results lead to the proposal that the lymph pump is important in the control of interstitial volume. In normal circumstances, the interstitial fluid volume is held constant by a balance between capillary filtration and the rate of filling of the initial lymphatic plexus. This in turn determines the degree of distension, the rate and

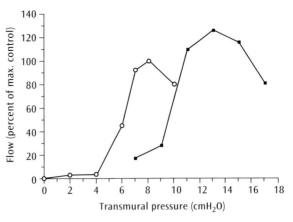

Figure 3.13 *Comparison of effects of lymph taken from a donor sheep before (open circles) and after (closed squares) endotoxin administration on the pumping activity in an 'isolated' doubly cannulated lymphatic in a second sheep. Reproduced with permission from reference 114.*

force of contraction of the collecting vessels and thus the lymph flow. If the lymph pump could be made more sensitive to distension, this would result in the same lymph flow being achieved at a lower filling pressure; thus, the interstitial fluid volume could be set to a lower value. In other words, the tissues would be maintained in a relatively dehydrated condition. This would be consistent with the body adjusting its set point for interstitial fluid volume to a lower value during a 'fight or flight' emergency in order to increase the available circulating fluid volume. The same mechanism might help to explain the increased lymph flow observed in response to haemorrhage.[113] Recently, an increase in lymphatic ejection fraction has also been reported after haemorrhage (see Fig. 3.10 above).

Conversely, the lymph pump can be made less sensitive to distension, a condition that might be called lymphatic pump failure. Elias and Johnston[114] showed that the effect of distension on flow in a doubly cannulated sheep mesenteric lymphatic vessel was shifted to the right when the vessels were perfused with lymph taken from a sheep that had been treated with endotoxin. Figure 3.13 shows the dependence of flow on transmural pressure in a doubly cannulated 'isolated' intestinal lymphatic of a recipient sheep that was pumping lymph taken from a donor sheep. The open circles on the left form the pressure flow curve before the donor sheep was treated with endotoxin, the closed squares on the right indicating the corresponding curve after endotoxin treatment.

LYMPHATIC ELECTROPHYSIOLOGY: IONIC CURRENTS AND PACEMAKERS

Origin of lymphatic rhythmicity

The above account of the lymph pump suggests that it is a relatively simple system that adjusts its output in response

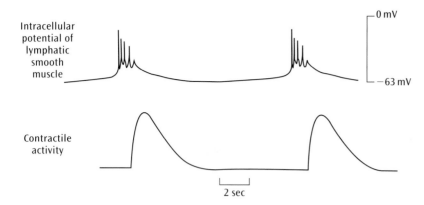

Figure 3.14 *Relation between electrical and contractile activity in isolated bovine lymphatic vessel. Depolarization and a cluster of action potentials precede each contraction. Redrawn from reference 119.*

to the amount of fluid delivered to it. The mechanism by which this is achieved was at first considered to be quite simple. Horstmann[115,116] suggested that the initiation of lymphatic contractions and their propagation were purely mechanical events. He argued that the functional pumping unit of a guinea-pig mesenteric lymph duct was the segment between two valves, because smooth muscle was scanty or absent in the valvular region of these particular vessels; such a segment has been called a lymphangion. Distension of a segment as it filled, it was argued, initiated a contraction that propelled lymph into the adjacent segment. This responded to stretch by contracting, and the process was repeated.

This simple explanation, however intuitively appealing, is not consistent with much of the evidence now available. The general existence of a 'lymphangion' is itself questionable as such isolated functional units certainly do not exist in the lymphatic vessels of large animals and may not exist in those of rats and guinea-pigs. It is true that longitudinal sections through the mesenteric lymphatic vessels of rats and guinea-pigs show regions devoid of smooth muscle, but careful examination in three dimensions using confocal microscopy frequently reveals smooth muscle continuity from one segment to the next.

The physiological evidence against Horstmann's hypothesis is even more compelling than the anatomical evidence. Isolated, longitudinal strips of bovine mesenteric lymphatic contract regularly for many hours under conditions exhibiting a lack of intraluminal distending force.[117] Similarly, McHale and Thornbury[104] observed that mesenteric lymphatic vessels in the conscious sheep continued to contract for more than 10 minutes after their fluid input was cut off, showing that luminal distension is not essential for contraction in these vessels. These results are consistent with an electrical pacemaker capable of generating a regular rhythm even when vessels are empty.

If Horstmann's simple hypothesis is rejected and it is accepted that pacemaking in lymphatic vessels is essentially an electrical phenomenon, we are still confronted by many difficult questions. What is the nature of the pacemaker mechanism? Are all lymphatic cells equally capable of initiating pacemaker activity? How is the electrical activity co-ordinated so that efficient pumping can occur? There

are as yet no clear answers to these questions, but evidence has recently been accumulating that provides some clues.

Electrophysiology of lymphatic action potentials and repolarization

Lymphatic smooth muscle is capable of very regular and well-coordinated phasic contractions that propel fluid efficiently in the direction determined by the orientation of the valves. Each contraction is preceded by a single action potential[118] or by an action potential complex,[119] as illustrated in Fig. 3.14. The repeating pattern of contraction triggered by spontaneous, rhythmic, electrical excitation is more akin to that of the heart than most smooth muscles.

A number of ionic currents have been characterized in sheep lymphatic smooth muscle that contribute to the membrane potential and action potentials. Outward currents include the calcium-activated potassium current and two delayed rectifier potassium currents.[120] Inward currents include calcium currents (both L- and T-type), the fast sodium current and a calcium-activated chloride current.[121–123] The exact roles of each current have yet to be elucidated. Preliminary evidence indicates that the L-type calcium current and fast sodium current generate the upstroke of the action potential. Some cells may have a predominance of calcium channels and thus have action potentials with a slow upstroke and propagation velocity; others may have a predominance of fast sodium channels, generating a faster upstroke and higher propagation velocity (lymphatic Purkinje fibres?). A calcium-activated potassium current makes an important contribution to the termination of the action potential complex and repolarization. After the action potential, the cell membrane potential repolarizes to a maximum hyperpolarized level, after which it slowly depolarizes until it reaches the threshold for firing the next action potential.

Pacemaker currents in lymphatic vessels

In a study of lymphatic vessels by the double sucrose gap technique, Allen and McHale[124] showed that the voltage deflection during a constant-current hyperpolarizing pulse sagged over seconds to a less hyperpolarized level. This indicated that membrane hyperpolarization switched on a slowly activating, depolarizing conductance. The voltage relaxation could be blocked with 10 mM caesium, an ion known to block the 'funny' pacemaker current I_f in cardiac pacemaker cells. It was suggested, therefore, that hyperpolarization can activate an inward current in lymphatic smooth muscle similar to the I_f of cardiac sino-atrial node cells.[125] McCloskey et al.[126] recently demonstrated such an inward current in isolated sheep lymphatic smooth muscle. Interestingly, the I_f current was found in only 5 per cent of the cells studied, indicating the existence of specialized pacemaker cells in these vessels.

Further support for this suggestion has been provided by the recent demonstration[127] of a subpopulation of cells lying below the endothelium in sheep mesenteric lymphatics. These cells show many of the immunohistochemical and ultrastructural features of the pacemaker cells found in the gastrointestinal tract[128,129] in that they react with antibodies against the intermediate filament vimentin and the proto-oncogene c-kit, they have many of the ultrastructural characteristics of pacemaker cells in other tissues and they are distinct from the bulk smooth muscle cells. It is probable, but not yet proven, that these are the same cells that possess the I_f current described above.

Although it is undoubtedly true that pacemaking in lymphatic vessels is electrical, it has proved difficult to establish its exact ionic basis. Experiments such as those described above[126] indicate a possible role for I_f in the generation of an electrical rhythm, perhaps by specialized pacemaker cells. Equally, however, calcium-activated chloride current[123] might be important in generating the electrical rhythm, as proposed by Van Helden.[130] In the latter model, the rhythmic release of calcium from the intracellular stores would activate chloride channels in the cell membrane to produce spontaneous transient depolarizations, which could in turn fire action potentials.

Integration of pacemakers, spread of excitation and contraction

Even if we understood the ionic basis of pacemaking, we would still have the problem of placing it in context, i.e. of defining its precise role in the function of the lymph pump. Where, anatomically, in the lymphatic vessel does pacemaking originate? Are all muscular segments equally capable of generating an electrical rhythm? If this is the case, why does one pacemaker dominate? (The random firing of a large number of pacemakers would result in 'lymphatic fibrillation' and pump failure.) How far does electrical activity originating in the dominant pacemaker propagate effectively? What happens when electrical waves collide at branch points? How is pacemaking modulated by stretch, by nerves and by circulating vasoactive substances?

We do not have clear answers to the above questions, but there are some pointers. McHale and Meharg[131] set up an 80 mm length of bovine mesenteric lymphatic in a three-compartment organ bath so that the temperature of each compartment could be independently controlled. Either the proximal or the distal end of the vessel could be made to initiate pacemaking by maintaining its temperature 1°C higher than the other end. The entire 80 mm length contracted synchronously under the influence of the dominant pacemaker. Interestingly, pumping was equally effective whether the pacemaker was at the proximal end, with the contractile wave propagating in the same direction as the fluid flow, or at the distal end, with the wave propagating against the direction of flow. When ice-cold Krebs solution was introduced into the central compartment, to prevent electrical but not mechanical propagation, the two ends of the vessel contracted at different frequencies and pumping became much less efficient (Fig. 3.15).

The propagation of the contractile wave is undoubtedly complex because the lymphatic network is highly branched and different amounts of lymph are produced in different parts of the network depending on variations in local blood flow and capillary permeability. This means that the degree of stretch can vary between two branches that are feeding into the same, higher-order vessel. The above experiments are important in that they demonstrate

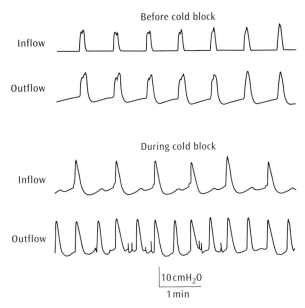

Figure 3.15 *Recordings of inflow and outflow pressure fluctuations before and during cold block produced by perfusing the central compartment with Krebs solution at 0–2°C. Prior to cold block, the outflow end (pacemaker) was contracting at a frequency of 1.43 contractions per minute, and the inflow end was faithfully following this. When cold Krebs solution was perfused through the central compartment, the frequency of the outflow end was increased to 2.56/min, whereas the inflow frequency fell to 1.27/min. Data from reference 131.*

that electrical propagation is essential and that retro-grade propagation does not impair pumping. It is thus conceivable that pacemaking may normally originate in the larger lymph ducts (which would be at a higher pressure than the branches that fed them) and then pass retrogradely to the smaller branches. This would avoid the problems that might arise at branch points if orthograde electrical waves were to collide. Nerves may play a role in propagation of the contractile wave, but propagation is unlikely to be undertaken purely by a local nerve network because pumping appears to be unaffected by tetrodotoxin.[132] It is more likely that sympathetic nerves can modulate excitability and thus the velocity of propagation. Much more work is needed to answer the questions posed above. It is clear, however, that the lymph pump is much more complex than was thought to be the case even a few years ago.

SUMMARY

1 Modern evidence shows that the microcirculation of most tissues is normally in a state of slight filtration, even in venules at heart level, leading to lymph generation. Microvessels can reabsorb interstitial fluid transiently, but there is little evidence of sustained venular reabsorption in most tissues, except the kidney, absorbing mucosa and lymph glands.

2 Tissue volume homeostasis thus depends critically on lymphatic drainage.

3 The rate of drainage of interstitial fluid into the initial lymphatic plexus is coupled to the microvascular filtration rate (e.g. in the dependent leg during orthostasis) through tissue hydration, interstitial fluid pressure/volume and extrinsic forces.

4 Lymphatic trunks are actively, rhythmically contractile, each contraction being initiated by an action potential complex. Efficient pumping depends on propagation of the electrical impulse.

5 Pacemaking initiates the action potential. Pacemaking is essentially electrical and appears to originate in specialized pacemaker cells.

6 The force and frequency of contractions are increased (up to a limit in the case of force) by distension. This allows coupling between the initial lymphatic plexus and the contractile vessels. The relation between frequency and distension can be enhanced by sympathetic nerve activity and can be enhanced/impaired by circulating vasoactive substances. Pumping can generate high pressures.

REFERENCES

1. Aukland K, Reed RK. Interstitial–lymphatic mechanisms in the control of extracellular fluid volume. *Physiological Reviews* 1993; **73**: 1–78.

2. Michel CC. Starling: The formulation of his hypothesis of microvascular fluid exchange and its significance after 100 years. *Experimental Physiology* 1997; **82**: 1–30.

3. Levick JR. Circulation of fluid between plasma, interstitium and lymph. In: Levick JR ed. *An introduction to cardiovascular physiology*. London: Arnold, 2003.

4. Yoffey JM, Courtice FC. *Lymphatics, lymph and the lymphomyeloid complex*. New York: Academic Press, 1970.

5. Nicoll PA, Taylor AE. Lymph formation and flow. *Annual Review of Physiology* 1977; **39**: 73–95.

6. Olszewski WL. *Peripheral lymph: formation and immune function*. Boca Ratan, FL: CRC Press, 1985.

7. Schmid-Schönbein GW. Microlymphatics and lymph flow. *Physiological Reviews* 1990; **70**: 987–1028.

8. McHale NG. Role of the lymph pump and its control. *News in Physiological Science* 1995; **10**: 112–17.

9. Garlic D, Renkin EM. Transport of large molecules from plasma to interstitial fluid and lymph in dogs. *American Journal of Physiology* 1970; **219**: 1595–605.

10. Nicolaysen G, Nicolaysen A, Staub NC. A quantitative radioautographic comparison of albumin concentration in different sized lymph vessels in normal mouse lung. *Microvascular Research* 1975; **10**: 138–52.

11. Rutili G, Arfors KE. Protein concentration in interstitial and lymphatic fluids from the subcutaneous tissue. *Acta Physiologica Scandinavica* 1977; **99**: 1–8.

12. Fokin AA, Robicsek F, Masters TN. Transport of viral-size particulate matter after intravenous versus lymphatic entry. *Microcirculation* 2000; **7**: 357–65.

13. Renkin EM. Some consequences of capillary permeability to macromolecules: Starling's hypothesis reconsidered. *American Journal of Physiology* 1986; **250**: H706–10.

14. Knox P, Pflug JJ. The effect of the canine popliteal node on the composition of lymph. *Journal of Physiology* 1983; **345**: 1–14.

15. Zweifach SS, Kramer GC, Renkin EM. Plasma to lymph transport of tracer albumin in the popliteal node of unanaesthetized sheep. *Microvascular Research* 1984; **27**: 271A.

16. Adair TH, Guyton AC. Modification of lymph by lymph nodes. III. Effect of increased lymph hydrostatic pressure. *American Journal of Physiology* 1985; **249**: H777–82.

17. Baldwin AL, Ferrer P, Rozum JS, Gore RW. Regulation of water balance between blood and lymph in the frog, *Rana pipens*. *Lymphology* 1993; **26**: 4–18.

18. Fraser JRE, Laurent TC. Hyaluronan. In: Comper WD ed. *Extracellular matrix*, Vol. 2. *Molecular components and interactions*. Amsterdam: Harwood Academic, 1996: 141–99.

19. Banerji S, Ni J, Wang SX, *et al.* LYVE-1, a new homologue of the CD44 glycoprotein, is a lymph-specific receptor for hyaluronan. *Journal of Cell Biology* 1999; **144:** 789–801.

20. Starling EH. On the absorption of fluids from the connective tissue spaces. *Journal of Physiology* 1896; **19:** 312–26.

21. Henriksen JH. *Ernest Henry Starling (1866–1927). Physician and physiologist – a short biography.* Copenhagen: Laegeforeningens, 2000.

22. Michel CC, Kendall S. Differing effects of histamine and serotonin on microvascular permeability in anaesthetized rats. *Journal of Physiology* 1997; **501:** 657–62.

23. Michel CC, Curry FE. Microvascular permeability. *Physiological Reviews* 1999; **79:** 703–61.

24. Landis EM, Pappenheimer JR. Exchange of substances through the capillary walls. In: Hamilton WF, Dow P eds. *Handbook of physiology, Section 2, Circulation II.* Washington, DC: American Physiological Society, 1963: 961–1034.

25. Rippe B, Haraldsson B. Transport of macromolecules across microvascular walls: the two-pore theory. *Physiological Reviews* 1994; **74:** 163–219.

26. Bates DO, Levick JR, Mortimer PS. Starling pressure imbalance in the human arm and alteration in postmastectomy oedema. *Journal of Physiology* 1994; **477:** 355–63.

27. Taylor AE, Townsley MI. Evaluation of the Starling fluid flux equation. *News in Physiological Science* 1987; **2:** 48–52.

28. Levick JR. Capillary filtration–absorption balance reconsidered in light of dynamic extravascular factors. *Experimental Physiology* 1991; **76:** 825–57.

29. Guyton AC, Granger HJ, Taylor AE. Interstitial fluid pressure. *Physiological Reviews* 1971; **51:** 527–63.

30. Michel CC, Phillips ME. Steady-state fluid filtration at different capillary pressures in perfused frog mesenteric capillaries. *Journal of Physiology* 1987; **388:** 421–35.

31. Levick JR, Mortimer PS. Fluid 'balance' between microcirculation and interstitium in skin and other tissues: revision of the classical filtration–reabsorption scheme. In: Messmer K ed. *Microcirculation in chronic venous insufficiency.* Basle: Karger, 1999: 42–62.

32. Engeset A, Olszewski WL, Jaeger PM, Sokolowski J, Theodorsen L. Twenty four hour variation in flow and composition of leg lymph in normal man. *Acta Physiologica Scandinavica* 1976; **99:** 140–5.

33. Intaglietta M, Gross JF. Vasomotion, tissue fluid flow and the formation of lymph. *International Journal of Microcirculation* 1982; **1:** 55–65.

34. Flynn MD, Hassan AAK, Tooke JE. Effect of postural change and thermoregulatory stress on the capillary microcirculation of the human toe. *Clinical Science* 1989; **76:** 231–6.

35. Levick JR. An analysis of the interaction between extravascular plasma protein, interstitial flow and capillary filtration; application to synovium. *Microvascular Research* 1994; **47:** 90–125.

36. Hu X, Weinbaum S. A new view of Starling's hypothesis at the microstructural level. *Microvascular Research* 1999; **58:** 281–304.

37. McDonald JN, Levick JR. Effect of extravascular plasma protein on pressure–flow relations across synovium in anaesthetized rabbits. *Journal of Physiology* 1993; **465:** 539–59.

38. Hu X, Adamson RH, Liu B, Curry FE, Weinbaum S. Starling forces that oppose filtration after tissue oncotic pressure is increased. *American Journal of Physiology* 2000; **279:** H1724–36.

39. Howarth DM, Southee AE, Whyte IM. Lymphatic flow rates and first aid in simulated peripheral snake or spider envenomation. *Medical Journal of Australia* 1994; **161:** 695–700.

40. Hargens AR, Zweifach BW. Transport between blood and peripheral lymph in intestine. *Microvascular Research* 1976; **11:** 89–101.

41. Aarli V, Reed RK, Aukland K. Effect of longstanding venous stasis and hypoproteinaemia on lymph flow in the rat tail. *Acta Physiologica Scandinavica* 1991; **142:** 1–9.

42. Olszewski WL, Engeset A, Jaeger PM, Sokolowski J, Theodorsen L. Flow and composition of leg lymph in normal men during venous stasis, muscular activity and local hyperthermia. *Acta Physiologica Scandinavica* 1977; **99:** 149–55.

43. Olszewski WL, Engeset A. Intrinsic contractility of prenodal lymph vessels and lymph flow in human leg. *American Journal of Physiology* 1980; **239:** H777–83.

44. Aas M, Skretting A, Engeset A, Westgaard R, Nicolaysen G. Lymphatic drainage from subcutaneous tissue in foot and leg in the sitting human. *Acta Physiologica Scandinavica* 1985; **125:** 505–11.

45. Havas E, Parviainen T, Vuorela J, Toivanen J, Nikula T, Vihko V. Lymph flow dynamics in exercising human skeletal muscle as detected by scintigraphy. *Journal of Physiology* 1997; **504:** 233–9.

46. Heidenhain R. Versuche und Fragen zur Lehre von der Lymphbildung. *Pflügers Archives* 1891; **49:** 209–301.

47. Renkin EM, Joyner WL, Sloop CH, Watson PD. Influence of venous pressure on plasma-lymph transport in the dog's paw: convective and dissipative mechanisms. *Microvascular Research* 1977; **14:** 191–204.

48. Levick JR, Michel CC. The effects of position and skin temperature on the capillary pressures in the fingers and toes. *Journal of Physiology* 1978; **274:** 97–109.

49. Franzeck UK, Fischer M, Costanzo U, Herrig I, Bollinger A. Effect of postural changes on human

lymphatic capillary pressure of the skin. *Journal of Physiology* 1996; **494:** 595–600.

50. Stanton AWB, Patel HS, Levick JR, Mortimer PS. Increased dermal lymphatic density in the human leg compared with the forearm. *Microvascular Research* 1999; **57:** 320–8.

51. Noddeland H, Omvik P, Lund-Johansen P, Ofstad J, Aukland K. Interstitial colloid osmotic and hydrostatic pressures in human subcutaneous tissue during early stages of heart failure. *Clinical Physiology* 1984; **4:** 283–97.

52. Zaugg-Vesti B, Dörffler-Melly J, Spiegel M, Wen S, Franzeck UK, Bollinger A. Lymphatic capillary pressure in patients with primary lymphoedema. *Microvascular Research* 1993; **46:** 128–34.

53. Gretener SB, Läuchli S, Leu AJ, Koppensteiner R, Franzeck UK. Effect of venous and lymphatic congestion on lymph capillary pressure of the skin in healthy volunteers and patients with lymph edema. *Journal of Vascular Research* 2000; **37:** 61–7.

54. Taylor AE, Grimbert F, Rutili G, Kvietys PR, Parker JC. Pulmonary oedema: changes in Starling forces and lymph flow. In: Hargens AR ed. *Tissue fluid pressure and composition.* Baltimore: Williams & Wilkins, 1981: 135–43.

55. Granger HJ. Role of the interstitial matrix and lymphatic pump in regulation of transcapillary fluid balance. *Microvascular Research* 1979; **18:** 209–16.

56. Levick JR. Flow through interstitium and other fibrous matrices. *Quarterly Journal of Experimental Physiology* 1987; **72:** 409–38.

57. Hogan RD. The initial lymphatics and interstitial fluid pressure. In: Hargens AR ed. *Tissue fluid pressure and composition.* Baltimore: Williams & Wilkins, 1981: 155–64.

58. Fischer M, Franzeck UK, Herrig I, *et al.* Flow velocity of single lymphatic capillaries in human skin. *American Journal of Physiology* 1996; **270:** H358–63.

59. Mellor RH, Stanton AWB, Azarbod P, Sheman MD, Levick JR, Mortimer PS. Enhanced cutaneous lymphatic network in the forearms of women with postmastectomy oedema. *Journal of Vascular Research* 2000; **37:** 501–12.

60. Ohshima N, Sato M. Mass transfer kinetics from blood to lymph in the mesenteric microcirculation studied by the fluorescent intravital microscope method. *Microvascular Research* 1987; **34:** 250–5.

61. Powers MR, Wallace JR, Bell DR. Initial equilibration of albumin in rabbit hindpaw skin and lymph. *American Journal of Physiology* 1988; **254:** H89–101.

62. Ogston AG, Preston BN, Wells JD. On the transport of compact particles through solutions of chain polymers. *Proceedings of the Royal Society A* 1973; **333:** 297–316.

63. Watson PD, Bell DR, Renkin EM. Early kinetics of large molecule transport between plasma and lymph in dogs. *American Journal of Physiology* 1980; **239:** H525–31.

64. Bell DR, Mullins RJ. Effects of increased venous pressure on albumin- and IgG-excluded volumes in skin. *American Journal of Physiology* 1982; **242:** 1038–43.

65. Hauck G, Bröcker W, Weigelt H. The prelymphatic transinterstitial pathway. *Journal of Lymphology* 1978; **2:** 70–4.

66. Casley-Smith JR, Földi-Börcsöck E, Földi M. A fine structural study of the tissue channels numbers and dimensions in normal and lymphoedematous tissues. *Journal of Lymphology* 1979; **3:** 49–58.

67. Levick JR, McDonald JN. Ultrastructure of transport pathways in stressed synovium of the knee in anaesthetized rabbits. *Journal of Physiology* 1989; **419:** 493–508.

68. Parker KH, Winlove CP. The macromolecular basis of the hydraulic conductivity of the arterial wall. *Biorheology* 1984; **21:** 181–96.

69. Rhodin JAG, Sue SL. Combined intravital microscopy and electron microscopy of the blind beginnings of the mesenteric lymphatic capillaries of the rat mesentery. *Acta Physiologica Scandinavica Supplement* 1979; **463:** 51–8.

70. Castenholz A. Functional microanatomy of initial lymphatics with special consideration of the extracellular matrix. *Lymphology* 1998; **31:** 101–18.

71. Fukuo Y, Shinohara H, Matsuda T. The distribution of lymphatic stomata in the diaphragm of the golden hamster. *Journal of Anatomy* 1990; **169:** 13–21.

72. Miserocchi G, Negrini D. Pleural space: pressures and fluid dynamics. In: Crystal RG, West JB eds. *The lung: scientific foundations,* 2nd edn. Philadelphia: Lippincott-Raven, 1997: 1217–25.

73. Negrini D, Del Fabbro M. Subatmospheric pressure in the rabbit pleural lymphatic network. *Journal of Physiology* 1999; **520:** 761–9.

74. Leak LV. Ultrastructure and function of the interstitial–lymphatic interface. In: Staub NC, Hogg JC, Hargens AR eds. *Interstitial–lymphatic liquid and solute movement.* Basle: Karger, 1986: 1–14.

75. McMaster PD. Changes in the cutaneous lymphatics of human beings and in lymph flow under normal and experimental conditions. *Journal of Experimental Medicine* 1937; **65:** 347–72.

76. Bollinger A. Microlymphatics of human skin. *International Journal of Microcirculation* 1993; **12:** 1–15.

77. Granger HJ. In: Staub NC, Taylor AE eds. *Edema.* New York: Raven Press, 1984.

78. Berk DA, Swartz MA, Leu AJ, Jain RK. Transport in lymphatic capillaries. II. Microscopic velocity

measurements with fluorescence photobleaching. *American Journal of Physiology* 1996; **270:** H330–7.

79. Hogan RD, Uthank JL. Mechanical control of initial lymphatic contractile behaviour in bat's wing. *American Journal of Physiology* 1986; **251:** H357–63.

80. Hogan RD, Uthank JL. The initial lymphatics as sensors of interstitial fluid volume. *Microvascular Research* 1986; **31:** 317–24.

81. Clough G, Smaje LH. Simultaneous measurements of pressure in the interstitium and the terminal lymphatics of the cat mesentery. *Journal of Physiology* 1978; **283:** 457–68.

82. Zweifach BW, Prather JW. Micromanipulation of pressure in terminal lymphatics in the mesentery. *American Journal of Physiology* 1975; **228:** 1326–35.

83. Wen S, Dörffler MJ, Herrig I, Schiesser M, Franzeck UK, Bollinger A. Fluctuations of skin lymphatic capillary pressure in controls and in patients with primary lymphedema. *International Journal of Microcirculation, Clinical and Experimental* 1994; **14:** 139–43.

84. McGeown JG, McHale NG, Thornbury KD. Effects of varying patterns of external compression on lymph flow in the hindlimb of the anaesthetised sheep. *Journal of Physiology* 1987; **397:** 449–57.

85. Skalak TC, Schmid-Schönbein GW, Zweifach BW. New morphological evidence for a mechanism of lymph formation in skeletal muscle. *Microvascular Research* 1984; **27:** 95–112.

86. Schmid-Schönbein GW, Zweifach BW. Fluid pump mechanisms in initial lymphatics. *News in Physiological Science* 1994; **9:** 67–71.

87. Casley-Smith JR. The functioning and interrelationships of blood capillaries and lymphatics. *Experientia* 1976; **32:** 1–12.

88. Brace RA, Power GG. Thoracic duct lymph flow and protein flux dynamics: responses to intravascular saline. *American Journal of Physiology* 1981; **240:** R282–8.

89. Drake RE, Scott RL, Gabel JC. Relationship between weight gain and lymph flow in dog lungs. *American Journal of Physiology* 1983; **245:** H125–30.

90. Casley-Smith JR. The influence of tissue hydrostatic pressure and protein concentration on fluid and protein uptake by diaphragmatic initial lymphatics: effect of calcium dobesilate. *Microcirculation, Endothelium and Lymphatics* 1985; **2:** 385–415.

91. Benoit JN, Zawieja DC, Goodman AH, Granger HJ. Characterization of intact mesenteric lymphatic pump and its responsiveness to acute edemagenic stress. *American Journal of Physiology* 1989; **257:** H2059–69.

92. Generisch H. Die Aufnahme der Lymphe durch die sehnen und Fascien der Skelettmuskeln. *Arbeiten aus der Physiologischen Anstalt* 1871; **5:** 53.

93. White JC, Field ME, Drinker CK. On the protein content and normal flow of lymph from the foot of the dog. *American Journal of Physiology* 1933; **103:** 34–44.

94. McCarrel JD. Cervical lymph pressure in the dog. *American Journal of Physiology* 1939; **127:** 154–60.

95. Morris B. Lymphatic contractility and its significance in lymph propulsion. In: Viamonte M ed. *Progress in Lymphology II.* Stuttgart: Georg Thieme Verlag, 1970.

96. Drinker CK, Yoffey JM. Lymph flow and lymph pressure. In: *Lymphatics, lymph and lymphoid tissue.* Cambridge, MA: Harvard University Press, 1941: 112–45.

97. Courtice FC, Simmonds WJ. Physiological significance of lymph drainage of the serous cavities and lungs. *Physiological Reviews* 1954; **34:** 419–48.

98. Hewson W. *A description of the lymphatic system. Experimental Enquiries Part II,* London, 1774.

99. Florey H. Observations on the contractility of lacteals. II. *Journal of Physiology* 1927; **63:** 1–18.

100. Carleton HM, Florey H. The mammalian lacteal: its histological structure in relation to its physiological properties. *Proceedings of the Royal Society B* 1927; **102:** 110–18.

101. Smith RO. Lymphatic contractility – a possible intrinsic mechanism of lymphatic vessels for the transport of lymph. *Journal of Experimental Medicine* 1949; **90:** 497–509.

102. McGeown JG, McHale NG, Thornbury KD. The role of external compression and movement in lymph propulsion in the sheep hind limb. *Journal of Physiology* 1987; **387:** 83–93.

103. Li B, Silver I, Sazalai JP, Johnston MG. Pressure–volume relationships in sheep mesenteric lymphatic vessels in situ: responses to hypovolaemia. *Microvascular Research* 1998; **56:** 127–38.

104. McHale NG, Thornbury KD. A method for studying lymphatic pumping activity in conscious and anaesthetised sheep. *Journal of Physiology* 1986; **378:** 109–18.

105. Todd GL, Bernard GR. The sympathetic innervation of the cervical lymph duct of the dog. *Anatomical Record* 1973; **177:** 303–16.

106. Alessandrini C, Gerli R, Sacchi G, Pucci AM, Fruschelli C. Cholinergic and adrenergic innervation of mesenterial lymph vessels in guinea pig. *Lymphology* 1981; **14:** 1–6.

107. McHale NG. Innervation of the lymphatic circulation. In: Johnston MG ed. *Experimental biology of the lymphatic circulation.* Elsevier Science, 1985: 121–40.

108. Hollywood MA, McHale NG. Mediation of excitatory neurotransmission by the release of ATP and noradrenaline in sheep mesenteric lymphatic vessels. *Journal of Physiology* 1994; **481:** 415–23.

109. Foy WL, Allen JM, McKillop JM, Goldsmith JP, Johnston CF, Buchanan KD. Substance P and gastrin releasing peptide in bovine mesenteric lymphatic vessels: chemical characterization and action. *Peptides* 1989; **10:** 533–37.

110. McGeown JG, McHale NG, Thornbury KD. The effect of electrical stimulation of the sympathetic chain on popliteal efferent lymph flow in the anaesthetised sheep. *Journal of Physiology* 1987; **393:** 123–33.

111. McHale NG, Adair TH. Reflex modulation of lymphatic pumping in sheep. *Circulation Research* 1989; **64:** 1165–71.

112. McCullough JS, McHale NG. Pressure flow relationships in isolated bovine mesenteric lymphatics during field stimulation. *Journal of Physiology* 1988; **396:** 177P.

113. Hayashi A, Johnston MG, Nelson W, Hamilton S, McHale NG. Increased intrinsic pumping of intestinal lymphatics following haemorrhage in anaesthetised sheep. *Circulation Research* 1987; **60:** 265–72.

114. Elias R, Johnston MG. Modulation of lymphatic pumping by lymph-borne factors following intravenous endotoxin administration in sheep. *Journal of Applied Physiology* 1990; **68:** 199–208.

115. Horstmann E. Über die functionelle Struktur des mesenterialen Lymphgefasse. *Morpholog Jahrbuch* 1952; **91:** 483.

116. Horstmann E. Beobachtungen zur Motorik der Lymphgefasse. *Pflügers Archives* 1959; **269:** 511–19.

117. Mawhinney HJD, Roddie IC. Spontaneous activity in isolated bovine mesenteric lymphatics. *Journal of Physiology* 1973; **229:** 339–48.

118. Kirkpatrick CT, McHale NG. Electrical and mechanical activity of isolated lymphatic vessels. *Journal of Physiology* 1977; **272:** 33–4P.

119. Ward SM, Sanders KM, Thornbury KD, McHale NG. Spontaneous electrical activity in isolated bovine lymphatics recorded by intracellular microelectrodes. *Journal of Physiology* 1991; **438:** 168P.

120. Cotton KD, Hollywood MA, McHale NG, Thornbury KD. Outward currents in smooth muscle cells isolated from sheep mesenteric lymphatics. *Journal of Physiology* 1997; **503:** 2–12.

121. Hollywood MA, Cotton KD, Thornbury KD, McHale NG. Tetrodotoxin sensitive sodium current in sheep lymphatic smooth muscle. *Journal of Physiology* 1997; **503:** 13–20.

122. Hollywood MA, Cotton KD, Thornbury KD, McHale NG. Isolated sheep mesenteric lymphatic smooth muscle cells possess both T and L-type calcium currents. *Journal of Physiology* 1997; **501:** 109–10P.

123. Toland HM, McCloskey KD, Thornbury KD, McHale NG, Hollywood MA. Calcium-activated chloride current in sheep lymphatic smooth muscle. *American Journal of Physiology* 2000; **279:** C1327–35.

124. Allen JM, McHale NG. The effects of known K^+ channel blockers on electrical activity in lymphatic smooth muscle. *Pflügers Archives* 1988; **411:** 167–72.

125. DiFrancesco D. The contribution of the 'pacemaker' current (i_f) to generation of spontaneous activity in rabbit sinoatrial node myocytes. *Journal of Physiology* 1991; **434:** 23–40.

126. McCloskey KD, Toland HM, Hollywood MA, Thornbury KD, McHale NG. Hyperpolarization-activated inward current in isolated sheep mesenteric lymphatic smooth muscle. *Journal of Physiology* 1999; **521:** 201–11.

127. McCloskey KD, Hollywood MA, Thornbury KD, Ward SM, McHale NG. C-kit positive cells in lymphatic vessels. *Journal of Physiology* 2000; **528:** 11P.

128. Sanders KM. A case for interstitial cells of Cajal as pacemakers and mediators of neurotransmission in the gastrointestinal tract. *Gastroenterology* 1996; **111:** 492–515.

129. Thuneberg L, Rumessen JJ, Mikkelsen HB. The interstitial cells of Cajal: intestinal pacemaker cells? In: Wienbeck M ed. *Motility of the digestive tract.* New York: Raven Press, 1982: 115–22.

130. Van Helden DF. Pacemaker potentials in lymphatic smooth muscle of the guinea-pig mesentery. *Journal of Physiology* 1993; **471:** 465–79.

131. McHale NG, Meharg MK. Co-ordination of pumping in isolated bovine lymphatic vessels. *Journal of Physiology* 1992; **450:** 503–12.

132. McHale NG, Roddie IC. The effect of transmural pressure on pumping activity in isolated bovine lymphatic vessels. *Journal of Physiology* 1976; **261:** 255–69.

4

Pathology

JUDIT DARÓCZY, JOHN WOLFE AND THOMAS MENTZEL

LYMPH VESSELS

The lymphatic system (lymph vessels and lymph glands) is responsible for transporting excess interstitial fluid and large molecular weight substances such as proteins, fat and waste materials from the interstitium to the central veins. In addition, it transports antigens, antibodies and leukocytes, thus also having an immunological surveillance function.

The substances destined to become lymph are absorbed by blind-ended lymph vessels in the periphery, a function made possible by their special morphological characteristics, namely the absence of a basal lamina, pericytes and smooth muscle cells in their walls and a lack of anchoring filaments. These vessels have been given various names – terminal lymphatics, initial lymphatics, small lymphatics – some of which can be misleading. We prefer to call them lymphatic capillaries or initial lymphatics. Their walls consist solely of endothelial cells. Valves in the lumen of the lymphatic capillaries ensure a one-way flow of lymph from them into the pre-collecting vessels.

Pre-collectors are present in the upper third of the dermis; their basal lamina is not continuous and they do not have a smooth muscle layer. Pre-collector lymphatics empty into the collecting lymphatics, the transition between pre-collectors and collectors being gradual.

Collecting lymphatics are present in the upper and middle third of the dermis. The structure of their wall is similar to that of blood vessels, comprising an inner layer of endothelial cells, a middle layer of smooth muscle cells and elastic fibres, and an outer loose network of fibroblasts. The collectors transport lymph from the pre-collectors to the larger lymph vessels in the subcutis and then to the central lymph trunks. A one-way flow of lymph is assisted by the regular contractions of the smooth muscle in their walls and by the valves. The walls of the central lymph trunks such as the thoracic duct have three distinct layers: a tunica intima, a tunica media and an adventitia similar to all blood vessels.

It is possible to demonstrate the skin lymphatics at light microscopy level, but the morphological details of any pathological changes remain undetectable (Fig. 4.1). Transmission electron microscopy, which displays the ultrastructure, is the best way of detecting and understanding the pathological changes that occur in chronic lymphoedema.[1,2]

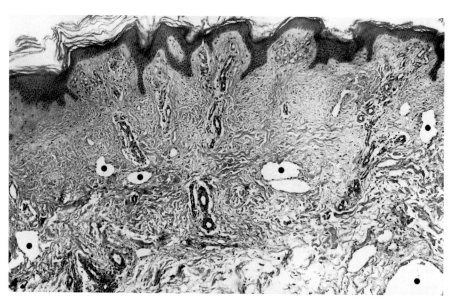

Figure 4.1 *The light microscopic features of chronic lymphoedematous skin. The acanthotic epidermis is covered by a hyperkeratotic stratum corneum. The number of blood vessels in the elongated dermal papillae is increased, and the lymph vessels are dilated (dotted). The connective tissue has a homogeneous appearance. The elastic fibres are missing. (Hematoxylin and eosin, ×150).*

The interstitial fluid, containing the products of the metabolic processes that take place in the extravascular space and cells, enters the lymph circulation through the initial lymph vessels. A fundamental issue in the physiology of lymphatics is the question of how interstitial fluid, proteins and cells find their way through the interstitium into the initial lymphatics (*see* Chapter 3). It is believed that local osmotic and hydrostatic pressure conditions, changes in the shape of the endothelial cells (actin) and the pulling of neighbouring fibres (anchoring filaments) induce gaps to form between the endothelial cells, these then opening interendothelial junctions that act as inlet or entrance valves.

ENDOTHELIAL CELLS

Normal structure

The shape of the endothelial cells of the initial lymphatics and pre-collectors changes. Under resting conditions, the endothelial cells are round and oval, their nuclei bulging into the vessel's lumen. When the vessel is transporting lymph, they become flattened. At rest, the endothelial cells are so close to each other that the lumen is hardly visible. Their cytoplasm is rich in organelles: a well-developed Golgi apparatus, an endoplasmic reticulum, mitochondria, cytoplasmic microfilaments and fuzzy-coated and smooth vesicles. Pinocytotic vesicles are marked on both the luminal and abluminal surface of the cells. In inactive cells, the shape of the nucleus is oval, whereas in actively budding cells it is deeply indented, and in active elongated cells the nucleus is comma shaped. The contractility of the endothelial cells is ensured by the presence of actin/myosin-type

microfilament bundles and microtubules. Bicuspid valves in the lumen ensure one-way centripetal flow.

There are no tight junctions between the endothelial cells. The interendothelial junctions of the initial lymphatics form interdigitations or overlapping areas that result from the change in the shape of the endothelial cells. A high degree of dilatation of the lumen is possible. Under increased interstitial pressure and a negative pressure in the lumen, the endothelial cells move apart. The gap that is formed between the endothelial cells is called the inlet or entrance valve or 'open junction'. This entrance valve is, in effect, the first element of a valved system that ensures the one-way movement of fluid and cells throughout the whole lymphatic system.

The number of microtubules and microfilaments in the cytoplasm varies according to the activity of the endothelial cell. Their function is to participate in the change of shape of the cell. There are two types of microfilament:

1 Some microfilaments of 6–7 nm in diameter display a longitudinal periodicity measuring approximately 10 nm. These filaments are arranged in bundles and run parallel to the luminal surface. They appear to be vimentin filaments.
2 Other microfilaments, also 6–7 nm in diameter, are like actin filaments. They are aggregated around the nuclei and along the abluminal membrane of the endothelial cells.

The microtubules, measuring 20–25 nm in diameter, are located around the nucleus of the cell.

The lymphatic capillaries do not have any nerve supply but lie in close apposition to sensory nerve endings.

The valves, which are covered by endothelial cells, have a 'backbone' of connective tissue fibres. The valves divide

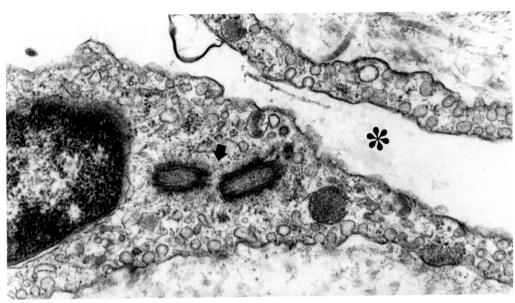

Figure 4.2 *The endothelial cells of the lymphatics in chronic lymphoedema. The cytoplasm of the endothelial cells contains ribosomes, and numerous pinocytotic vesicles around the lumen (starred) and along the abluminal membrane surface. The most characteristic organelles are the basal bodies of the cilia (arrowed). (×16 000).*

the lymphatic collectors into contractile segments called lymphangions. When the intraluminal pressure in a lymphangion rises above that of its immediate distal lymphangion, the valve between the two lymphangions closes and the cells at the tip seal the lumen to prevent reflux.

Structure in chronic lymphoedema

In chronic lymphoedema, the endothelial cells are elongated and their nuclei comma shaped. The number of vesicles in their thin cytoplasmic processes is increased, and there is significant pinocytotic activity to be seen along both the luminal and abluminal endothelial membranes (Fig. 4.2). The number of microtubules and actin-like microfilaments is considerably decreased.

Because the anchoring microfilaments and actin-like filaments are missing from the connective tissue surrounding the capillaries (the anchoring filaments in normal conditions being directly connected to the endothelial cell membranes), many of the interendothelial junctions are open and the active functioning of the inlet valves is hindered. There are frequent arch-like elevations of the endothelial cells from the connective tissue at which serial sections show the lumen to be open to the surrounding oedematous connective tissue (Fig. 4.3). Along the abluminal cell membrane, there are long and short stretches of a dense plate to which a large number of actin-like microfilaments adhere. The basal lamina grows along these dense plates.

In chronic lymphoedema, the endothelial cells contain lipid droplets, dense granules and various endothelial inclusions. These inclusions consist of reticularly arranged tubules 20–28 nm in diameter or crystal-like tubules (Fig. 4.4). The tubuloreticular inclusions are the

pathological variants of endoplasmic reticulum and have been described in immunodeficiency syndromes.[3]

BASEMENT LAMINA

Normal structure

The basement lamina around the initial lymphatics is missing or discontinuous. This makes possible the direct connections between the membranes of the endothelial cells and the perivascular microfilaments. (The collecting lymphatics have a continuous basal lamina.) The discontinuous basal lamina consists of very fine microfilaments embedded in a loose matrix. The basal lamina segments are usually found alongside the dense cytoplasmic plates of the abluminal endothelial membrane.

Structure in chronic lymphoedema

The basement laminar components are thicker around the lymph capillaries and the collecting lymphatics. The basement membrane may be reduplicated and multilamellar, and the granulofilamentous ground substance between the layers of the basal lamina is increased (*see* Figs 4.3 and 4.4).

PERICYTES

Normal structure

There are no pericytes around the initial lymphatics; these can be found around the collecting lymphatics.

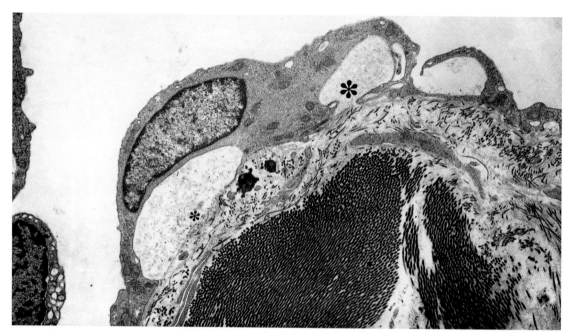

Figure 4.3 *Arched endothelial cells elevated from their connective tissue basis. The granulofilamentous protein-rich oedema fluid (starred) is directly connected to the lumen through the inlet valve (lock-gate) system of the endothelial cell processes. (×8200).*

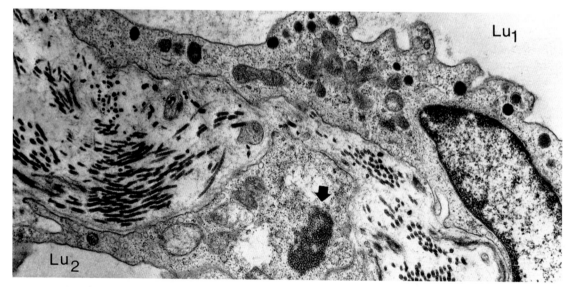

Figure 4.4 *Two lymphatic capillaries (Lu_1 and Lu_2) in close proximity. There are numerous dense granules in the endothelial cytoplasm of the Lu_1 capillary. A tubuloreticular inclusion (arrowed) composed of reticular aggregates of tubules measuring 25–28 nm in diameter can be seen in the Lu_2 capillary endothelial cell. (×7200).*

A few elongated fibroblasts with narrow cytoplasm or dendrite-shaped macrophages may be present.

Structure in chronic lymphoedema

A number of spindle-shaped cells – fibroblasts – similar to pericytes grow around the lymphatic capillaries. Their cytoplasm is rich in rough endoplasmatic reticulum and mitochondria (Fig. 4.5). The presence of myofibroblasts (fibroblasts that have modulated into contractile cells) around the capillaries is characteristic.[4] The myofibroblasts

contain actin-like microfilament bundles the transverse periodicity of which is similar to that of smooth muscle fibres (Fig. 4.6).

PERIVASCULAR FIBRES

One of the most important functional features of the lymph vessels of the skin is their great ability to dilate. When functioning efficiently, they are collapsed without a visible lumen, their interdigitating, overlapping

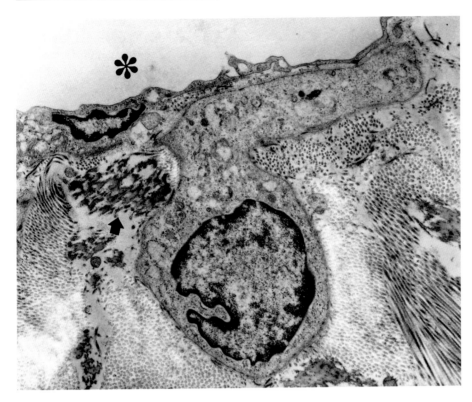

Figure 4.5 *A pericyte surrounded by basement membrane that seems to be in close contact with the endothelial cells of the dilated lymphatic capillary (starred). The perilymphatic elastic fibres (arrowed) have degenerated and fragmented. (×5000).*

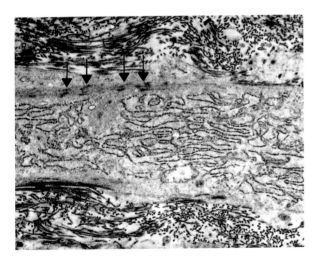

Figure 4.6 *Detail of an elongated perilymphatic myofibroblast. The rough endoplasmic reticulum is well developed. The bundles of actin-like microfilaments contain periodic densities (arrowed). (×5500).*

endothelial cells indistinguishible from the connective tissue fibroblasts. Depending on the lymph load, lymphatic capillaries can dilate 20–50-fold, changing their shape, connections and relationship to the surrounding connective tissue microfilaments.

Normal structure

The microfilaments with a diameter of 10–12 nm that run directly to the abluminal endothelial cell membrane connect to an elastic matrix. They have the same

morphological features as elastic microfilaments, i.e. hollow-profile initiating tubules, and the same longitudinal periodicity.

These are the anchoring microfilaments that anchor the lymphatic capillaries to the connective tissue. The elastic microfilaments and the elastic matrix together make up the elastic fibre. Some of the fine connective tissue microfilaments are 4–6 nm in diameter and lie in bundles parallel to the long axis of the lymphatic capillary wall. These microfilament bundles may connect to the dense cytoplasmic plate that is situated along the abluminal endothelial surface.

Structure in chronic lymphoedema

The number of anchoring microfilaments is decreased in chronic lymphoedema. Neither collagen nor elastic microfilaments connect directly to the endothelial cells. The ground substance around the lymphatic capillaries and small collecting lymph vessels is increased. This zone, of varying width, contains modified collagen and degenerated elastic fibres and appears to be pushing the normal perivascular collagen and elastic fibres away from the lymphatic endothelial cells, thus decreasing the direct contact between the endothelial cells and the connective tissue fibres (Fig. 4.7).

VALVES

Lymphatic capillaries and collecting lymphatics both possess valves that facilitate the flow of lymph from the periphery towards the central lymph vessels. The valve system includes the interendothelial inlet valves and the intraluminal valves.

Inlet valves

Normal structure

The entrance or inlet valves appear between overlapping endothelial cells.[1,2] They are inconstant, transitory

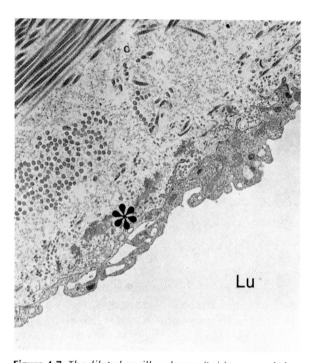

Figure 4.7 *The dilated capillary lumen (Lu) is surrounded by elongated endothelial cells. The anchoring elastic filaments are missing. Fragments of the collagen fibres and the degenerated remnants of the elastic fibres (starred) are embedded in the granulofilamentous material that fills the wide perilymphatic space. (×26 500).*

structures that develop between the cytoplasmic projections of neighbouring endothelial cells and respond to local pressure variations and intraluminal/interstitial pressure gradients.

Structure in chronic lymphoedema

In chronic lymphoedema, the permanently increased pressure in the connective tissue drives a large amount of fluid into the lymphatic capillaries, the subsequent increased intraluminal pressure preventing the gap between the endothelial cells closing (Fig. 4.8). The number of elastic microfilaments decreases, and the anchoring filaments may be missing. The opening/closing function of the inlet valve is disturbed because the pull/push mechanism of the anchoring filaments is lost.

Intraluminal valves

Normal structure

Intraluminal valves consist of folds of connective tissue that extend into the lumen and are covered by modified endothelial cells. On the tip of the valves lie similarly modified endothelial cells called tip cells.

Structure in chronic lymphoedema

In chronic lymphoedema, the connective tissue 'backbone' of the valves becomes fibrotic, presumably as a consequence of permanently abnormal conditions of flow. The number of collagen fibres and tubular microfilaments of 10–12 nm diameter is increased, as is the number of dense cytoplasm plaques on the abluminal surface of the endothelial cells. Lipid droplets and dark pigment granules bordered by membranes appear in the cytoplasm of the endothelial cells; these being degeneration products. The tip cells of the valves generate a large

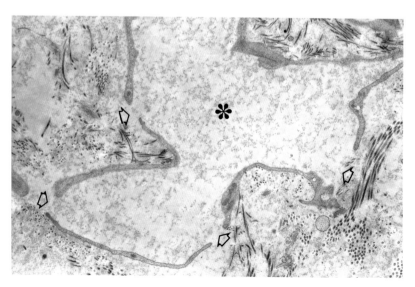

Figure 4.8 *The lumen (starred) of this dilated lymphatic capillary contains protein-rich granulofilamentous oedema fluid and is directly connected to the perivascular space through open junctions between the endothelial cell processes (arrowed), these interendothelial junctions acting as inlet valves. (×10 200).*

number of pseudopodia. As a result of a high degree of lymphatic dilatation, the valves can become incompetent, and reflux may occur.

COLLECTING LYMPHATICS

Normal structure

The endothelial cells of the collecting lymphatics are connected to each other by desmosomes and some tight junctions, the basal lamina being continuous. Elastic fibres surround the vessels in a spiral arrangement. Pericytes and smooth muscle fibres capable of spontaneous rhythmic contraction are also present around the basal lamina.

Structure in chronic lymphoedema

In chronic lymphoedema, the collecting vessels are usually dilated and incompetent. Lipid inclusions can be seen in the endothelial cells. Dense plaques grow on the abluminal surface to which an increased number of actin filaments connect. The substance of the perivascular basal lamina grows and becomes multilaminated.

A mixed cellular infiltration develops around the collecting vessels, consisting primarily of mast cells and lymphocytes. Fibrin rings, together with pericytes and myofibroblasts, are frequently seen around the connective tissue fibres. The myofibroblasts are recognizable by their elongated cytoplasm, oblong nuclei and a rich rough endoplasmic reticular content. Parallel to the longitudinal axis of the cell lie actin-like microfilament bundles. The periodic density of the microfilament bundles is characteristic of actin-containing microfilaments.

The elastic fibres around the vessel degenerate and develop into an elastotic material characterized by a decreased number of elastic microfilaments and a large amount of the granulofilamentous substance that, being darkly pigmented in the light-coloured elastin matrix, makes the fibres look like tiger skin. Collagen and elastic fibres as well as inflammatory, enzyme and other proteins produced by inflammatory cells are part of this degenerated product. Extravasated red blood cells are mixed in with the cells of the infiltration.

The chondroitin-6-sulphate and hyaluronic acid content of the ground substance is increased. This increased glycosaminoglycan content influences the polymerization of microfilaments in the connective tissue, so thin and thick collagen fibres are frequent.

CONNECTIVE TISSUE

The density of the lymphatic network in the skin is low in comparison with the density of the vascular network.

The fluid filtered from the vasculature therefore needs to be carried over relatively long distances in the interstitial space before it can enter the initial lymphatic pathways. The substances to be transported from the interstitium are carried through the so-called prelymphatic gaps between the fibres of the connective tissue. Thus, the state and composition of the connective tissue – the collagen, elastic fibres and granulofilamentous ground substance – play an important role in the commencement of lymph flow.[5]

Collagen fibres

There is a tight connection between the walls of the initial lymphatics and the surrounding collagen and elastic fibres. These connections between the collagen and elastic fibres and the fibroblasts and membrane-binding (anchoring) filaments play an important role in the control of the working of the lymphatic capillaries.

Normal structure

The collagen fibres in the pericapillary space are embedded in the granulofilamentous ground substance. Microfilaments of collagen fibres may make direct contact with the endothelial cells. The polymerization of the tropocollagen chains produces the 64–68 nm diameter and 63–64 nm longitudinal periodicity of the mature collagen fibres.

Structure in chronic lymphoedema

The changes in the amino acid composition of the dermal collagen fibres affect its ultrastructural morphology. The stability of the collagen is dependent on its hydroxyproline level, the hydroxyl residue being able to participate in hydrogen linkages. The lysine and hydroxylysine components behave as targets for enzymatic reactions. In chronic lymphoedema, the reshaping of the collagen chains is influenced by inflammatory enzymes such as hydrolases and collagenases.

In chronic lymphoedema, the collagen fibres become deformed. Three main morphological changes are visible.

Thick and thin variants
The diameter of normal collagen fibres varies from 25 to 200 nm. In lymphoedema, a pathological polymerization of the microfibrils causes the thickness of the fibres to vary, but the transverse periodicity of the fibres remains unchanged at 63 nm (Fig. 4.9). The thin and thick collagen variants can be mostly seen in the lower third of the dermis and in the subcutis.[6]

Flower-like collagen
The diameter of this collagen variant varies from about 60 to 400 nm. The surface of the fibre is uneven, and in

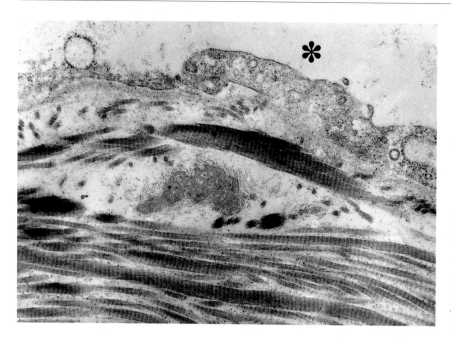

Figure 4.9 *The perilymphatic region of this dilated lymphatic capillary (starred) contains extremely thick collagen bundles mixed with thin collagen variants and elastic fibres. The longitudinal periodicity of the twisting collagen fibres remains unchanged. (×7200).*

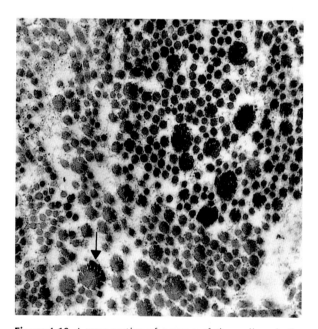

Figure 4.10 *A cross-section of a group of the perilymphatic collagen fibres shown in Fig. 4.9, demonstrating their different diameters (20–200 nm) and the flower-like surface (arrowed) of the thick collagen variants. (×10 600).*

cross-section the irregular contours of the fibre looks like a flower. There is no change in the transverse periodicity of 63 nm (Figs 4.9 and 4.10). The causes of development of flower-like collagen fibres – a similar phenomenon to that which has been described in inherited connective tissue disorders[7] – are abnormal fibrillogenesis, an altered connective tissue ground substance and pathological polymerization. Modified collagen fibres are found in the upper and middle thirds of the dermis.[8]

Long-spacing collagen

In human skin, the long-spacing collagen variant is observed around dermal nerves. The appearance of this collagen variant independently from neural tissue can be explained by the accumulation of a large amount of glycosaminoglycan-rich ground substance and the altered conditions for microfilament polymerization. Long-spacing collagen is characterized by an 80–120 nm longitudinal periodicity. These filaments are embedded in the increased volume of the granulofilamentous ground substance (Fig. 4.11). The long-spacing collagen is located in the perilymphatic space and loose connective tissue surrounding the blood vessels in the upper and middle thirds of the oedematous dermis.[9]

There is a considerable degree of phagocytosis in the macrophages of the middle and lower thirds of the dermis. Many pieces of fragmented collagen fibres lie in the cytoplasm of the dendritic connective tissue cells. The fibres in the phagosomes are in various phases of decomposition (Fig. 4.12). Collagen phagocytosis is frequent in disorders that characteristically involve the degeneration of the connective tissue. Collagen phagocytosis in lymphoedema is a sign of increased collagen rebuilding.

Elastic fibres

Normal structure

Lymph vessels are surrounded by elastic fibres. Elastic microfilaments connect directly to the endothelium of the lymph capillaries. This connection to the elastic fibres is indispensable for the normal functioning of the lymph vessels.

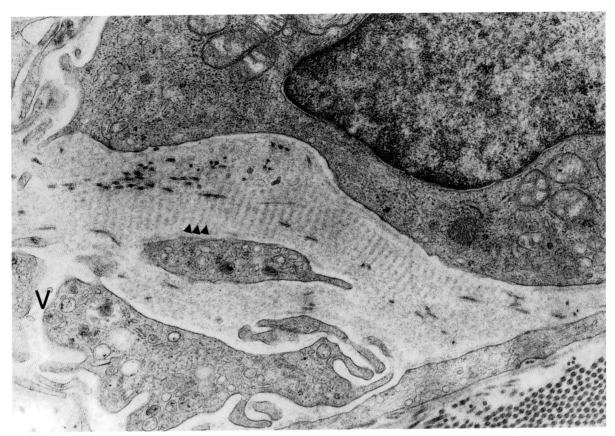

Figure 4.11 *A bundle of long-spacing collagen embedded in the granulofilamentous ground substance of the perivascular space around a postcapillary venule (V). The long-spacing collagen is characterized by 80–120 nm periodicity (arrowheads). (×25 000).*

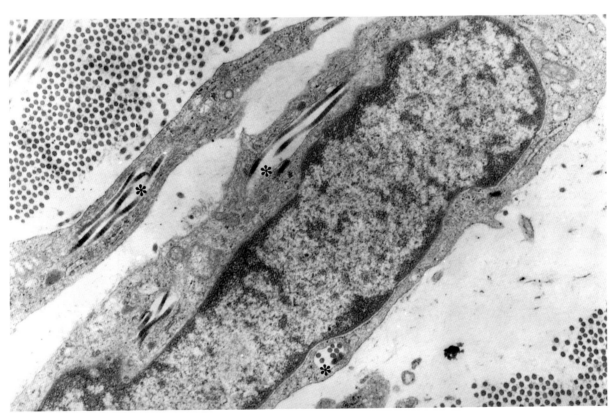

Figure 4.12 *Detail of a connective tissue histiocyte. There are numerous intracellular fragments of collagen fibres in the cytoplasm (starred), the longitudinal periodicity of these fibres being seen. The inclusions are membrane bound. (×20 000).*

The dermal lymphatic capillaries are also surrounded by elastic fibres.[10,11] These elastic fibres are arranged in a spiral pattern but do not form a continuous elastic lamina around the capillaries.[2] Because of the anchoring elastic microtubules, the elastic fibres can connect directly to the abluminal endothelial membrane of the initial lymphatics.

Structure in chronic lymphoedema

In this situation, the elastic fibres are fragmented and degenerating. A feature of chronic oedema, in which inflammatory infiltration plays an important role, is the destruction of elastic fibres. Enzymes (elastase) released from infiltrating neutrophil leukocytes disintegrate the elastic fibres and encourage the development of the elastotic substance.

The number of 10–12 nm elastic anchoring microfilaments directly attached to the lymphatic endothelial cells decreases in chronic lymphoedema.[12] In the late fibrotic stage of lymphoedema, the direct connections of the peri-endothelial elastic microfilaments to the capillary endothelial membrane are lost. The degeneration of elastic fibres is morphologically characterized by an alteration in the proportion and structure of elastic microfilaments and elastin. The number of elastic microfilaments decreases, and the matrix displays a fine granular structure with dense granules in it. This alteration is called elastotic degeneration, a consequence of which is to make the elastic fibres look like Gruyère cheese (Fig. 4.13). In chronic lymphoedema, these changes are also found in the subcutis.

Interfibrillar ground substance

The ground substance is capable of absorbing a large amount of interstitial fluid. Any alteration of the ground substance changes its capability to absorb water so the glycosaminoglycan component of the ground substance has a significant effect on the movement of interstitial fluid. Sclerosis decreases the ability to absorb water.

Normal structure

The dermal microfilaments have different origins. They are embedded in the connective tissue ground substance, which consists of different glycosaminoglycans, mainly hyaluronic acid and dermatan sulphate. Since the glycosaminoglycans are polyanionic molecules, they are very sensitive to local and environmental ionic and

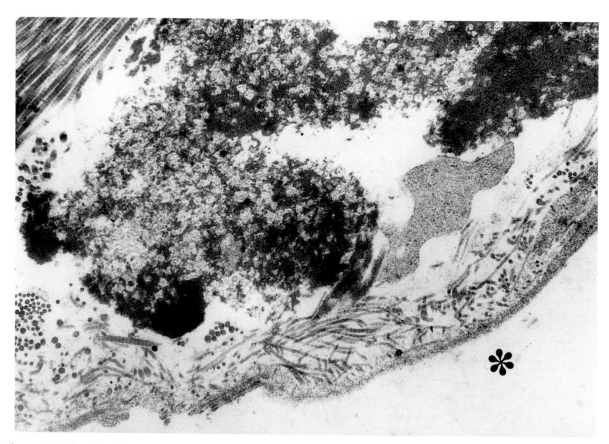

Figure 4.13 *The dilated lumen of this lymphatic capillary (starred) is surrounded by a very thin endothelial layer. The continuous basal lamina is missing, and the perivascular elastic fibres have degenerated. The dense fragmented elastin is intermingled with a granulofilamentous material, making it look like Gruyère cheese. (×6400).*

chemical changes. Staining with ruthenium red highlights connective tissue microfilaments 5–50 nm in diameter communicating with both the collagen and the elastic microfilaments. This explains the ruthenium red surface positivity of the collagen and elastic fibres.

The collagen-associated chondroitin sulphate resists digestion by hyaluronidase and accounts for the appearance of a ruthenium red-positive coat around the collagen fibres.[13,14] The addition of glycosaminoglycans to a native collagen preparation in vitro results in the formation of long-spacing collagen.[15]

Structure in chronic lymphoedema

The heparin sulphate and dermatan sulphate content of the ground substance varies, changes influencing the structure of the various extracellularly polymerized connective tissue microfilaments (collagen and elastin). In chronic lymphoedema, the quantity of dermatan sulphate and heparin sulphate falls, although the amount of hyaluronic acid remains unchanged for a long time.[16] The anastomosing so-called hyaluronate microfilaments[17] are hyaluronic acid–protein complexes and are digestable by hyaluronidase. They have diameters in the range 20–40 nm and are found in bundles dispersed in the granulomatous ground substance, intermingled with collagen microfilaments forming long-spacing collagen fibres. The appearance of long-spacing collagen in the dermis of different disorders is connected with the increased amount of the granulofilamentous interfibrillar material[9] and the fall in the level of normal collagen and elastin microfilaments.

Fibrosis

Fibrosis develops in the dermis in chronic lymphoedema at the end-stage of the pathological processes in the connective tissue. The number of fibroblasts and macrophages showing hyperactivity is decreased, and a few star-shaped cells with enormous elongated dendritic processes represent the histiocytes. These are surrounded by featureless hyalin-like material. Fibrosis is characterized by the ultrastructural deposition of material that appears amorphous on light microscopy (Fig. 4.14) but in fact represents a mixture of two types of microfilament embedded in finely granulated substances. These are microfilaments 1–2 nm in diameter that are rigid and short and presumably represent an abnormal product of the fibroblast rather than degenerated collagen, and hyalin microfilaments 5–10 nm in diameter that are not digested by hyaluronidase but are partially digested by trypsin. Whether hyalin is a product of degenerated collagen or a pathological cell product of chronic inflammation remains to be proved.[14]

The relative mass of collagen is increased in fibrosis. Thin and thick collagen variants and flower-like collagen are intermingled with the interstitial granulofilamentous material, the elastic fibres disappearing. Necrotic remnants of degenerated cells can be detected in the hyalin-like material (Fig. 4.15).

Dilated lymphatic vessels surrounded by granulofilamentous ground substance are rare. The inlet valves between the endothelial cells are usually open, and the intraluminal valves become shortened by the fibrosis of

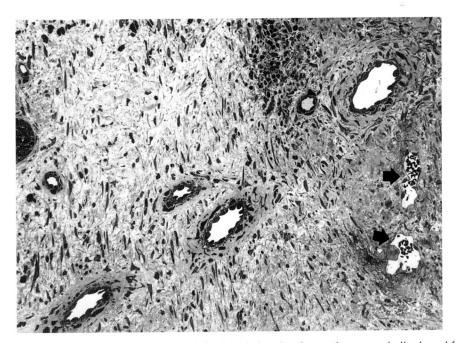

Figure 4.14 *The light microscopic features of the dermis in chronic lymphoedema. There are spindle-shaped fibroblasts and inflammatory cells embedded in an increased amount of oedematous ground substance. The endothelial cells of the blood vessels are swollen and protrude into the lumen, the perivascular tissue being fibrotic. The dilated lymphatic vessels (arrowed) are filled by red blood cells. (Haematoxylin and eosin, ×250).*

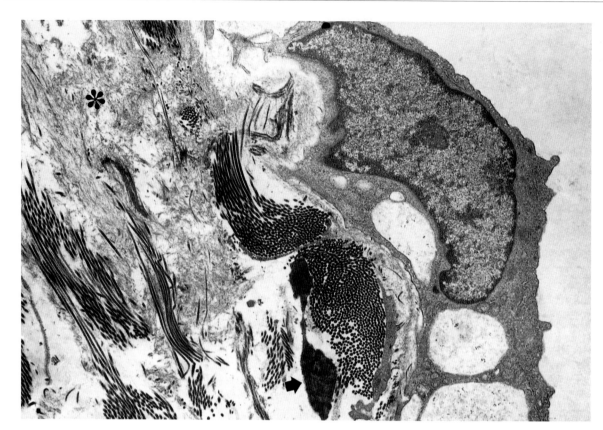

Figure 4.15 *Detail of an arch-like lymphatic endothelial cell. The amount of perivascular basal lamina material is increased. The remnants of the degenerated elastic and collagen fibres (arrowed) are embedded in large amounts of connective tissue microfilaments (starred). (×8200).*

their connective tissue skeleton. A decrease occurs in the cellular elements in the dermis.

CELLULAR COMPONENTS

Chronic inflammation in lymphoedema

Histologically, chronic lymphoedema can be diagnosed by the appearance of inflammatory cells in the dermis (Fig. 4.16) – mast cells, polymorphonuclear leukocytes, macrophages, lymphocytes, plasma cells and histiocytes (Fig. 4.17). The mononuclear cell infiltrate initiates the cytokine cascade that accompanies the release of the proteases and local tissue destruction. One of the proteins damaged early in these events is the elastic fibre.

The well-developed rough endoplasmic reticulum contains histiocytes with elongated cytoplasmic processes, these containing crystal-like inclusions and the phagocytosed remnants of red blood cells in their cytoplasm (Fig. 4.18). A large number of fragmented collagen fibres stored in the dendritic histiocytes can be seen in the mid-dermis. Collagen phagocytosis, which characterizes the cutaneous diseases accompanied by connective tissue degeneration, can be a sign of increased collagen rebuilding in lymphoedema (*see* Fig. 4.12, p. 73).

Lipid clearance from the dermis is impaired in chronic lymphoedema, stored lipid droplets being a characteristic feature of the macrophages. The origin of the lipid droplets is either the fat-like materials in the lymph fluid of the interstitium or the digested cell components of degenerate tissue. In the late stage of lymphoedema, the number of cells is diminished.

BLOOD VESSELS

Blood vessel–lymph vessel shunts

Normal structure

Red blood cells are often seen in the lumen of the lymphatics, arriving there via blood vessel–lymphatic shunts (Fig. 4.19). The existence of these communications in the human dermis has been documented by serial sections (Fig. 4.20, p. 79).

Structure in chronic lymphoedema

The number of communications between the blood vessels and the lymphatic capillaries increases in chronic inflammation. These probably represent preformed or acquired structures that compensate for the failure of lymphatic transport in chronic lymphoedema.

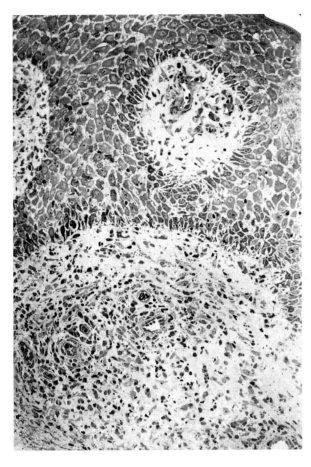

Lymphostatic haemangiopathy

In chronic lymphoedema, the accumulation of protein-rich oedema fluid in the dermis changes the metabolism of dermal connective tissue and adversely affects the venous and arterial microcirculation. The morphological changes that develop in both the venous and arterial microcirculation are called lymphostatic haemangiopathy.[18]

The arteriolar and venular lumens become filled with red blood cells, the numerous extravasated red blood cells in the upper and mid-dermis being a well-recognized feature of raised venous pressure (Fig. 4.21, p. 79).

Structure of the small arteries in chronic lymphoedema

The endothelial cells of the small arteries are swollen and protrude into the lumen, possessing cushion-like forms.

Figure 4.16 *Chronic inflammation in lymphoedematous skin. The acanthotic epidermis is oedematous, and haemostasis has caused the dermal perivascular infiltration to become intermingled with extravasated red blood cells. Exocytotic inflammatory cells are present among the basal keratinocytes. (Haematoxylin and eosin, ×250).*

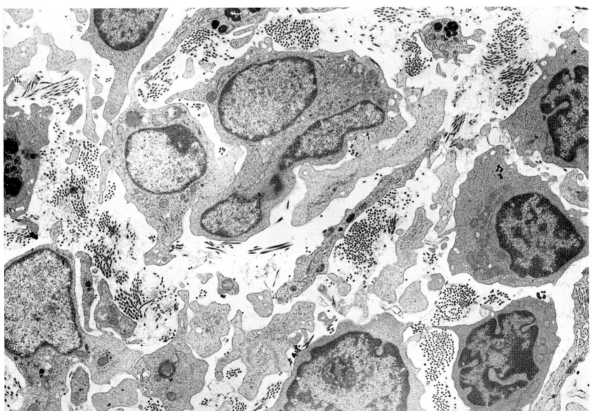

Figure 4.17 *An example of the mixed cellular infiltrate of lymphocytes, histiocytes and macrophages in the oedematous interstitium that is seen in chronic inflammation. (×8200).*

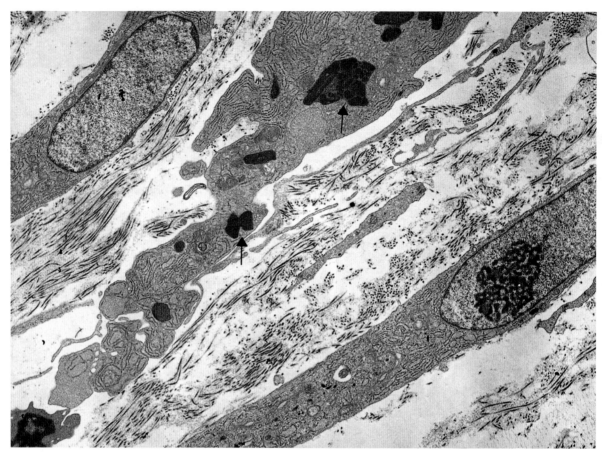

Figure 4.18 *The histiocytes, connective tissue macrophages with well-developed endoplasmic reticulum and phagosomes of different sizes seen in chronic inflammation. The bizarrely shaped phagosomes (arrowed) are partly membrane bound and show uneven density. (×8200).*

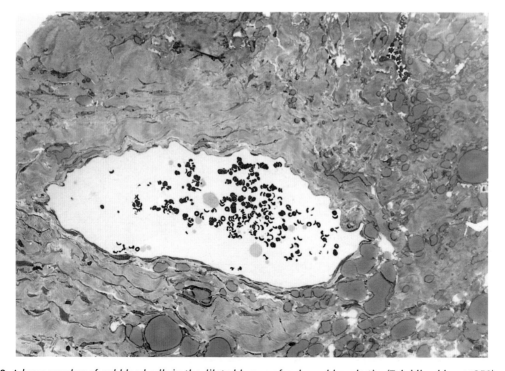

Figure 4.19 *A large number of red blood cells in the dilated lumen of a dermal lymphatic. (Toluidine blue, ×250).*

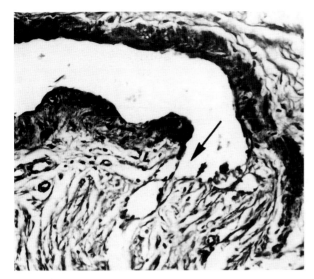

Figure 4.20 *A demonstration of the existence of blood vessel-to-lymph vessel shunts between a dermal vein and a lymphatic (arrowed). (Haematoxylin and eosin, ×250).*

Their cytoplasm is rich in mitochondria, ribosomes and glycogen. In some regions, the lumen is filled with red blood cells, whose shape, because of the increased luminal pressure, becomes faceted (Fig. 4.22).

The basement lamina is duplicated around the small arteries. The number of pericytes is increased, their basement laminae being thick and reduplicated. Large numbers of mast cells, lymphocytes, histiocytes and fibroblasts can be seen in the peri-arteriolar space (Fig. 4.23).

Structure of the small veins in chronic lymphoedema

The endothelial cells of the small veins protrude into the lumen, sometimes making the lumen very narrow. There are two types of endothelial cell:

1 Some have an electron-dense cytoplasm because of the large number of ribosomes, mitochondria, Weibel–Palade bodies and endoplasmic reticulum. The presence of a centriole, as a modified mitotic centre, is not uncommon. The nuclei are lobulated.
2 The so-called pale endothelial cells, with only a few mitochondria and microfilaments about 3–5 nm in diameter, run to the plate-like densities on the abluminal cell membrane. This microfilamentous bundle contains periodic densities like those of actinomyosin filaments. These pale endothelial cells probably function as baroreceptors. Lipid droplets and phagosomes varying in size and density can be seen in the endothelial cells. The pericytes surrounded by multilayered basement lamina are arranged in reduplicated layers.

The cytoplasmic membranes are accompanied by a large number of pinocytotic vesicles. Fragments of degenerated collagen and elastic fibres can be seen among the

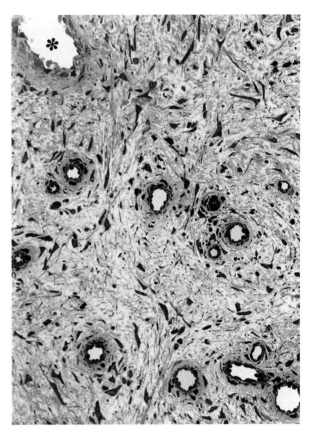

Figure 4.21 *The perivascular spaces of the blood vessels and lymph vessels (starred) in lymphostatic haemangiopathy characteristically contain extravasated red blood cells and an increased number of pericytes and spindle-shaped fibrocytes. (Haematoxylin and eosin, ×250).*

layers of the elongated pseudopodia of the pericytes and in the multilayered basement laminae. A great number of red blood cells can be found in the perivascular spaces. The connective tissue here is very loose because of the increased amount of interfibrillar ground substance and microfilaments.

Endothelial cells can become detached from the pericytes and oedema fluid and inflammatory cells can be captured in the widened subendothelial space (Fig. 4.24). The vascular wall is frequently infiltrated by inflammatory cells.

Angiogenesis

Numerous newly formed vessel buds can be seen in the papillary and upper part of the dermis. These newly formed blood vessels have narrow, slit-like, star-shaped lumens. The vascular buds composed of endothelial cells can hardly be differentiated from groups of histiocytes or other inflammatory cells (Fig. 4.25). It is likely that the growth of these new vessels is stimulated by local inflammatory agents, vascular endothelial growth factor and growth factor C,[19] but the exact cause is not known.[5,20]

Oedema fluid in itself does not facilitate angiogenesis. In cases of dermatosclerosis, atrophy, post-thrombotic syndrome and chronic venous insufficiency, for example, there is elongation and tortuosity of the blood vessels but no new capillaries.

It should be noted that benign and malignant vascular tumors, including angiosarcoma, are complications of chronic lymphoedema.

EPIDERMAL CHANGES

Acanthosis–papillomatosis

The epidermis is acanthotic (Fig. 4.26), the proliferation of the keratinocytes being influenced by cytokines released from the cellular elements of chronic dermal infiltration,

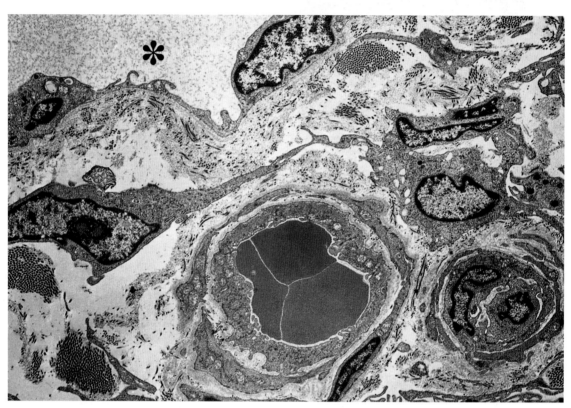

Figure 4.22 *Red blood cells become trapped in the arteriolar lumen in chronic lymphoedema because of the haemostasis, their shapes become faceted. The amount of basement lamina material is increased. Mastocytes and fibrocytes are seen in the perivascular space. The granulofilamentous substance around the dilated lymphatic capillary (starred) has become intermingled with collagen fibres. (×8200).*

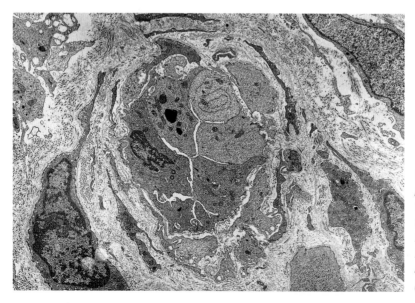

Figure 4.23 *Swollen endothelial cells protruding into the lumen of a blood vessel in lymphoedematous skin, giving the lumen a split-like appearance. The reduplicated layers of the basement laminae and dendritic pericytes are characteristic of a postcapillary venule. (×8200).*

hypertrophic vascular endothelial cells and epidermal cells. The intercellular spaces are expanded and filled with protein-rich, oedema fluid. This protein-rich fluid is filtered from the dermis through the dermo-epidermal junction. The keratinocytes become vacuolated because of the intracellular oedema and show numerous elongated pseudopodia. Tonofilaments and desmosomes are decreased in number. There is epidermal migration of

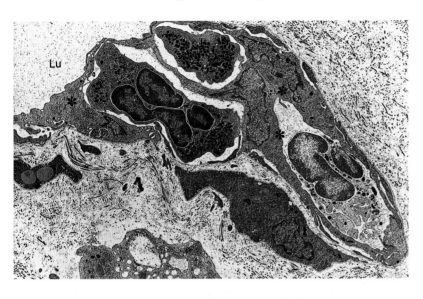

Figure 4.24 *A dermal vein in chronic lymphoedema. Polymorphonuclear granulocytes and monocytes are captured between the endothelial cells and pericytes (starred). Lu, lumen. (×8200).*

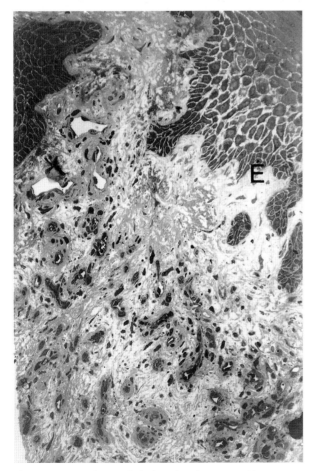

Figure 4.25 *Angiogenesis in lymphoedematous skin. Beneath the acanthotic epidermis (E), the papillary dermis is oedematous. The mid-dermis contains a large number of thick-walled venules, arteries and dilated lymphatic capillaries. (Haematoxylin and eosin, ×250).*

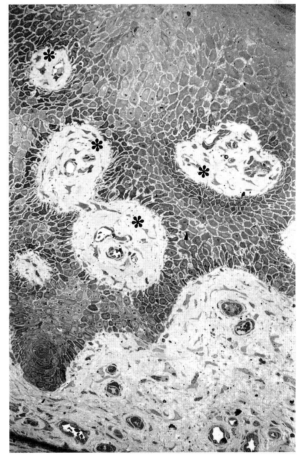

Figure 4.26 *Acanthosis in lymphoedematous skin. The elongated dermal papillae (starred) are surrounded by acanthotic epidermis. The thick-walled arteries and venules are embedded in the homogeneous connective tissue. (Haematoxylin and eosin, ×250).*

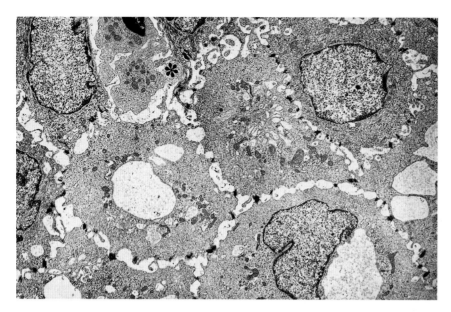

Figure 4.27 *Detail of lymphoedematous epidermis. Lymphocytes are seen in the wide intercellular spaces (starred). There is a decreased number of tonofilaments and desmosomes in the vacuolated keratinocytes. (×19 600).*

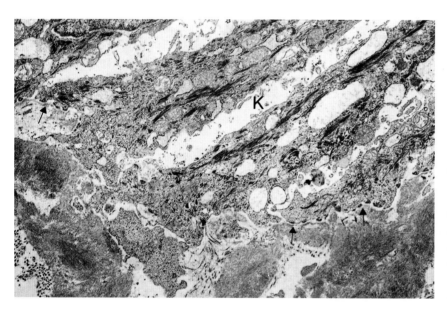

Figure 4.28 *The dermo-epidermal junction in lymphoedema. A large number of connective tissue microfilaments, of different origins, are deposited in the region of the basal lamina. The basal lamina material (arrowed) is intermingled with the connective tissue microfilaments. K, keratinocytes. (×27 500).*

inflammatory cells (exocytosis) from the papillary dermis into the epidermis (Fig. 4.27).

Papillomatosis (the pseudotumour-like proliferation of the skin) may develop in those cases in which there is epidermal acanthosis, hyperkeratosis, an increased amount of dermal ground substance, proliferation of the connective tissue and an increased number of newly formed blood vessels. These papillomata contain a very small number of dilated lymphatics.

Dermo-epidermal junction

The epidermal basement lamina is thickened or multi-layered, and epidermal anchoring collagen filaments are missing or decreased in number. Microfilaments of different origin, such as fibrin, colloid bodies (degenerated keratinocytes) and collagen microfilaments, are deposited in this region (Fig. 4.28).

Fibrin deposition may be produced by the increased plasma protein filtration from the blood vessels and the vascular congestion. The identification of fibrin is easy in those cases in which its characteristic 20–25 nm periodicity has already developed. The colloid bodies, which are of keratinocytic origin, contain microfilaments 7–10 nm in diameter, melanosomes and cell remnants. The tonofilaments of the degenerated, oedematous, vacuolated keratinocytes migrate down into the dermis. The collagen microfilaments are thin collagen fibres 15–20 nm in diameter with longitudinal periodicity. There are dilated lymphatic capillaries in close contact with the dermo-epidermal junction.

HISTOLOGY OF THE LYMPH GLANDS IN LYMPHOEDEMA

We owe to Virchow the origin of the concept that lymph glands act as a barrier when he stated, 'the elements lie crowded together like the particles of a charcoal filter so that the lymph trickles out again on the other side in a more or less purified state'. It was therefore logical for Mowlem to suggest, in 1948,[21] that intrinsic lymph gland disease might be the cause of primary lymphoedema, but this hypothesis was not critically examined until the 1970s.

In 1976, Kinmonth and Eustace[22] hypothesized, on the basis of a thorough investigation of patients with primary lymphoedema by lymphography, that abnormalities in the lymph glands were as important a cause of lymphoedema as were abnormalities in the lymphatics. At this time, similar suggestions were being made to explain the high incidence of elephantiasis in the continent of Africa. There is little doubt that benign lymph gland disease can cause lymphoedema, filariasis being the prime example, but there is a very low incidence of filariasis in Uganda, Ethiopia, Kenya and Rwanda Barundi, areas where lymphoedema is endemic. At first onchocerciasis was suggested to be the cause, but this was conclusively refuted by Teneych.[23] Then Price and colleagues,[24–26] having analysed the contents of the lymph glands of African patients with lymphoedema and found silica particles surrounded by a dense fibrotic reaction, suggested that the lymphoedema was caused by a fibrosis initiated by particles of silica in the lymphatics and lymph glands that had entered from the soil via splits in the skin of damaged feet.

This hypothesis gained support when Price found a relationship between the geographical incidence of lymphoedema and the silica content of the soil. At the same time, Price also reported that the tribesmen of Rwanda Barundi considered lymphoedema to be a familial condition, which they considered barred a girl from marriage. One third of the patients he questioned gave a clear history of another member of the family with the disease. This, he hypothesized, indicated that lymph gland fibrosis caused by silica could precipitate or hasten the appearance of lymphoedema in patients with a predisposition to the condition. He also suggested that the African cases of lymphoedema were caused by a spectrum of primary and secondary causes, mainly genetic and silica, which overlapped and exacerbated each other.

Lymphographic evidence that changes in the lymph glands strangled the drainage of lymph from the limb and affected the distal lymphatics came from a 1982 study based on sequential lymphograms performed in patients with lymphoedema by Fyfe et al.[27] This showed that patients who had lymphographically abnormal inguinal lymph glands showed a gradual occlusion of their peripheral lymphatics, a process these authors called 'die-back'. They concluded that the primary proximal abnormality was causing an aquired obliteration of

more distal glands and lymphatics. Similar changes have been found in the peripheral lymphatics following the surgical excision of lymph glands.[28]

Reproducing any form of clincal lymphoedema is a notoriously difficult exercise, but in 1983 Wolfe et al.[29] attempted to produce lymph gland fibrosis in the hind leg of the rabbit by occluding either the afferent or efferent lymphatics of the popliteal lymph node,[29] the effects on the gland being assessed lymphographically and histologically. Unfortunately, they were unable to produce convincing fibrosis because of the regenerative capacity of the lymphatic collecting ducts, suggesting that, in most circumstances, the lymphatics are able to regenerate and bypass an occluded lymph gland.

In 1985, Fyfe and Price[30] injected the lymphatics of rabbits' limbs with silica. This produced a severe inflammatory reaction follwed by fibrosis in the lymphatics, and to a lesser degree the lymph glands, suggesting that the lymphatic obstruction caused by silica entering the tissues through the foot may result more from the effect of the silica on the lymph vessels than the lymph glands.

These studies were accompanied by a histological study of 74 patients with established primary lymphoedema that compared inguinal gland pathology with high-quality lymphadenography.[31] The glands were removed with great care to avoid damage to the surrounding tissues and cause as little interference as possible with lymphatic collateral vessels. The histology of the glands was compared with that of normal lymph glands. In many glands, there was a dense, extensive fibrosis with occlusion of both the cortical and medullary lymphatic channels, but in other lymph glands the degree of fibrosis was small. The area of fibrosis was measured in a series of histological sections from each gland and expressed as a proportion of the whole. The mean area of fibrosis in each clinical group was as follows:

- normal non-oedematous limbs – 10 per cent;
- limbs with distal hypoplasia/obliteration – 11 per cent;
- limbs with distal and proximal hypoplasia/ obliteration – 34 per cent;
- limbs with proximal obstruction/obliteration only – 41 per cent;
- limbs with bilateral numerical hyperplasia – 28 per cent;
- limbs with megalymphatics (all unilateral) – 11 per cent.

From these results, it was concluded that patients with evidence of distal lymphatic disease and no proximal disease and patients with congenital megalymphatics had a normal amount of inguinal lymph gland fibrous tissue, whereas patients with lymphographic evidence of proximal obstruction (obliteration) had a significantly greater quantity of fibrous tissue in their inguinal lymph glands. It thus became apparent that the abnormal lymphadenographic findings reported by Kinmonth and Eustace[22] were caused by fibrosis in the lymph glands and that fibrosis was associated with the more severe forms of primary lymphoedema because the patients with a large amount of inguinal lymph node fibrosis were found to be those with lymphoedema affecting the whole limb and a poor prognosis.[32]

LIGHT MICROSCOPY OF INGUINAL LYMPH GLANDS IN PRIMARY LYMPHOEDEMA

Macroscopic appearance

Normal inguinal lymph glands are usually oval and the afferent lymphatics discernible as strands attached to the capsule of the node. Tiny vessels entering the capsule may also be apparent. The major vessels supplying and draining them enter and leave at a hilum. Normal lymph glands are surrounded by a loose capsule of connective tissue. The afferent lymphatics penetrate this capsule over its convex surface, the efferent lymphatics leaving via the hilum. The main blood vessels also enter the gland at the hilum. The lymph entering the gland flows into the subcapsular sinus before permeating through the cortex into the medulla and thence to the efferent lymphatics at the hilum. Macroscopically, the inguinal lymph glands of patients with lymphoedema of the lower limb look normal or sometimes slightly smaller than normal.

Microscopic appearance

The framework of the lymph node is made up of a network of reticulin fibres that connect with the capsule and also with the connective tissue trabeculae that extend into the node from both the capsule and the hilum to provide support. The reticulin fibre network varies in density, being almost non-existent in areas of active lymphocyte differentiation in the cortex. The germinal centres lie in pyramidal areas of reticulin with their base lying close to the capsule. The areas between the pyramids contain few reticulin fibres, and this is the region of the lymph sinuses. At the apex of the pyramids, these merge into the medullary cords, which interconnect. This framework forms a lattice supporting the lymphocytes packed into the pyramidal areas (Fig. 4.29). Perinodal fibrosis is the result of previous episodes of lymphangitis. Hyaline thickening of the fibrous network also increases with age and is attributed to episodes of non-specific lymphadenitis.

Taking these changes and the involutionary changes that occur with age into consideration, the most striking abnormality that was seen in the patients with lymphoedema[31] was the large amount of central and hilar fibrous tissue. This was different from the findings in perinodal fibrosis, which may be seen as a feature of previous episodes of lymphangitis. It is well recognized that

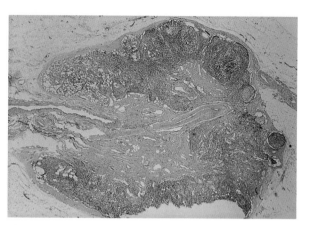

Figure 4.29 *A cross-section through the hilum of a normal lymph gland showing a normal amount of fibrous tissue around the blood vessels and normal germinal follicles. (Haematoxylin and eosin).*

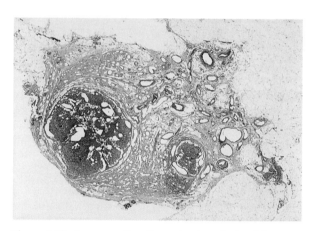

Figure 4.30 *A cross-section through a lymph gland from a woman with primary proximal obstructive lymphoedema. The gland is almost entirely replaced with fibrous tissue, only three small germinal follicles remaining. The vacuoles are artefacts caused by the presence of Lipiodol in the gland. (Trichrome).*

inguinal lymph nodes are difficult to interpret histologically because normal inguinal lymph nodes contain some central fibrous tissue. Although varying degrees of hilar fibrosis were present in the inguinal lymph glands taken from control patients, none had the extensive fibrosis seen in patients with lymphoedema. In the patients with lymphoedema, the hilar fibrosis extended into the medulla, the paracortical area and even large areas of the cortex.

In those lymph glands which were least affected, there was a small amount of perivascular hilar fibrosis. In the moderately affected lymph glands, larger areas of hilar and medullary fibrosis were present that extended through the cortex between the lymphoid follicles to the capsule. In the most severely fibrosed glands, only small islands of lymphoid tissue remained, the gland being almost totally replaced by fibrous tissue (Fig. 4.30). These lymph glands were barely recognizable as lymph glands, and the fibrous tissue was often highly vascular. The fibrosis was usually associated with an infiltrate of mast cells, cells known to promote the proliferation of fibroblasts. Any remaining cortical lymphoid tissue appeared to be normal. Fibrin deposition is known to lead to fibroblastic proliferation and fibrosis, but there was no evidence in these lymph glands of an increased amount of fibrin.

Inguinal lymph node biopsies were taken from two patients with Milroy's disease who, by definition, had a congenital maldevelopment of their lymphatic system. In the first, a male 58 years of age, there was extensive lipomatosis and dilated lymphatics in a normally sized lymph node containing a moderate amount of cortical lymphoid tissue. In the second, a female aged 18 years, the inguinal lymph nodes were smaller with more dense fibrosis associated with thick-walled and obliterated lymphatics. It was not possible to differentiate between the findings in these two patients and the other categories of patient studied.

CONCLUSION

- Patients with primary lymphoedema may show marked fibrosis of their lymph glands.
- The distribution and appearance of the fibrosis is quite different from that known to follow acute inflammation.

- The amount of fibrosis varies between different clinical and lymphographic groups, being greatest in patients with lymphographic evidence of proximal obstruction to lymph flow. Clinically, the lymphoedema is worse in those patients with a proximal obstruction of their lymphatics.
- Clinically, the lymphoedema is less widespread and less severe in patients with a distal obliteration of their lymphatics and normal inguinal lymph glands.

There are two ways in which fibrosis within a lymph gland may obstruct lymph flow. It almost certainly strangles and blocks the lymphatic channels within the gland, but it may also prevent the gland expanding to accommodate the increased lymph flow generated by exercise. It has been shown[33] that the resistance of a lymph gland to lymph flow is high at a low rate of flow but falls when the flow increases because, as the gland fills and expands, the flow pathways within the gland dilate. Intraglandular fibrosis will abolish this natural adjustment to an increased lymph flow.

The cause of fibrosis in the lymph glands and the obliteration of peripheral lymphatics,[34] which may be different facets of the same process, needs further study because it is possible that it may be preventable. Unfortunately, the advent of lymphoscintigraphy has reduced the number of X-ray lymphograms performed and the number of occasions on which direct injection into an inguinal lymphatic or gland is needed, so that biopsy of the inguinal glands hardly ever occurs, making it extremely difficult to continue this avenue of research.

BENIGN AND MALIGNANT LYMPHATIC TUMOURS OF SKIN AND SOFT TISSUE

Benign vascular neoplasms are relatively frequent, especially in children and adolescents, in whom they account for approximately 25 per cent of all mesenchymal lesions,[35] whereas angiosarcomata of the skin and soft tissues are uncommon and constitute fewer than 1 per cent of all sarcomata.[36] In striking contrast, true tumours of lymphatic vessels, i.e. vascular neoplasms with an endothelium showing a lymphatic line of differentiation, are uncommon, comprising only 4 per cent of all vascular neoplasms.[37] This difference between the incidence of haemangiomata and angiosarcomata, and lymphangiomata and lymphangiosarcomata, may represent our previous inability to reliably differentiate lymphatic from capillary vascular endothelium, rather than being a true difference. In addition, there is in some lesions a combination of both vessel and endothelial types, these consequently being called haemolymphangiomata.

Histologically, neoplastic lymphatic vessels tend to be lined by endothelial cells with plump, prominent, match stick-like nuclei (in contrast to the flat or epithelioid endothelial cells that line the vascular spaces of haemangiomata; Fig. 4.31) that often show variations in the thickness of their vessel walls and are not completely surrounded by actin-positive (myo)pericytes. In addition, endothelial cells in lymphatic neoplasms tend to be negative for CD34 or stain only focally positive for this endothelial marker, which is uniformly positive in most blood vessels and angiomata as well as in a number of angiosarcomata.

It was until recently held that no immunohistochemical marker could precisely distinguish lymphatic and blood vessel endothelium, but in the past few years it has been speculated that the expression of the vascular endothelial growth factor-C receptor (VEGFR-3) and of podoplanin is limited mainly to lymphatic endothelium.[38,39] Subsequently, in studies of a large number of vascular neoplasms using these immunohistochemical markers, it has been shown that, in addition to traditional lymphatic neoplasms, some of the following distinctive clinicopathological vascular entities – hobnail haemangioma, papillary intralymphatic angioendothelioma (so called Dabska's tumour), retiform haemangioendothelioma, Kaposi's

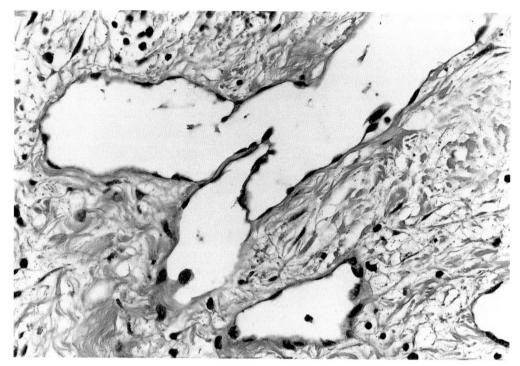

Figure 4.31 *Dilated lymphatic vascular structures lined by flat but also enlarged endothelial cells with prominent, matchstick-like nuclei. In contrast to small blood vessels, these vessels contain thin valves. (Haematoxylin and eosin).*

sarcoma, kaposiform haemangioendothelioma and a subset of angiosarcomata – are probably lymphatic lesions.[38–42]

This section describes the traditional lymphatic neoplasms: lymphangioma circumscriptum, cavernous lymphangioma/cystic hygroma, benign lymphangio-endothelioma (acquired progressive lymphangioma), lymphangiomatosis and lymphangiosarcoma. Entities with a questionable lymphatic line of differentiation are mentioned and illustrated only briefly in the differential diagnosis. The reader is also referred to Chapter 19.

LYMPHANGIOMA CIRCUMSCRIPTUM

Clinical features

Lymphangioma circumscriptum is a developmental malformation of equal sex incidence that presents in infancy or adult life. The cutaneous lesions are invariably associated with cavernous lymphangiomata/cystic hygromata in the subcutaneous tissues beneath them. The fact that the cutaneous vesicles connect with the deeper cavernous lymphatics is responsible for the high rate of local recurrence after superficial cutaneous excisions. Clinically, lymphangioma circumscriptum may occur at any anatomical site, although it shows a predilection for the limb girdles and proximal extremities. The skin lesions present as groups of small vesicles containing clear fluid, but secondary bleeding is occasionally noted (Fig. 4.32). A rare association of cutaneous lymphangioma with dyschondroplasia (Maffucci's syndrome) has been reported.[43]

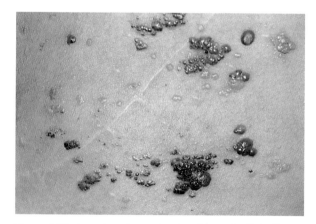

Figure 4.32 *Lymphangioma circumscriptum is clinically characterized by groups of small vesicles containing clear fluid. In this case, secondary bleeding has turned the vesicles reddish-purple.*

Cutaneous lymph-filled vesicles that present in adult life are often mistakenly called lymphangioma circumscriptum. These should, however, be designated as lymphangiectasia because they do not represent a true neoplasm and are seen mainly in association with chronic lymphoedema caused by reflux or radiotherapy.[44,45]

Pathological features

Lymphangioma circumscriptum is composed of numerous dilated, thin-walled lymphatic vascular structures

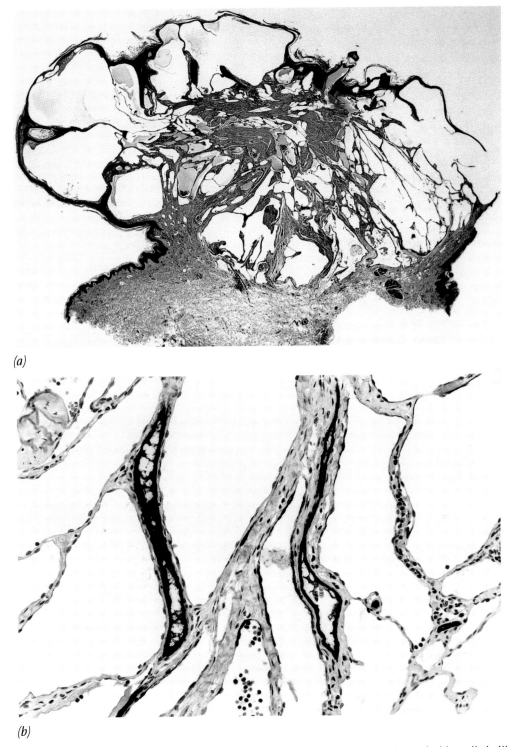

(a)

(b)

Figure 4.33 *(a) Low-power view of a lymphangioma circumscriptum showing superficially located, thin-walled, dilated vascular structures containing proteinaceous fluid. (Haematoxylin and eosin). (b) In contrast to what is seen with haemangiomata, the endothelial cells in lymphangioma circumscriptum stain only focally positive for CD34. (Labelled streptavidin biotin technique).*

located in the superficial dermis. In some cases, a verruciform epithelial hyperplasia is noted. The cysts and channels contain a proteinaceous fluid with few erythrocytes and are lined by a single layer of cytologically bland endothelial cells that contain often slightly enlarged and prominent nuclei with an evenly distributed chromatin lacking mitotic figures (Fig. 4.33). Secondary features include a lymphocytic infiltrate in the surrounding stroma. The endothelial cells of lymphangioma circumscriptum stain positively for CD31, VEGFR-3 and podoplanin,[39] but are inconsistently positive for CD34 (Fig. 4.33b) and are not surrounded completely by actin-positive pericytes, a striking contrast to most haemangiomata. Recent extended immunohistochemical studies have further emphasized that lymphangiomata resemble vascular malformations more than haemangiomata.[46]

Differential diagnosis

In contrast to lymphangioma circumscriptum, hobnail haemangioma (targetoid haemosiderotic haemangioma) presents clinically as a solitary vascular neoplasm in adults and is characterized by a biphasic growth of superficial dilated and, in deeper parts, rather narrow vascular structures that are lined by enlarged endothelial cells with prominent hobnail-like nuclei (Fig. 4.34). The vascular structures of a typical hobnail haemangioma are set in a dense collagenous stroma with abundant haemosiderin deposits. Similarities in immunohistochemical features and overlapping histological findings suggest, however, that hobnail haemangioma belongs probably to the spectrum of benign lymphatic lesions.[40]

Importantly, lymphangioma circumscriptum has to be distinguished from lymphangioma-like cutaneous angiosarcoma and lymphangioma-like Kaposi's sarcoma. Lymphangioma-like cutaneous angiosarcoma contains anastomosing vascular spaces lined by atypical and proliferative active endothelial cells. The rare lymphangioma-like Kaposi's sarcoma, which typically occurs as multifocal vascular lesions on the lower legs of elderly patients of Jewish or Mediterranean origin, contains focal areas of a spindle cell proliferation.[47,48]

CAVERNOUS LYMPHANGIOMA/CYSTIC HYGROMA

Clinical features

Cavernous lymphangioma and cystic hygroma represent variants of the same hamartomatous lesion. They are present at birth or develop within the first years of life and have an equal sex incidence.[49] Whereas cavernous lymphangiomata arise predominantly in the oral cavity, the extremities and the mesentery, cystic hygromata tend to occur in the neck, groin and axillae. Rare sites such as the retroperitoneum, mediastinum and scrotum, as well as multifocal lesions, have been described.[50]

Complete resection is the treatment of choice; extensive lesions may cause clinical problems such as progressive dyspnoea with mediastinal lesions, and bowel obstruction with intra-abdominal/mesenteric lesions.[51]

Pathological features

Cavernous lymphangiomata/cystic hygromata are composed of dilated lymphatic vascular structures with

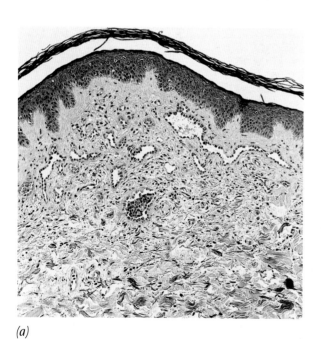

(a)

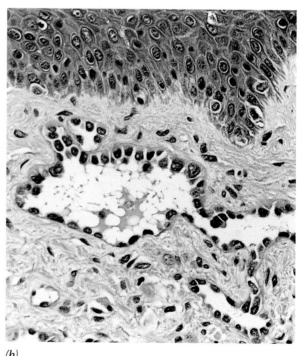

(b)

Figure 4.34 *Cases of hobnail haemangioma are characterized histologically by a biphasic growth of superficial dilated and, in deeper parts, rather narrow vascular spaces (a) lined by endothelial cells with enlarged, prominent nuclei (b). (Haematoxylin and eosin).*

variably thick walls (Fig. 4.35). Their rim of actin-positive pericytes is often incomplete. Their lining endothelial cells are typically attenuated and cytologically bland, rarely being enlarged cuboidal or epithelioid.[52] The vascular lumens are either empty or full of a proteinaceous material and scattered erythrocytes.

Lymphocytes and lymphoid aggregates are frequently present in the surrounding stroma. The immunopositivity of the endothelial cells of an intrapericardial lesion for podoplanin has been reported.[53] As in lymphangioma circumscriptum, long-standing lesions may show stromal fibrosis.

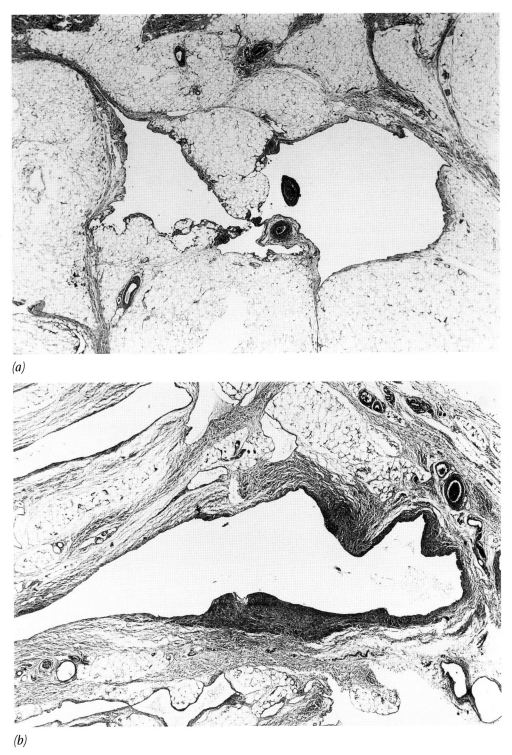

(a)

(b)

Figure 4.35 *The dilated lymphatic vascular structures characteristic of cavernous lymphangioma/cystic hygroma (a). Note the variable thickness of the vessel walls, a frequent finding in these lesions (b). (Haematoxylin and eosin).*

Differential diagnosis

The distinction of cavernous lymphangioma/cystic hygroma from cavernous haemangioma on histological grounds may be impossible, but the presence of stromal lymphocytes and lymphoid aggregates tends to be associated with cavernous lymphangioma/cystic hygroma. Intra-abdominal and scrotal lesions have to be separated from cystic mesotheliomata, but the latter are composed of variably sized cysts lined by cytokeratin-positive cells that are negative for endothelial immunohistochemial markers.

BENIGN LYMPHANGIOENDOTHELIOMA (ACQUIRED PROGRESSIVE LYMPHANGIOMA)

Clinical features

Benign lymphangioendothelioma was first described and delineated by Wilson Jones and collegues[54,55] and recently further characterized by Guillou and Fletcher.[56] It is a rare cutaneous vascular neoplasm affecting patients over a broad age range (5–90 years in 35 reported cases). It frequently occurs on the limbs, being next most commonly seen on the trunk and the head and neck. Clinically, individual lesions present usually as slowly but progressively enlarging, asymptomatic, well-demarcated macules or plaques that are pink-to-reddish brown in colour (Fig. 4.36) and may reach a considerable size. Lesions of more than 30 cm maximum diameter have been reported.[55] Multifocal lesions are rare.[56]

Benign lymphangioendothelioma is a benign vascular proliferation with an excellent clinical prognosis. Complete excision is the treatment of choice, but the complete removal of large lesions can be difficult or impossible. Despite the large size of a number of lesions, only a few have been shown to recur locally after complete excision,[56] and metastases, tumour-related deaths and sarcomatous progression have not been recorded.

Pathological features

The histological hallmark of benign lymphangioendothelioma is the presence of delicate, thin-walled vascular spaces orientated horizontally in the dermis (Fig. 4.37), involvement of the underlying subcutis being uncommon. The dilated vascular spaces in the superficial dermis often separate the dermal collagen in an angiosarcomatous fashion and may show a Kaposi-like peri-adnexal growth. In the deeper parts of the dermis, the vascular spaces tend to become narrower. The vascular spaces are normally empty or contain a pale, eosinophilic, proteinaceous material with scattered erythrocytes. The lining endothelial cells are relatively flat with generally slightly enlarged ovoid and hyperchromatic nuclei (Fig. 4.37). An

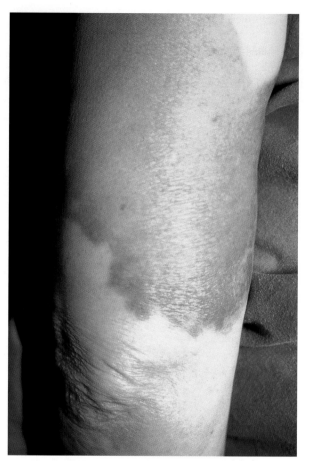

Figure 4.36 *Benign lymphangioendotheliomata often present clinically as progressive enlarging reddish-brown plaques.*

occasionally hobnail cytomorphology of the endothelial cells with prominent hyperchromatic nuclei and endothelium-lined papillary stromal projections has been reported.[56] Prominent endothelial multilayering and mitotic figures are not seen. The surrounding stroma may show hyalinization and contain lymphocytes and/or plasma cells. Haemosiderin deposits are usually not found. The endothelial cells stain variably positive for CD31, CD34 and von Willebrand factor. As in other lymphatic lesions, the layer of actin-positive cells surrounding the vascular spaces is incomplete.

Differential diagnosis

The histopathological differential diagnosis of benign lymphangioendothelioma includes lymphangioma circumscriptum, lymphangiomatosis involving the skin, hobnail haemangioma, retiform haemangioendothelioma, papillary intralymphatic angioendothelioma (Dabska's tumour), cutaneous angiosarcoma and patch-stage Kaposi's sarcoma.

Lymphangioma circumscriptum differs clinically and shows separated small vesicular, clear or blood-filled lesions. Histologically, the reported dissection of collagen

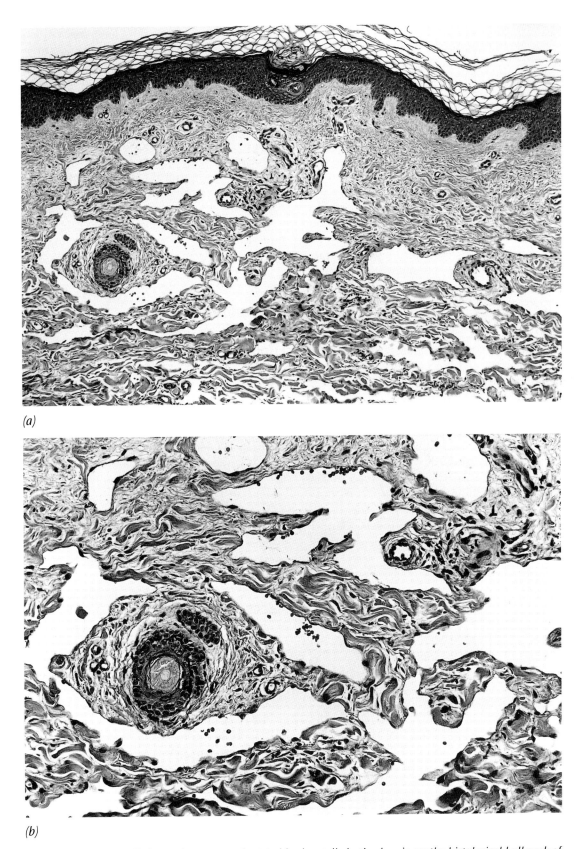

(a)

(b)

Figure 4.37 *Dilated, thin-walled vascular spaces orientated horizontally in the dermis are the histological hallmark of benign lymphangioendothelioma (a). Note the peri-adnexal growth of vascular spaces, lined by flat endothelial cells with slightly enlarged nuclei (b). (Haematoxylin and eosin).*

by proliferative lymphatic vessels in cases of benign lymphangioendothelioma is absent in lymphangioma circumsciptum. Lymphangiomatosis (see below) differs mainly clinically, since in lymphangiomatosis a diffuse involvement of skin, soft tissues and bone as well as parenchymal organs is seen. The two entities, however, share some histological features, and it has been speculated that benign lymphangioendothelioma might be considered to be a localized form of lymphangiomatosis.[56]

Hobnail haemangioma presents clinically as a solitary small papule or nodule and is histologically characterized by a biphasic growth pattern, hobnail endothelial cells and prominent stromal fibrosis with haemosiderin deposits.[40]

Retiform haemangioendothelioma represents a further distinctive vascular neoplasm with similarities to benign lymphangioendothelioma that usually arises in the distal extremities of adolescents and young adults. Clinically, retiform haemangioendothelioma is characterized by a locally aggressive growth, a high rate of local recurrence and, in rare cases, metastases, fulfilling the criteria for a low-grade malignant vascular neoplasm.[57] In contrast to benign lymphangioendothelioma, the dissecting vascular spaces of retiform haemangioendothelioma are not orientated horizontally in the dermis, show an infiltrative growth similar to the pattern of the rete testis and are lined by prominent hobnail endothelial cells (Fig. 4.38). On the other hand, the reported positivity of neoplastic cells for the lymphatic marker VEGFR-3[41] suggests that retiform haemangioendothelioma probably represents a low-grade malignant neoplasm of the lymphatic vessels.

Papillary intralymphatic angioendothelioma is a further low-grade, malignant vascular neoplasm with phenotypic features of lymphatic vessels.[41] Originally described in 1969,[58] papillary intralymphatic angioendothelioma, which occurs in children and adults, shows a broad anatomical distribution. Histologically, the condition is characterized by dilated and infiltrating lymphatic spaces containing prominent papillary proliferations composed of hyaline cores and columnar hobnail or matchstick-like endothelial cells with enlarged nuclei (Fig. 4.39). The neoplastic cells stain positively for CD31, von Willebrand factor and VEGFR-3, whereas CD34 is positive only focally.[41] Intraluminal and stromal lymphocytes, as well as the adjacent features of a pre-existing lymphangioma in a number of cases, add further support to the interpretation of papillary intralymphatic angioendothelioma as a neoplasm of the lymphatic vessels.[41]

Cutaneous angiosarcoma and patch-stage Kaposi's sarcoma. It is important to distinguish benign lymphangioendothelioma from cutaneous angiosarcoma and patch-stage Kaposi's sarcoma. Clinically, cutaneous angiosarcoma occurs frequently (but not exclusively) on the face, neck and scalp of elderly patients. Even histologically well-differentiated cases are characterized by a poor clinical outcome. In contrast to benign lymphangioendothelioma, the anastomosing vascular spaces of cutaneous angiosarcoma are lined by atypical and proliferative active endothelial cells, which may show tufts and multilayering, the stroma often containing small areas of spindle-shaped and/or epithelioid neoplastic cells. The clinical presentation of patch-stage Kaposi's sarcoma and the rare lymphangioma-like variant of Kaposi's sarcoma differs from that of benign lymphangioendothelioma in that cases of Kaposi's sarcoma usually present as widespread multiple lesions in immunocompromised patients or elderly people of Jewish or Mediterranean origin. The rare lymphangioma-like variant of Kaposi's sarcoma has widely dilated vascular spaces that, together with a lymphoplasmacellular infiltrate, extravasated erythrocytes and haemosiderin deposits, help to distinguish it from benign lymphangioendothelioma.

LYMPHANGIOMATOSIS

Clinical features

Lymphangiomatosis is a very rare developmental disorder characterized by proliferating lymphatic vascular channels that diffusely involve bone, dermis, soft tissue and parenchymal organs. It typically presents at birth but also occurs in children and adolescents, with no sex predilection.[59–61] The lung, pleura, spleen and liver are the parenchymal organs most commonly affected, the thymus, breast, kidney and heart rarely being involved.[60,62–64] As in other vascular lesions, there may be a clinical and histological overlap with angiomatosis and other forms of vascular malformation, the diagnosis often having to be confirmed by lymphangiography.

The clinical outcome of a diffuse multifocal lymphangiomatosis is strongly related to the extent of the disease. The involvement of visceral organs (especially the pleura and lung) is usually associated with a poor clinical outcome, whereas cases confined to the soft tissues and bones are characterized by a more favourable prognosis.[63] A rare variant of lymphangiomatosis with predominant or exclusive involvement of the soft tissues of one limb and concomitant skeletal involvement, associated with a good clinical prognosis, has recently been reported (*see* Chapter 19).[65] Lymphangiomatosis of the soft tissues presents as an ill-defined, spongy, sometimes brown-to-purple lesion with variably sized vascular spaces lacking blood in their lumina. Lymphangiomatosis of the skin and soft tissues is occasionally associated with the rare kaposiform haemangioendothelioma.[66]

Pathological features

Lymphangiomatosis of the skin and soft tissues shows histological features similar to those of benign lymphangioendothelioma, with an extensive dissection of

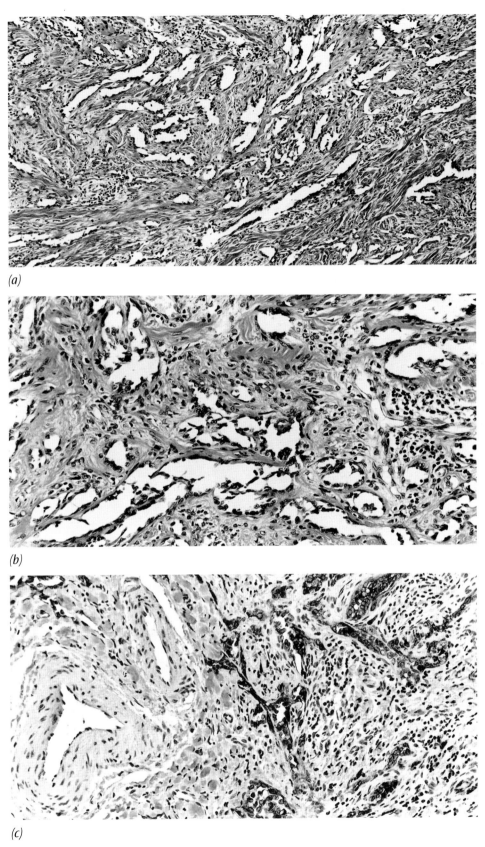

Figure 4.38 *Retiform haemangioendothelioma is characterized by infiltrating vascular spaces (a) lined by prominent hobnail endothelial cells, which may form small intravascular papillary structures (b). (Haematoxylin and eosin) In contrast to pre-existing blood vessels (c, left), neoplastic endothelial cells in retiform haemangioendothelioma express VEGFR-3. (Labelled streptavidin biotin technique).*

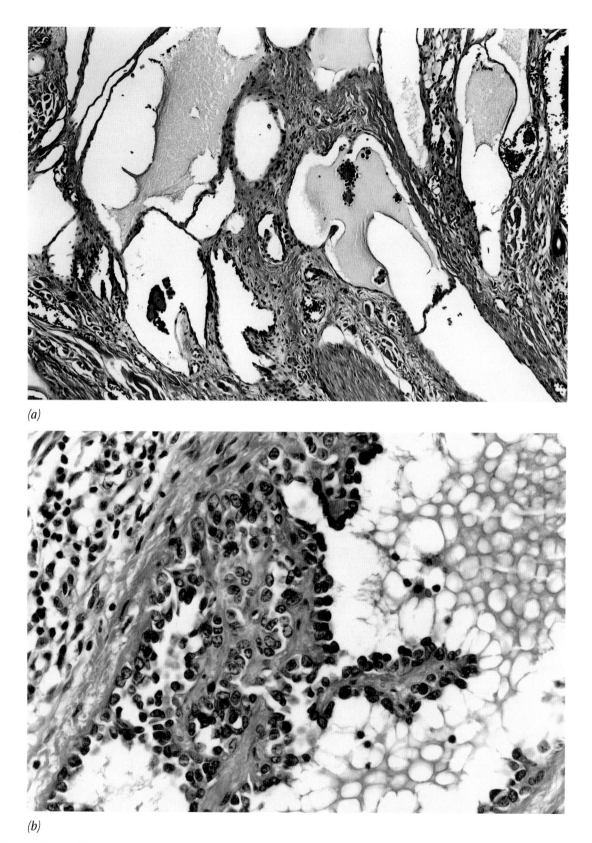

(a)

(b)

Figure 4.39 *Papillary intralymphatic angioendothelioma (so-called Dabska's tumour) is composed of infiltrating, dilated lymphatic channels (a) containing prominent intravascular papillary proliferations with a hyaline core and enlarged hobnail endothelial tumour cells (b). (Haematoxylin and eosin).*

pre-existing structures by interconnected and mainly dilated lymphatic channels lined by a single layer of attenuated endothelial cells without atypia and proliferative activity (Fig. 4.40). The separation of the tissues of the skin and soft tissues may be very prominent and is imaginatively described as a 'hair-dryer effect'.[65] The larger vascular spaces may have muscular walls of varying thickness (Fig. 4.40). Lymphoid aggregates are frequently seen

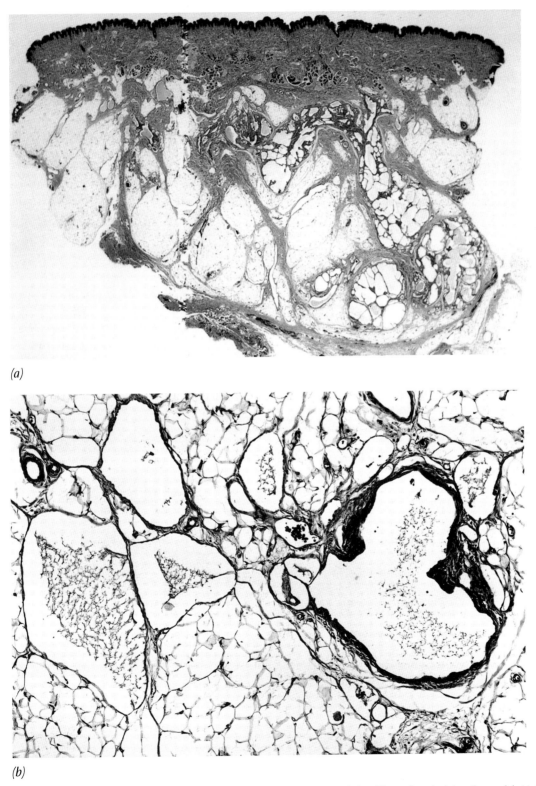

(a)

(b)

Figure 4.40 *An example of lymphangiomatosis showing diffuse involvement of the skin and underlying tissues (a). Note the dilated vascular spaces containing muscle walls of varying thickness (b, right). (Haematoxylin and eosin).*

in the surrounding stroma, which may show prominent fibrosis in long-standing lesions. In contrast to benign lymphangioendothelioma, a wider involvement of subcutaneous and deep soft tissues is seen in lymphangiomatosis of the skin and soft tissues. Despite the absence of erythrocytes in the vascular spaces of lymphangiomatosis, abundant haemosiderin deposits have been noted in a considerable number of cases.[65] In bone and parenchymatous organs, the numerous thin-walled dilated or collapsed lymphatic spaces form an anastomosing network and split up pre-existing structures. The lining endothelial cells stain positively for von Willebrand factor and CD31. CD34 is negative or only weakly and focally positive.[63,65]

Differential diagnosis

Generally speaking, lymphangiomatosis has to be distinguished from angiomatosis, lymphangiomyomatosis and well-differentiated angiosarcoma. Although angiomatosis of the soft tissues can resemble lymph-angiomatosis, the former is characterized by a mixture of thin-walled capillaries with thick-walled blood vessels and prominent mature adipocytes.[67]

Lymphangiomyomatosis represents a rare hamartomatous condition and occurs almost exclusively in women of reproductive age.[52] Lymphangiomyomatosis is histologically characterized by a diffuse proliferation of specific myoid cells within the lymphatic channels and lymph nodes (Fig. 4.41). Cytologically, the bland, spindle-shaped myoid cells in lymphangiomyomatosis are arranged in clusters and short fascicles, and stain immunohistochemically positive for desmin and muscle-specific actin. In addition, these cells are consistently positive for HMB-45 (Fig. 4.41), an interesting immunophenotype shared by muscle cells in angiomyolipoma.[68,69] Even in cases of well-differentiated angiosarcoma, the anastomosing vascular spaces are lined by variably pleomorphic and proliferative active endothelial cells that frequently show multilayering, tufts and papillary formations.

The differential diagnosis of pulmonary lymphangiomatosis also includes pulmonary lymphangiectasia, persistent interstitial pulmonary emphysema and pulmonary capillary haemangioma.

Pulmonary lymphangiectasia represents a dilatation of the pre-existing lymphatic structures in the interlobular septa and pleura, resulting in massive cystic changes. It presents most frequently at birth or in young children, only rarely affecting adults.[70] In pulmonary lymphangiomatosis, the numerous small lymphatic spaces are not limited to pre-existing structures.[71]

Persistent interstitial pulmonary emphysema is found in newborns treated with artificial oxygen and/or ventilation, and anastomosing cystic spaces lined by multinucleated giant cells that are negative for endothelial markers can be seen in bronchopulmonary dysplasia.[72] Pulmonary

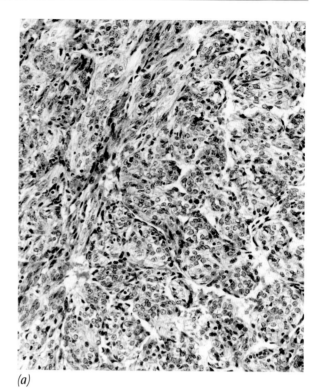

(a)

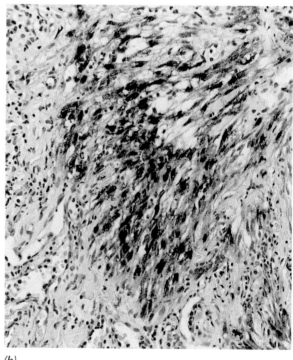

(b)

Figure 4.41 *(a) In lymphangiomyomatosis, a proliferation of plump, spindled and round myoid cells is seen in association with lymphatic channels. (Haematoxylin and eosin).*
(b) Interestingly, these specific myoid cells stain positively for HMB-45. (Labelled streptavidin biotin technique).

capillary haemangioma/haemangiomatosis arises in older patients, is associated with pulmonary hypertension and is composed of multiple, thin-walled capillaries lacking a smooth muscle component.[73]

In cases of lymphangiomatosis involving the skeletal structures, the differential diagnosis includes Gorham's disease, a condition characterized by progressive osteolysis by thin-walled vascular channels with secondary extension into the soft tissues.[74]

LYMPHANGIOSARCOMA

Clinical features

Angiosarcoma occurs as four main clinical pictures:

1 angiosarcoma of the parenchymal organs;
2 idiopathic angiosarcoma of the skin and soft tissues unassociated with lymphoedema;
3 post-irradiation angiosarcoma;
4 the rare lymphoedematous angiosarcoma.

The latter has traditionally been designated as lymphangiosarcoma, but, as stated above, it has been tentatively suggested that lesions such as retiform haemangioendothelioma, papillary intralymphatic angioendothelioma and a subset of angiosarcomata may also show a lymphatic line of differentiation.[42,75,76]

Ninety per cent of cases of angiosarcoma associated with lymphoedema occur in patients who have been treated for carcinoma of the breast with mastectomy and/or radiotherapy and who have developed a significant degree of chronic oedema.[77–80] Lymphangiosarcoma is more rarely seen in lymphoedema after radiotherapy,[81] or in congential/hereditary as well as idiopathic lymphoedema (Fig. 4.42).[82–85] Irrespective of the clinical picture, angiosarcomata associated with lymphoedema often develop as multicentric sarcomata with rapid spread and are characterized by a poor clinical prognosis with a high incidence of systemic metastases.[79,80]

Pathological features

Lymphangiosarcoma in the skin and soft tissues is composed of irregularly anastomosing vascular spaces that diffusely dissect and infiltrate pre-existing structures. As with typical angiosarcomata,[86] they have a wide morphological spectrum ranging from obvious vasoformative neoplasms to poorly differentiated sarcomata with solid, spindled and epithelioid features (Fig. 4.43). The vascular lumens may be empty or contain a pale eosinophilic proteinaecous fluid as well as erythrocytes. Lymphocytes and lymphoid aggregates are frequently found around the neoplastic vessels. Neoplastic vascular channels are lined by variably pleomorphic endothelial cells with enlarged and hyperchromatic nuclei showing multilayering, tufts and papillary formation, and are not surrounded completely by actin-positive pericytes. Mitoses including abnormal mitotic figures are frequently found. Electron microscopy[87] and immunohistochemistry confirm the endothelial line of differentiation in these neoplasms.

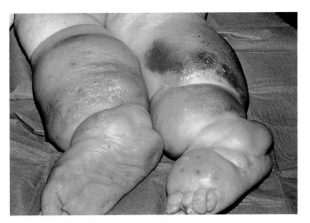

Figure 4.42 *This patient with long-standing lymphoedema has developed a lymphangiosarcoma.*

Differential diagnosis

The clinical and histological features that distinguish a well-differentiated angiosarcoma from a benign neoplasm of the lymphatic vessels have been discussed above. A benign lymphangiomatous papule of the skin following surgery and radiotherapy that may mimic lymphangiosarcoma as well as cutaneous angiosarcoma has been described.[88,89] These lesions occur as solitary or multiple papules and are composed of dilated, sometimes anastomosing vascular spaces lined by slightly atypical endothelial cells. They have intravascular small papillae reminiscent of those seen in papillary intralymphatic angioendothelioma, and a stromal lymphoplasmocytic inflammatory infiltrate.

Lymphangiosarcomata are characterized by an irregular, diffusely infiltrative growth, prominent cellular atypia with focal multilayering and the presence of more solid areas, and increased proliferative activity. In addition to their immunohistochemical differences from angiosarcomata, lymphangiosarcomata are often associated with areas of so-called 'lymphangiomatosis',[78] in striking contrast to conventional angiosarcomata of the skin and soft tissues. These 'lymphangiomatous' changes probably represent a premalignant change of small lymphatic vessels as they form a diffuse vascular network lined by endothelial cells with hyperchromatic nuclei.

Poorly differentiated lymphangiosarcomata have to be distinguished from other sarcomata and acantholytic, pseudovascular carcinomata by the aid of special (silver) stains and immunohistochemistry.

NOTE

The first sections of this chapter were written by Professor Judit Daróczy, Second Dermatology Unit, St Stephan Hospital, Budapest, Hungary, the section on the histology of the lymph glands in lymphoedema by Mr John Wolfe, St Mary's Hospital, London, UK, and the section on

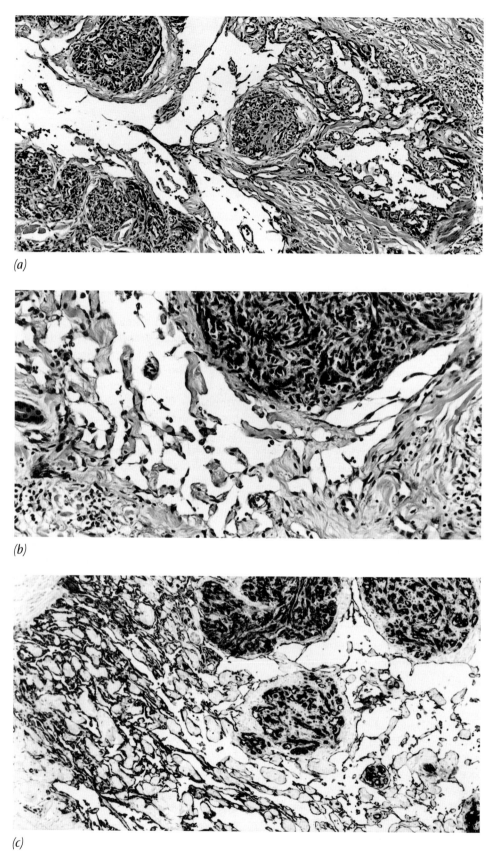

Figure 4.43 *(a) A lymphangiosarcoma showing characteristic well-differentiated and poorly differentiated sarcomatous areas. (Haematoxylin and eosin). (b) The high-power view reveals nuclear atypia even in well-differentiated areas. (Haematoxylin and eosin). (c) Staining with the endothelial antibody CD31 confirms the presence of irregularly anastomosing vascular spaces. (Labelled streptavidin biotin technique).*

cardiovascular, craniofacial and vertebral abnormalities similar to those seen in lymphoedema–distichiasis syndrome but without lymphoedema.[23] A mutational analysis of 14 families with lymphoedema–distichiasis syndrome by the group at St George's Hospital Medical School, London, demonstrated that all but one of the pedigrees had small insertions or deletions in the *FOXC2* gene that seems likely to produce haplo-insufficiency.[24]

There is no obvious correlation between mutation and phenotype. Nevertheless although lymphoedema–distichiasis syndrome has a variable phenotype, it appears to be 95 per cent penetrant. Considering the data so far, if distichiasis is the main manifestation, there are only three out of 67 gene carriers who have no apparent disease phenotype. The lymphoedema in this condition has an earlier age of onset in males, who are also more likely to have episodes of cellulitis.[15] Nevertheless, when *FOXC2* gene was sequenced in 86 lymphoedema families to identify mutations, 11 families were identified with mutations suggesting heterogeneity.[25] Care must be taken, however, before excluding lymphoedema–distichiasis syndrome because distichiasis may easily be missed.

It seems likely that lymphoedema and ptosis (MIM 153000) is part of the lymphoedema–distichiasis syndrome.

Incontinentia pigmenti (MIM 308300)

Incontinentia pigmenti is a rare, X-linked dominant condition that is not usually associated with lymphoedema in surviving females. Only the second liveborn male to be reported recently led to the identification of an NF-κB essential modulator (*NEMO*) stop codon mutation in the affected child and his mother, who had classical incontinentia pigmenti.[26] The baby had features of hypohidrotic ectodermal dysplasia with immune deficiency, recurrent infections and lower limb lymphoedema that developed at a few weeks of age. A lymphoscintigram showed severe lymphatic obstruction. Magnetic resonance imaging suggested a lymphangiomatous malformation. Cutaneous capillary angiomata and possible vascular malformations co-existed in the gut.[27] Further males with similar phenotypes were reported with *NEMO* mutations and the term 'OL-EDA-ID' (osteopetrosis, lymphoedema, ectodermal dysplasia anhydrotic and immune deficiency) has been applied to these patients.[28] NF-κB has a documented role in endothelial cell survival and may influence lymphatic development.

Other genetic forms of lymphoedema with likely germline mutations

Meige's disease (MIM 153200)

In 1898, eight years after Milroy described congenital lymphoedema, Henri Meige[29] described the pedigree of a family with a distinct history of lymphoedema appearing at puberty. The eponym 'Meige's disease' has therefore come to be associated with this, the most common variety of primary lymphoedema (Kinmonth's lymphoedema praecox), which affects adolescent females three times more often than males and has a genetic predisposition in only 30 per cent of cases.[30] This variety of lymphoedema is usually mild, rarely extends above the knee and is generally bilateral. Kinmonth found, by lymphography, that this disorder is invariably associated with a reduced number of distal lymphatics (Kinmonth's hypoplasia), the proximal lymphatic channels remaining patent. Browse and Stewart[31] have suggested that this disorder represents a peripheral lymphatic occlusion rather than a true congenital hypo- or aplasia. The term 'Meige's disease' should be reserved for familial lymphoedema developing at or soon after puberty in which there are no associated abnormalities, for example distichiasis.

Identifying the location of the gene underlying this condition has proved difficult. This may be because of genetic heterogeneity within this group of patients: there may be more than one gene causing Meige's disease. These are important genes to identify as Meige's disease is the most common cause of primary lymphoedema of pubertal onset.

It should be noted that Meige's disease is not related to Meigs' disease, in which there is ascites and hydrothorax together with an ovarian fibroma.[32]

Turner's syndrome

This well-known congenital abnormality is caused by the absence of one X chromosome, early spontaneous abortion occurring in over 95 per cent of fetuses. Severely affected fetuses who survive to the second trimester can be detected on ultrasonography, which may reveal cystic hygroma, chylothorax, ascites and hydrops. The diagnosis may be suggested in the newborn by redundant neck skin and peripheral oedema. Surviving children have webbed necks (Fig. 5.5) from involuted cystic hygromata and may exhibit mild peripheral oedema that often diminishes as the child grows older. The peripheral oedema sometimes persists and may very occasionally present later in life. The most common manifestations are short stature and primary amenorrhoea. Both lymphatic hypoplasia and hyperplasia have been described in Turner's syndrome.[33]

Chromosomal abnormality testing should always be undertaken in neonates or young children with primary lymphoedema, particularly if a Turner phenotype is present. When 37 unselected patients with primary lymphoedema were investigated, three out of 32 phenotypic females had ovarian dysgenesis (the karyotype being X0 in two and XY in one). One patient had testicular feminization, as had a previously reported case.[34] All cases with chromosomal abnormalities showed hypoplasia of the leg lymphatics on lymphangiography.

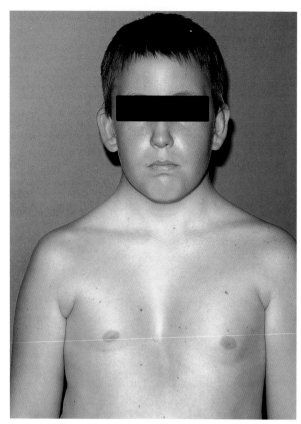

Figure 5.5 *Neck webbing (pterygium colli), a feature of Turner's syndrome, suggests the presence of cystic hygromata in utero.*

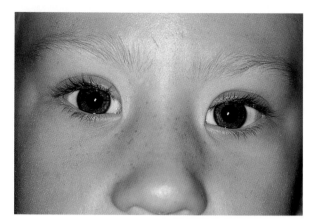

Figure 5.6 *Medial epicanthic folds: a remnant of intra-uterine oedema.*

There may be a gene on the X chromosome that is responsible for the lymphoedema of Turner's syndrome. Some work has already been carried out to identify a lymphoedema-critical region on chromosome X.[35]

Noonan syndrome

Noonan syndrome is a multiple congenital anomaly syndrome. It may occur on a sporadic basis or in a pattern consistent with autosomal dominant inheritance. It is therefore thought to be caused by a mutation in a single gene, which was located to chromosome 12q in 1994[36] and has recently been identified as *PTPN11*, a protein tyrosine phosphatase gene.[37]

Phenotypic characteristics include short stature, ptosis, low-set ears and posterior hairline, neck webbing and congenital cardiac anomalies, typically pulmonary stenosis or cardiomyopathy. Lymphoedema is usually present at birth, but the age of onset may vary from the prenatal period to adulthood. Many affected cases have no evidence of lymphoedema at birth, but the presence of webbed neck with a low hairline suggests the presence of a cystic hygroma in utero. Cystic hygromata are thought to be caused by a failure of maturation of the lymphatic vessels.[38] Lymphoedema tends to affect the lower limbs,[39] but there have been reports of testicular, pulmonary and intestinal lymphangiectasia.[38]

Hennekam lymphangiectasia–lymphoedema syndrome (MIM 235510)

In 1989, Hennekam *et al.* described a syndrome of intestinal lymphangiectasia with severe lymphoedema of the limbs, genitalia and face associated with mental retardation.[40] The intestinal lymphangiectasia causes hypoproteinaemia, hypogammaglobulinaemia and lymphocytopenia. Facial anomalies are characteristic, the flat face appearing somewhat oriental, with a flat nasal bridge, epicanthic folds (Fig. 5.6), hypertelorism, a small mouth, tooth anomalies and small ears. Seizures are not uncommon. An autosomal recessive inheritance appears probable. The onset of the lymphoedema usually occurs between one and 12 years, but in some cases the oedema is present at birth. The lymphoedema is progressive and may be asymmetrical.

Cholestasis–lymphoedema syndrome (Aagenaes syndrome, MIM 214900)

In 1998, Aagenaes *et al.*[41] described two Norwegian kindreds demonstrating a syndrome of hereditary recurrent cholestasis and lymphoedema. Jaundice became evident soon after birth and recurred in episodes throughout life. Oedema of the leg, which was caused by hypoplasia of the lymphatic vessels, began at school age and progressed. Liver histology showed giant cell transformation in infancy and some fibrosis or cirrhosis in later childhood. Of 21 patients born before 1970, 11 died in early childhood, mainly from bleeding because of unavailability of vitamin K at that time. Two died from cirrhosis. Consanguinity was frequent, and an autosomal recessive inheritance was proposed. The genetic cause is unknown but a locus has now been mapped to a 6.6 CM interval on chromosome 15q.[42]

Proteus syndrome (MIM 176920)

This very rare syndrome causes many varied (protean) abnormalities. Characteristic features are asymmetrical overgrowth of almost any part of the body, including the face, and macrodactyly with rugose or cerebriform overgrowth of the plantar or palmar soft tissue. 'Overgrowth' can also include verrucous epidermal naevi, angiomata lipoma-like hamartomata and lymphangiomatous swelling. A recent paper has suggested that Proteus syndrome is caused by mutations in the *P10* gene. This gene was originally discovered as the cause of Cowden syndrome and Bannayan–Riley–Ruvalcaba syndrome, which are other hereditary hamartoma syndromes. Two out of ten patients with Proteus syndrome, and three out of five of those with Proteus-like syndrome, were found to have a germline mutation in *P10*.[43]

Microcephaly–lymphoedema–chorioretinal dysplasia (MIM 152950)

In 1986, Crowe and Dickerman[44] described a male and his maternal uncle who both had microcephaly and peripheral oedema, the child's mother, maternal grandmother and maternal aunt all having lymphoedema. There is an association between lymphoedema and microcephaly in an autosomal dominant syndrome described by Jarmas et al.[45] in which falciform retinal folds are also present. The current view is that all cases described with microcephaly and lymphoedema are linked to chorioretinopathy.

Pes cavus and lymphoedema

Bilateral pes cavus and lymphoedema has been described in two unrelated patients, one of whom possessed a family history. The patient's mother, maternal grandfather and uncle had right-sided pes cavus, and an aunt and a cousin had a combination of bilateral pes cavus and lymphoedema. In the propositus, lymphangiography revealed hypoplasia of leg lymphatics with no dermal backflow and a failure to opacify lymphatics on the dorsum of the foot.[46]

Yellow nail syndrome (MIM 153300)

The relationship between yellow nail syndrome (yellow nails (Fig. 5.7), chronic sinusitis, bronchiectasis and pleural effusions) and lymphoedema is not clear cut. In most cases, the peripheral oedema does not bear the hallmarks of lymphoedema clinically in that there are no characteristic skin changes, the oedema can resolve (as can the nails) and lymphoscintigraphy reveals minimal lymphatic insufficiency.[47] Conventional lymphography has nevertheless demonstrated megalymphatics accompanying pleural effusions and ascites.

One of the current authors has seen in excess of 30 cases, but not one patient has had a family history. Yellow nail syndrome is, however, described in Online Mendelian Inheritance in Man as an autosomal dominant condition. This appears to be based on only two case reports. One describes yellow nail syndrome with familial primary hypoplasia of the lymphatics manifesting late in life,[48]

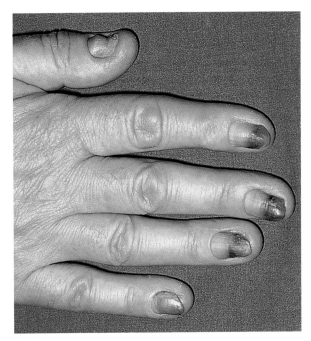

Figure 5.7 *Yellow nail syndrome. The nails are thickened and overcurved in the transverse plane. They are slow to grow, are hard to cut and can shed. The yellow colour is probably an optical effect, whereas the black discolouration has arisen secondary to bacterial infection.*

the other a fetus with unexplained fetal hydrops and recurrent chylothorax born to a mother with yellow nail syndrome.[49] In addition, a recent report of *FOXC2* mutations in 11 lymphoedema families revealed one family possessing three members with yellow nails.[25]

Congenital, non-hereditary forms of lymphoedema

There are a number of sporadic forms of lymphoedema, usually presenting at birth or during childhood, in which there is no family history and the defect is likely to be caused by a somatic rather than a germline mutation. The most common type is Klippel–Trenaunay syndrome, in which lymphoedema may be the presenting abnormality. More characteristic features, such as limb overgrowth, cutaneous angioma and venous disease may subsequently develop (*see* Chapter 18).

Another, albeit poorly understood, form of congenital lymphoedema is that associated with amniotic bands.[50] These bands, which allegedly wrap around digits or limbs, cause circumferential fibrosis and scarring. This can lead to auto-amputation of digits or lymphoedema of a limb distal to the band.

Maffucci's syndrome (dyschondroplasia with haemangiomata) usually manifests with venous cavernous malformations in infancy, but cavernous lymphangiomata giving rise to limb swelling are often seen and may be the sole manifestation.[51] Hard nodules arise from the bones, especially of the fingers and toes, which are pathologically enchondromata and radiologically translucent. The malignant potential of the syndrome is high. A familial occurrence has not been recorded.

REFERENCES

1. Ferrara N. Molecular and biological properties of vascular endothelial growth factor. *Journal of Molecular Medicine* 1999; **77:** 527–43.

2. Kaipainen A, *et al*. Expression of the fms-like tyrosine kinase FLT4 gene becomes restricted to lymphatic endothelium during development. *Proceedings of the National Academy of Sciences of the USA* 1995; **92:** 3566–70.

3. Jeltsch M, *et al*. Hyperplasia of lymphatic vessels in VEGF-C transgenic mice. *Science* 1997; **276:** 1423–5.

4. Dumont DJ, *et al*. Cardiovascular failure in mouse embryos deficient in VEGF receptor-3. *Science* 1998; **282:** 946–9.

5. Makinen T, *et al*. Inhibition of lymphangiogenesis with resulting lymphedema in transgenic mice expressing soluble VEGF receptor-3. *Nature Medicine* 2001; **7:** 199–205.

6. Wigle JT, Oliver G. Prox 1 function is required for the development of the murine lymphatic system. *Cell* 1999; **98:** 769–78.

7. Milroy WF. An undescribed variety of hereditary oedema. *New York Medical Journal* 1892; **56 (Nov.):** 505–8.

8. Nonne M. Vier Falle von Elephantiasis Congenita Hereditaria. *Virchow's Archives of Pathology and Anatomy* 1891; **125:** 189–96.

9. Lettessier EE. De L'éléphantiasis des Arabes et de son Hérédite. Thesis, University of Strasbourg, 1895.

10. Ferrell RE, *et al*. Hereditary lymphoedema: evidence for linkage and genetic heterogeneity. *Human Molecular Genetics* 1998; **7:** 2073–8.

11. Evans AL, *et al*. Mapping of primary congenital lymphoedema to the 5q35.3 region. *American Journal of Human Genetics* 1999; **64:** 547–55.

12. Karkkainen MJ, *et al*. Missense mutations interfere with VEGFR-3 signalling in primary lymphoedema. *Nature Genetics* 2000; **25:** 153–9.

13. Falls HE, Kertesz ED. A new syndrome combining pterygium colli with developmental abnormalities of the eyelids and lymphatics of the lower limbs. *Transactions of the American Ophthalmic Society* 1964; **62:** 248–75.

14. Pap Z, Biro T, Szabo L, *et al*. Syndrome of lymphoedema and distichiasis. *Human Genetics* 1980; **53:** 309–10.

15. Brice G, Mansour S, Bell R, *et al*. Analysis of the phenotypic abnormalities in lymphoedema–distichiasis syndrome in 74 patients with *FOXC2* mutations or linkage to 16q.24. *Journal of Medical Genetics* 2002; **39:** 472–83.

16. Goldstein S, *et al*. Distichiasis, congenital heart defects and mixed peripheral vascular anomalies. *American Journal of Medical Genetics* 1985; **20:** 283–94.

17. Bartley GB, Jackson IT. Distichiasis and cleft palate. *Plastic and Reconstructive Surgery* 1989; **84:** 129–32.

18. Schwartz JF, *et al*. Hereditary spinal arachnoid cyst, distichiasis and lymphoedema. *Annals of Neurology* 1980; **7:** 340–3.

19. Rosbotham J, *et al*. Distichiasis–lymphoedema: clinical features, venous function and lymphoscintigraphy. *British Journal of Dermatology* 2000; **142:** 148–52.

20. Dale RF. Primary lymphoedema when found with distichiasis is of the type defined as bilateral hyperplasia by lymphography. *Journal of Medical Genetics* 1987; **24:** 170–1.

21. Mangion J, *et al*. A gene for lymphedema–distichiasis maps to 16q24.3. *American Journal of Human Genetics* 1999; **65:** 427–32.

22. Fang J. Mutations in FOXC2 (MFH-1), a forkhead family transcription factor, are responsible for hereditary lymphedema–distichiasis syndrome. *American Journal of Human Genetics* 2000; **67:** 1382–8.

23. Kume T, *et al*. The murine winged helix transcription factors, Foxc1 and Foxc2, are both required for cardiovascular development and somatogenesis. *Genes and Development* 2001; **67:** 2470–82.

24. Bell R, *et al*. Analysis of lymphoedema–distichiasis families for FOXC2 mutations reveals small insertions and deletions throughout the gene. *Human Genetics* 2001; **108:** 546–51.

25. Finegold D, *et al*. Truncating mutations in FOXC2 cause multiple lymphedema syndromes. *Human Molecular Genetics* 2001; **10:** 1185–9.

26. Smahi A, *et al*. Genomic rearrangement in NEMO impairs NF-κB activation and is a cause of incontinentia pigmenti. *Nature* 2000; **405:** 466–72.

27. Mansour S. Incontinentia pigmenti in a surviving male is accompanied by hypodidrotic ectodermal dysplasia and recurrent infection. *American Journal of Medical Genetics* 2001; **99:** 172–7.

28. Doffinger R, *et al*. X-linked anhidrotic ectodermal dysplasia with immunodeficiency is caused by impaired NF-κB signalling. *Nature Genetics* 2001; **27:** 277–85.

29. Meige H. Dystrophie oedemateuse héréditaire. *Presse Médicale* 1898; **6:** 341–3.

30. Dale RF. The inheritance of primary lymphoedema. *Journal of Medical Genetics* 1985; **22:** 274–8.

31. Browse NL, Stewart G. Lymphoedema: pathophysiology and classification. *Journal of Cardiovascular Surgery* 1985; **26:** 91–106.

32. Meigs JV. Fibroma of the ovary with ascites and hydrothorax: Meigs syndrome. *American Journal of Obstetrics and Gynecology* 1954; **67:** 962–85.

33. Alvin A, *et al.* Lymph vessel hypoplasia and chromosome aberrations in six patients with Turner's syndrome. *Acta Dermatologica et Venereologica* 1967; **47:** 25–33.

34. Benson PF, *et al.* Chromosome anomalies in primary lymphoedema. *Lancet* 1967; **i:** 461–2.

35. Boucher CA, *et al.* Breakpoint analysis of Turner patients with partial Xp deletions: implications for the lymphoedema gene location. *Journal of Medical Genetics* 2001; **38:** 591–8.

36. Jamieson CR, *et al.* Mapping a gene for Noonan syndrome to the long arm of chromosome 12. *Nature Genetics* 1994; **8:** 357–60.

37. Tartaglia M, Mehler EL, Goldberg R, *et al.* Mutations in *PTPN11* encoding the protein tyrosine phosphatase SHP-2, cause Noonan syndrome. *Nature Genetics* 2001; **29:** 465–8.

38. Witt DR, *et al.* Lymphedema in Noonan syndrome: clues to pathogenesis and prenatal diagnosis and review of the literature. *American Journal of Medical Genetics* 1987; **27:** 841–56.

39. Minikin W, *et al.* Lymphedema in Noonan's syndrome. *International Journal of Dermatology* 1974; **13:** 179–83.

40. Hennekam RCM, Geerdink RA, Hamel BCJ, *et al.* Autosomal recessive intestinal lymphangiectasia and lymphedema, with facial anomalies and mental retardation. *American Journal of Medical Genetics* 1989; **34:** 593–600.

41. Aagenaes O, *et al.* Hereditary cholestasis with lymphoedema (Aagenaes syndrome, cholestasis–lymphoedema syndrome): new cases and follow-up from infancy to adult age. *Scandinavian Journal of Gastroenterology* 1998; **33:** 335–45.

42. Bull LN. Mapping of the locus for cholestasis–lymphedema syndrome (Aagenaes syndrome) to a 6.6-CM interval on chromosome 15q. *American Journal of Human Genetics* 2000; **67:** 994–9.

43. Zhou X-P, *et al.* Association of germline mutation in the PTEN tumour suppressor gene and Proteus and Proteus-like syndromes. *Lancet* 2001; **358:** 210–11.

44. Crowe CA, Dickerman LH. A genetic association between microcephaly and lymphedema. *American Journal of Medical Genetics* 1986; **24:** 131–5.

45. Jarmas AL, Weaver DD, Ellis FD, Davis A. Microcephaly, microphthalmia, falciform retinal folds and blindness. A new syndrome. *American Journal of Diseases of Children* 1981; **135:** 930–3.

46. Jackson BT, Kinmonth JB. Pes cavus and lymphoedema. *Journal of Bone and Joint Surgery* 1970; **52B:** 518–20.

47. Bull RH. Lymphatic function in the yellow nail syndrome. *British Journal of Dermatology* 1996; **134:** 307–12.

48. Wells GC. Yellow nail syndrome with familial primary hypoplasia of lymphatics, manifest late in life. *Proceedings of the Royal Society of Medicine* 1966; **59:** 447.

49. Govaert P, Leroy JG, Pauwels R, *et al.* Perinatal manifestations of maternal yellow nail syndrome. *Pediatrics* 1992; **89:** 1016–18.

50. Coady NS, Moor MH, Wallis K. Amniotic band syndrome: the association between rare facial clefts and limb ring constrictions. *Plastic and Reconstructive Surgery* 1998; **101:** 640–9.

51. Carlton A, Elkington J St. C, Greenfield JG, *et al.* Maffucci's Syndrome. *Quarterly Journal of Medicine* 1942; **11:** 203–28.

6

Diagnosis and investigation of lymphoedema

WITH A CONTRIBUTION FROM HUGO PARTSCH

CLINICAL FEATURES

Advanced forms of lymphoedema develop characteristic clinical features resulting from changes in the skin and subcutaneous tissues. In the early stages of lymphoedema, however, the swelling may be clinically indistinguishable from other forms of oedema in which only pitting is evident.

Swelling

The swelling of lymphoedema (Fig. 6.1) usually begins insidiously, worsening slowly over months and years, although it may occasionally develop suddenly, for example overnight. In such circumstances, pain may be a feature, and other diagnoses such as venous thrombosis, soft tissue injury or acute cellulitis should be considered. The pain usually settles once the lymphoedema has become established, although the swelling may be intermittent before it becomes permanent. Pain is a rare symptom of uncomplicated lymphoedema; if it is a significant complaint, other causes must be excluded.

Unlike all other forms of chronic oedema caused by increased capillary filtration, lymphoedema tends to reduce very slowly with elevation. This is presumably related to the fact that elevation reduces venous pressure, and to some extent, the lymphatic load arising from capillary filtration, but does little to enhance lymph flow, which requires limb movement. Similarly, diuretics do not have much effect on lymphoedema. A dramatic improvement with diuretics suggests that the cause of the swelling is not solely lymphoedema.

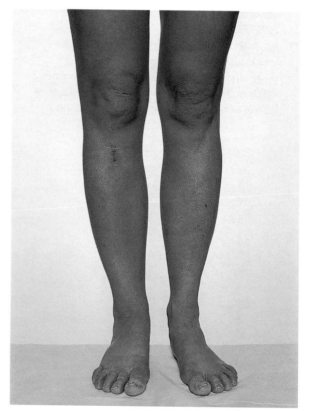

(a)

Figure 6.1 *Lymphoedema of the lower limb and trunk. (a) Mild unilateral oedema confined to the right lower leg, ankle and foot of a young woman.*

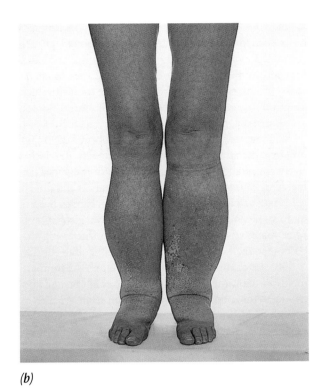

(b)

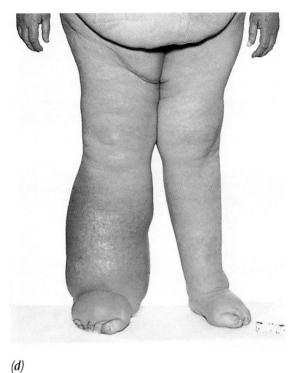

(d)

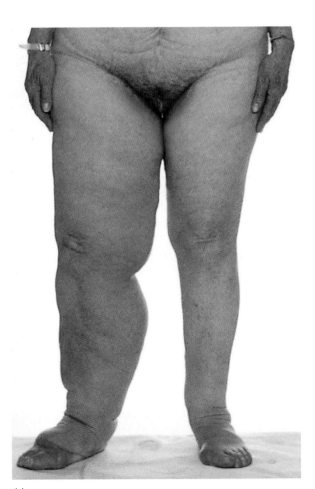

(c)

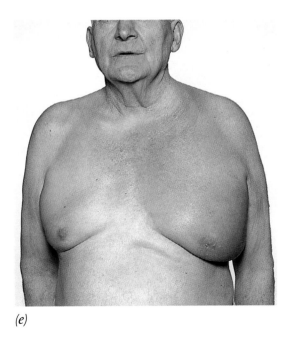

(e)

Figure 6.1 *(b) Moderate oedema of both lower legs with early skin thickening and hyperkeratosis. (c) Swelling of the whole of one leg with some oedema of the lower abdomen and mons veneris. (d) Gross lymphoedema that interferes with walking. (e) An example of lymphoedema of the anterior chest wall and arm caused by a lymphoma in the axillary lymph glands.*

Skin changes

At an early stage in the development of lymphoedema, the skin thickens, making it more difficult to pick up or pinch a fold of skin. In the lower limb, this is most noticeable at the base of the second toe – the Kaposi–Stemmer sign (Fig. 6.2a).[1] A positive Kaposi–Stemmer sign is highly specific for lymphoedema but not very sensitive.

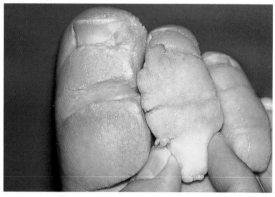

(a)

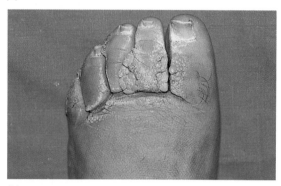

(b)

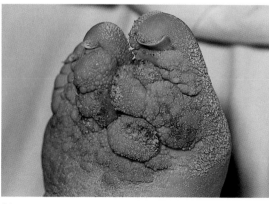

(c)

Figure 6.2 *Signs of lymphoedema in the foot. (a) Kaposi–Stemmer sign. The thickened skin, particularly at the base of the second toe, prevents pinching of a skin fold. This sign invariably indicates the presence of lymphoedema, but its absence does not exclude it. (b) Square toes with thick keratotic edges and papillomatosis indicates lymphoedema. (c) Hyperkeratotic 'warty' skin.*

Whole-leg lymphoedema with relative foot sparing may be associated with a negative Kaposi–Stemmer sign. The combined effect of swelling, skin thickening and compression by the adjacent toes makes the toes square in cross-section rather than circular. Square toes with thick, longitudinal, keratotic edges along their dorsal borders are almost diagnostic of lymphoedema (Fig. 6.2b).

Skin creases become enhanced as a horny scale builds up (hyperkeratosis) and the skin eventually develops a warty appearance (Fig. 6.2c). Dilatation of the upper dermal lymphatics with consequent organization and fibrosis gives rise to papillomatosis. These skin changes become more marked with time and are referred to as elephantiasis. After many years, the tissue fibrosis and thickening may become so marked that pitting may be difficult to ellicit.

Fibrotic changes occur in the subcutaneous compartment, which is the site of most of the swelling, and contribute to the solid or brawny tissue consistency. Excessive subcutaneous swelling results in large folds or bulges separated by deep crevices. In severe cases, such folds can become dependent and thus incur additional oedema from increased capillary filtration. The process then becomes self-perpetuating (*see* Fig. 6.1d).

Lymph may leak though the skin via superficial vesicles connected to dilated dermal lymphatics. White-to-yellow vesicles that discharge milky fluid suggest that chylous reflux is occuring (Fig. 6.3). Lymphangiomata, which may also present as soft, compressible vesicles bulging out of the skin surface (*see* Chapter 19), are not fibrotic, do not have hyperkeratotic papillomatous skin and must not be confused with the dilated (ectatic) dermal lymphatics sometimes found in long-standing lymphoedema.

Symptoms

Symptoms may be few with lymphoedema. Mention has been made of the pain that may be associated with a sudden onset of swelling, but this lasts only a few days. Established lymphoedema tends to cause aching and heaviness rather than pain, and the skin feels tight. Functional impairment is slight until the swelling becomes severe. In the lower limb, severe swelling eventually compromises mobility, and as exercise is the main stimulus for lymph flow, a vicious cycle of deterioration develops.

Psychological morbidity is significant in lymphoedema. Primary lymphoedema develops most commonly in females in their late teens or early adulthood at a time when social pressures are high. An inability to wear fashionable clothes or shoes can create problems with relationships. The disfigurement can result in reclusiveness and a reluctance to take part in sporting activities such as swimming, a pursuit beneficial to lymphoedema.

A study of patients with breast cancer-related lymphoedema has demonstrated significant psychosocial maladjustment to their illness over and above any effect arising from the breast cancer. Arm swelling affected

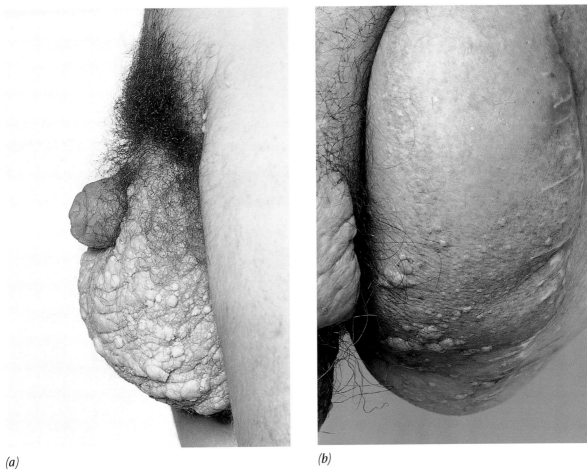

(a) *(b)*

Figure 6.3 *Lymphatic vesicles in the skin. (a) Vesicles on the scrotum full of white chyle. (b) Lymph-filled vesicles on the flaps of a high thigh amputation. The leg had been amputated because of an excessive discharge of lymph from vesicles all over the leg. No attempt had been made to stop the lymph reflux.*

vocation and domestic issues such as cooking and cleaning, as well as causing disruption to sexual relationships.[2]

Distribution

Lymphoedema most commonly affects the lower, and less often the upper, limbs. This predilection is related to the limited collateral drainage available at the root of a limb. Careful examination often reveals extension of the swelling into the associated quadrant of the trunk (*see* Fig. 6.1e). The lymphatic basin draining to the axilla, for example, includes the upper quadrant of the trunk as well as the upper limb. Oedema of the posterior axillary fold frequently accompanies arm swelling. Less oedema is present at the medial and inferior boundaries of the lymphatic basin because of greater opportunity for lymph to drain across the watershed into the adjoining basin.

The distribution of swelling in lymphoedema depends on the site of the anatomical defect. Hypoplasia or obliteration of the distal lymphatics in the lower limb often

presents with oedema of one foot but is usually bilateral; consequently, both feet eventually swell, one side usually being worse than the other. The oedema then tends to spread up the leg. Conversely, an obstruction to the lower limb's lymph drainage in the ilio-inguinal region tends to cause swelling of the whole limb, which progresses down, rather than up, the leg, with the bulk of the oedema being located in the thigh. One of the mysteries of lymphoedema of the arm following breast cancer treatment is why some women develop swelling predominantly in the upper arm whereas in others the hand is most severely affected despite (apparently) similar surgery and radiotherapy. Judging the probable site of the fault from the clinical features is therefore not straightforward.

Cellulitis, infection and inflammation

The classic signs of inflammation – rubor, tumor, calor and dolor – often appear in lymphoedematous limbs. Uncertainty as to whether all acute inflammatory attacks represent acute cellulitis of bacterial origin has led to the introduction of a variety of confusing terms. Many acute attacks are clearly episodes of classical cellulitis of bacterial origin, but on other occasions episodes of acute inflammation occur without any obvious portal of entry, without the characteristic cellulitic rash or a detectable pathogen.

The International Society of Lymphology has proposed that these episodes, which appear in all forms of lymphoedema, including those caused by filariasis, onchocerciasis and podoconiosis (which arises from the uptake of microparticles of aluminosalicates through the soles of the feet)[3] be called 'secondary acute inflammation'.[4] In the UK, the term 'acute inflammatory episodes' has been introduced. Worldwide, a multitude of other names are used to describe the same process: acute dermatolymphangioadenitis,[5] erysipelas, pseudo-erysipelas and lymphangitis. The concept underlying the term 'acute inflammatory episode' is that the adjective 'acute' distinguishes the condition from the ever-present low-grade chronic inflammation caused by the presence of the proteinaceous lymph in the tissues, and that the adjective 'inflammatory' allows for the absence of infection. For the sake of simplicity, we will use the term cellulitis (from the Latin *cellula* meaning cell and 'itis' referring to inflammation), which refers to inflammation of tissue in general as it is impossible to determine whether the predominant site affected is lymphatic vessel, interstitium or lymph gland (if present).

Acute inflammation in filariasis

Parasitologists recognize two types of acute inflammation in filariasis, both associated with systemic upset. The first type – the so-called 'filarial fever' – is characterized by high fever and rigors, lymphadenitis and retrograde lymphangitis in the absence of any injury or entry site for bacterial infection. Such attacks respond well to diethylcabarmazine, indicating that microfilaraemia is the cause. The second type is usually a bacterial cellulitis or one of the other forms of inflammation described below and is a consequence of the impaired lymphatic drainage rather than the filariasis per se.[6]

Cellulitis in non-filarial lymphoedema

Attacks of 'cellulitis' frequently complicate both the primary and secondary forms of non-filarial lymphoedema seen in the Western world.

Acute cellulitis of bacterial origin (erysipelas)

Whenever a patient presents with the classical clinical signs of acute inflammation in a lymphoedematous limb, the clinician's first task is to decide whether the inflammation has been caused by an infecting organism. Acute streptococcal cellulitis, the most common infection, presents with a history of 12–24 hours of general malaise and headache (which the patient often thinks is influenza) followed by

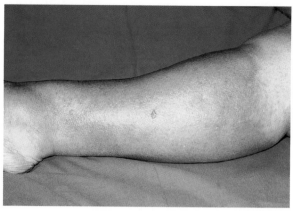

(a)

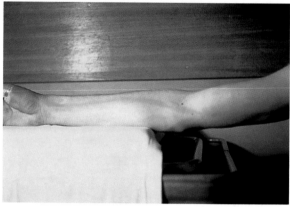

(b)

Figure 6.4 *(a) An acute inflammatory episode (cellulitis, erysipelas). Erysipelas is, strictly speaking, a more superficial infection than cellulitis. Erysipelas causes blistering of the skin, whereas cellulitis involves predominantly the deeper subcutaneous layer, as illustrated here. (b) The red streaks of lymphangitis.*

the appearance on the swollen limb of a raised, red, hot, tender patch of skin oedema with a visible and palpable edge (Fig. 6.4a). The whole leg becomes painful, and the patient has a pyrexia and tachycardia. Red streaks (lymphangitis; Fig. 6.4b) may develop proximal to the red patch of skin, and the lymph glands at the root of the limb may become tender and swollen. A blood culture may be positive, but there are times, even if all the clinical diagnostic features are present, when an infecting organism cannot be found on the skin or in the bloodstream. Patients who have had a previous attack may start taking antibiotics when the prodromal malaise begins, thus making the successful culture of the infecting organism most unlikely.

Many patients have streptococcal infections with only a few of the symptoms and signs described above. Pain may occur without any obvious inflammation. The constitutional upset may be minimal, and the condition can sometimes 'grumble' on in a subacute manner for days or weeks. Nevertheless, if the clinical features are suggestive of an acute streptococcal infection, a suitable antibiotic should be administered (*see* Chapter 9) even when laboratory tests fail to detect a causative organism, the diagnosis being made retrospectively if there is a favourable therapeutic response.

Cellulitis in lymphoedema tends to recur. The interval between episodes may be more than 12 months or as short as three weeks. There is often a stepwise deterioration in the lymphoedema with each attack, thus setting up a vicious cycle of worsening swelling and more frequent attacks of cellulitis.

Non-specific inflammatory episodes

A number of inflammatory episodes do not fit into any recognizable clinical pattern, and the clinician is forced to admit that their cause is unknown. Some of the patients involved may have a coincidental unrelated dermatological problem. Some have a hidden collection of pus, often sterile, in their subcutaneous tissues, and others may have a low-grade atypical latent infection in the skin which flares up as their general health and immunological status fluctuates. The term 'episodic dermato-lymphangio-adenitis' has been coined to describe this mixed clinical syndrome, which ranges from skin changes to cellulitis to inflamed lymph nodes.[5]

If radiological investigations, skin biopsies and tissue cultures fail to detect a cause, the clinician has to rely solely upon symptomatic treatment.

Chronic inflammatory changes (lipodermatosclerosis) without infection

This condition lies at the opposite end of the inflammation spectrum. It is chronic, long lasting and clearly not caused by a bacterial infection. It occurs in the lower half of lymphoedematous legs and is similar to the lipodermatosclerosis associated with venous disease. At first, the condition causes a red discoloration of the skin that is initially tender but this slowly changes over many months to reddish-brown pigmentation with thickening of the skin and subcutaneous tissues, hyperkeratosis and occasionally a very superficial ulceration that becomes secondarily infected. The fibrosed skin and subcutaneous tissues may contract and narrow the lower third of the leg. This change may impede lymph drainage from the foot and exacerbate the oedema in the foot. There is no specific treatment.

Fungal infections

Fungal infections, particularly tinea pedis, are difficult to avoid because of web space skin maceration arising from swollen toes. Local immune deficiency may also be a contributing factor, as suggested by a case of cryptococcosis complicating congenital lymphoedema.[7] The maceration and splits in the skin provide bacteria with a convenient portal of entry into the subcutaneous tissues. A high proportion of patients who present with cellulitis have active tinea pedis.

MEASUREMENT OF LYMPHOEDEMA

Most clinicians assess limb volume from circumference measurements or by water displacement, but these methods are not applicable to lymphoedema of the face, genitalia or trunk. Measurements of volume can be misleading, particularly when the swelling of an obviously oedematous limb is restricted by tissue resection or contraction from fibrosis. Furthermore, volume measurements are prone to error because all oedema varies widely according to the time of day, the stage of the menstrual cycle and physical activity.

Measurement of limb size

Limb size[8] is the main outcome measure used for lymphoedema management and in clinical trials. The accurate measurement of limb size is also important in studies on the pathophysiology of lymphoedema, as demonstrated in breast cancer-related lymphoedema, in which unexpected relationships were revealed between arm volume and interstitial fluid protein concentration[9] and between skin surface area and capillary density.[10]

Circumference

The simplest measure of swelling is circumference using a tape-measure at fixed points, for example 15 cm above and below the olecranon or patella, but this approach tends to be prone to error because it is difficult to ensure that the tape-measure is in exactly the same place and held at the same tension on successive days. It is not as sensitive for detecting differences between limbs as is volume measurement.[11]

Water displacement volumetry

Water displacement volumetry is considered to be the most accurate method of measurement, with a small standard deviation of 1.5–3.9 per cent, but the procedure is messy, and hygiene considerations limit its use.[12] It is, however, the best method for accurately determining hand and foot volume.

Calculated limb volume

Limb volume can be indirectly calculated from multiple circumference measurements. Measurement intervals accurately marked from a fixed point, for example the ulnar styloid or tip of the middle finger, serve as the points for circumference recording. Measurements are made every 4 cm along the axis of the limb (not along the surface), and volume is calculated from the formula for a frustum of a cone (i.e. a truncated cone):

$$V_{limb} = \frac{\sum x^2 + y^2 + xy}{3\pi}$$

or for a cylinder:

$$V_{limb} = \frac{\sum z^2}{\pi}$$

In these equations, χ is the circumference at one point on the limb, for example the ulnar styloid, and y the circumference at a point 4 cm up the limb from χ. Z is the circumference of the 4 cm annulus taken from one point, preferably the mid-point. Close agreement has been reported for the tape/cylinder method (based on circumference measurements taken every 3 cm) and water displacement for the healthy lower limb.[13] The accuracy of each method depends on the shape of the limb. The greater the deviation of the shape of the limb from the assumed cylinder or truncated cone, the greater the potential for error for the spacing, for example 4 cm, measurements. Either method of calculation is accurate providing the measurements are accurate.

Optoelectronic volumetry

Optoelectronic volumetry, for example with the Perometer, depends on the interruption of infrared light beams by the limb. The arm or leg is positioned inside a vertically orientated square frame that contains rows of infrared-emitting diodes on two adjacent sides, and rows of corresponding sensors on the opposite two sides (Fig. 6.5a). The limb casts shadows in two planes, and when the frame is moved on its tracks along the length of the limb, the volume is automatically calculated from a large number of vertical and horizontal diameter measurements at 3.1 mm intervals.

Optoelectronic volumetry is probably the most accurate method of limb volume measurement and is also the best method for recording limb shape.[14] Another application of this method is the measurement of dynamic events, for example following venous occlusion for plethysmography.[15] A small overestimation seems to occur with the tape-measure when compared with either water displacement or the Perometer.

Measurement of limb shape

Distortions in limb shape are characteristic of lymphoedema. The large folds with deep intervening creases that form around the ankle can, for example, be a major complaint of the patient by contributing to the disfigurement. Indeed, the shape of a lymphoedematous limb can be abnormal yet the volume normal because of tissue fibrosis. Shape also determines the success of treatment, particularly with elastic hosiery. Off-the-shelf hosiery is designed for 'normally' shaped legs or arms and does not produce graduated pressure if the limb is misshapen.

The measurement of limb shape is best performed by electronic volumetry, which produces a visual display of

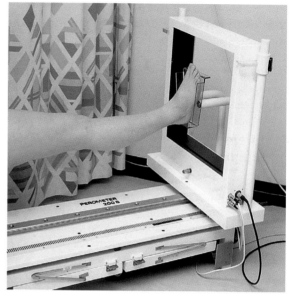

(a)

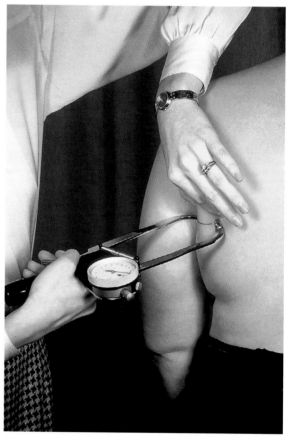

(b)

Figure 6.5 *The measurement of lymphoedema. (a) Optoelectronic volumetry. The arm or leg is positioned inside a square frame containing rows of infrared-emitting diodes on two adjacent sides and rows of corresponding sensors on the opposite two sides. The volume is calculated when the frame is moved on its tracks along the length of the limb. (b) Modified Harpenden skinfold calipers for the measurement of truncal oedema.*

the limb's profile or outline. Converting a subjective image into a quantifiable measure of shape is not straightforward. Badger[16] discovered that the ratio of proximal to distal limb volume (P:D ratio) gave the best indicator of shape distortion. This ratio reflects the relative proportions of the proximal, for example thigh, to distal, for example leg, segments of a limb.

Measurement of physical characteristics of lymphoedematous tissues

Tonometry

Pitting is the pathognomonic sign of peripheral oedema and results because external pressure displaces interstitial fluid to leave a depression or pit. Lymphoedema does not (generally) pit as easily as other forms of oedema. The objective measurement of the depth of pitting in lymphoedema has been described using a tonometer,[17] which registers the depth of tissue compression by a known mass over a fixed time interval. It has been shown, using an electronic tonometer that recorded the initial deformation and the time constant of the subsequent slow indentation, that the latter slow deformation component of the graph was fourfold greater in a lymphoedematous arm than in its contralateral normal control.[18] The sensitivity and specificity of this methodology has, however, yet to be established.

Measurement of truncal swelling

The involvement of the adjoining quadrant of the trunk is not unusual with limb lymphoedema. The measurement of this involvement is desirable, particularly as compression therapy to a limb can push fluid into that quadrant, where it can remain. A reduction in limb volume may therefore not necessarily mean an improvement in the lymphoedema overall.

In the upper limb, the posterior axillary fold is most commonly affected by lymphoedema. Roberts et al.[19] described an objective means of assessing post-axillary fold oedema using modified Harpenden skinfold calipers (Fig. 6.5b). A sustained application of the calipers demonstrated 'creep', i.e. a decrease in the measured fold thickness with time, caused by the displacement of fluid. Creep proved to be a more sensitive indicator of truncal oedema than skinfold thickness alone.

Measurement of extracellular water

Bioelectrical impedance

Multiple frequency bio-electrical impedance measurements have been used to study the volume of lymphoedematous limbs. A value for impedance can be calculated from a fixed-strength alternating current being passed through the body, the value being inversely proportional to the amount of fluid. Impedance at 50 KHz is indicative of total water content, whereas the extrapolated impedance at 0 KHz is a measure of extracellular fluid alone. In a study monitoring the effect of a four week programme of compression therapy and massage, extracellular water volume measured by this technique reduced relatively more than arm volume.[20] One drawback is the uncertainty of the volume of the body region investigated, i.e. the volume of tissue studied.

LYMPHOGRAPHY

Many interchangeable terms are used to describe the techniques used to obtain images of the lymphatics, so the following definitions may be helpful:

- *Lymphography*: technique that produces images of all parts of the lymphatic system.
- *Lymphangiography*: techniques that produce images of the lymph vessels.
- *Lymphadenography*: techniques that produce images of the lymph glands.
- *Lymphogram*: the technique used to produce images of the lymphatic system.
- *Lymphograph*: the image (picture) of the lymphatic system.

These five terms should all be preceded by an adjective that describes the method used to obtain the images, for example:

- the eye: visual lymphography;
- radioactivity: isotope lymphography or lymphoscintigraphy;
- X-rays: X-ray or radiological lymphography.

Lymphoscintigraphy

Lymphoscintigraphy (radionuclide or isotope lymphography) and indirect lymphography (see below) are based on a similar principle: lymphatic drainage is assessed after the '*indirect*' injection of a tracer into the subcutaneous tissues or skin, in contrast to the '*direct*' injection of a radio-opaque material into a lymphatic as performed during conventional lymphangiography. Labelled compounds are used for scintigraphy and newly developed, water-soluble contrast media for indirect lymphography.

Although lymphoscintigraphy has become a very important tool for diagnosing compromised lymph drainage,[21] indirect lymphography has become established in only a few centres, where it is used for scientific research. Much of the research that has been performed on the various scintigraphic methods is summarised in references.[22–26]

The essential capability of the lymphatics to clear large molecules from the interstitium can be tested by introducing labelled proteins or colloids into the tissue.[27]

Scintigraphy using a gamma camera provides an assessment of the distribution of the tracer in the leg and its uptake into the lymph glands, images of the lymph glands and the collecting lymphatics. New high-resolution techniques ('lymphangioscintigraphy, LAS') can now provide high-quality images.[28–40] The lymphatic drainage in a limb can be assessed by comparing the uptake of radioactivity in the lymph glands at the root of the limb with the injected dose.[41–48]

Lymph gland scintigraphy has become an important part of the assessment of sentinel lymph gland drainage in some types of cancer surgery.[49,50]

Labelled tracers

It has been suggested that the optimal particle size for a lymphatic tracer is in the range of 10 nm. After injection into the tissue, some of these particles are incorporated into macrophages although the majority enter the initial lymphatics and are transported towards the lymph glands. The compounds most commonly used are antimony sulphide colloid, rhenium sulphate, human serum albumin nanocolloid and DTPA serum albumin, all labelled with technetium (^{99m}Tc).[51] Labelled gold colloids are no longer used.[27]

Injection

The volume injected should be small (0.1–0.2 mL) and should have a high specific activity. Subcutaneous injections are made into the web space between the first and second toes or the first and second fingers. Using several subcutaneous injections may improve diagnostic accuracy.[47] Injections may be placed into other areas of interest, for example around leg ulcers or into the scrotum, in order to assess the lymphatic drainage of these sites. Subfascial lymph transport can be assessed after an intramuscular injection of the tracer into the distal third of the calf or forearm.[42,44,46,52]

Stress tests

Lymph transport is enhanced by active movement, for example exercise with a foot ergometer or walking on a treadmill. Exercise during the test is important if the assessment of lymphatic drainage is to be based on the amount of radioactivity taken up by the regional lymph glands. It has been shown that the sensitivity and specificity of static images obtained 1 hour after the pedal injection of the tracer are increased by muscular exercise.[53] Some authors still, however, prefer to assess static images taken at different time intervals after the injection without any stress test.[28,33]

Measurement of radioactivity

A number of different techniques have been described to measure the uptake of the isotope. Time–activity curves over the injection site reflect the local clearance of the tracer, but it has been shown that there is a poor correlation

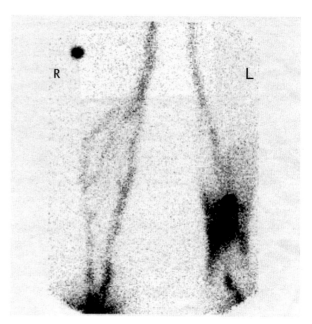

Figure 6.6 *Lymphangioscintigraphy of the lower legs after subcutaneous injections of ^{99m}Tc-labelled colloid (nanocoll) into the web spaces of both feet of a patient with lymphoedema of the left leg. Only one lymphatic can be seen and there is dermal backflow. Nodal uptake: (left) 2.5 percentile activity of injected dose (D%); (right) 8.4 D%. Marker at the right lateral knee.*

between the clearance of the tracer from the depot and its uptake into the lymph glands.[46] This method of assessment has nevertheless been used to demonstrate therapeutic effects.[54] Gamma camera images of the whole extremity and torso may show a pathological distribution of the isotope within the skin from dermal backflow caused by an obstruction in the main collecting lymphatics.[31,32,55] Figure 6.6 shows an abnormal leg scan in a patient with lymphoedema praecox and Fig. 6.7 an example of lymphangioscintigraphy in a patient with venous ulcers.

The uptake of radioactivity by the lymph glands is the most reliable measurement of lymph transport. It can be documented by simple scintigraphy using a scintillation probe or gamma camera, or by combining the transmission and emission measurements to correct for the different depths of the inguinal and iliac lymph nodes. The injected dose is then compared with the corrected lymph gland activity to provide quantitative information about lymph transport.[46] The time taken for the isotope to appear in the lymph glands after the injection of the tracer in the web space, which should be less than 40 minutes under normal conditions, is not a reliable measure of lymph transportation.

A number of semi-quantitative scoring systems have been proposed that take account of the different characteristics of tracer kinetics and calculate a transport index,[31,56] but a visual interpretation of the gamma camera images is sufficient for routine diagnosis in the majority of cases.[30]

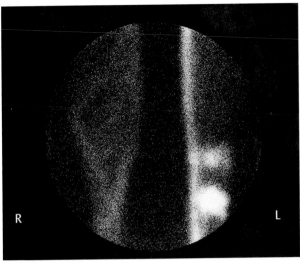
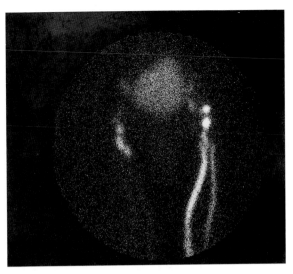

Figure 6.7 *Lymphangioscintigraphy of the lower legs (left) and of both thighs (right) after intracutaneous injection of* ^{99m}Tc*-labelled dextran into the dorsum of the feet of a patient with chronic venous insufficiency and two ulcers above the left medial malleolus. There is extravasation of the tracer in the region of the ulcers and an increased visualization of enlarged collectors and inguinal lymph nodes.*

Table 6.1 *Tracer uptake in the inguinal lymph nodes measured by quantitative lymphoscintigraphy*

	Prefascial lymph transport (subcutaneous injection)		Subfascial lymph transport (intramuscular injection)	
	Normal	Lymphoedema	Normal	Post-thrombotic syndrome
n	25	25	9	6
D%	14.3 ± 4.2	2.0 ± 2.5	1.1 ± 0.3	0.2 ± 0.16
Statistical difference	$P < 0.001$		$P < 0.02$	

D% = percentile activity of injected dose.
Adapted from reference 46.

Results

Based on visual interpretation, the sensitivity of isotope lymphography for diagnosing lymphoedema has been reported to be 97 per cent with a specificity of 100 per cent.[48] Some of the results obtained using quantitative lymphoscintigraphy[46] are shown in Table 6.1.

Figure 6.8 demonstrates that the intracutaneous tracer injection technique is not able to distinguish lymphoedema from other varieties of oedema. The lymph gland storage values after intracutaneous tracer injection in patients with lymphoedema, even when caused by metastases in the lymph glands, are normal, demonstrating that the intracutaneous networks of initial lymphatics act as an effective collateral pathway. Therefore although the intracutaneous injection of the tracer is useful to detect sentinel lymph glands or to visualize pathological skin lymphatics filled by dermal backflow (as achieved by the LAS technique), subcutaneous injection is the method of choice for any quantitative measurement of lymph gland activity. It has been shown that lymphatic function declines with age, markedly so after the age of 65 years.[43,45]

Table 6.2 summarizes the results of the findings in different conditions that have been reported in the literature.

Comment

Isotope lymphoscintigraphy is the best screening technique available for confirming a clinical suspicion of lymphoedema, is easy to perform and is minimally invasive. It is also useful for excluding lymphatic involvement as a cause of an unexplained swollen limb. The technique is most effective when used by clinicians interested in lymphology who can, with their colleagues in the department of nuclear medicine, interpret the scintigraphic findings in the light of their clinical findings.

Indirect X-ray lymphography

Skin lymphatics can be opacified by the intradermal injection of newly developed contrast media, which provides valuable information about the local dermal lymphatics in the region of interest and important clues to the state of the lymphatic drainage of the whole limb. The lymph glands are rarely opacified so this method is not a substitute for conventional, direct lymphoscintigraphy.

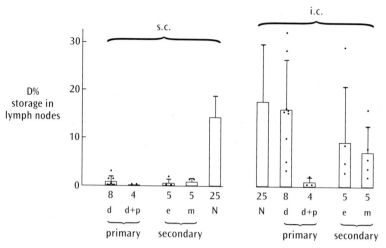

Figure 6.8 *Lymph node storage after subcutaneous (left, s.c.) and intracutaneous (right, i.c.) injection in lymphoedema patients. There is no significant difference in normal individuals (centre). Patients with the distal type of primary lymphoedema, and also those with secondary lymphoedema caused by metastases, may show 'normal' nodal uptake after intracutaneous injection. N = normal limbs; d = limbs with distal oedema; d + p = limbs with distal and proximal oedema; e = limbs with oedema secondary to infection; m = limbs with oedema secondary to lymph node metastases. Adapted from reference 46.*

Table 6.2 *Lymph drainage in different conditions: summarized findings reported in the literature*

	Lymph transport		References
	Prefascial	**Subfascial**	
Lymphoedema	⇓	⇓	21, 27, 28, 30, 32–38, 44–48, 53
Venous oedema	⇑	⇓	41, 44, 46
	⇓	⇓	43, 45
Deep vein thrombosis	⇑	⇓	52
Post-thrombotic syndrome	⇑	⇓	42, 44, 52
Leg ulcers	⇓	⇓	45, 52
Lipoedema	⇔		41

Method

Non-ionic, water-soluble, dimeric, hexa-iodinated contrast media such as Iotasul or Iotrolan are constantly infused into the dermis using a motorized injection pump (0.12 mL/min) through thin, butterfly needles. A total of 2–4 mL can be infused at each injection site.[57–61] The tip of the needle has to be situated in the uppermost part of the dermis so that the injection produces a bluish wheal with a glassy appearance. Under normal conditions, the lymphatics begin to fill with contrast after a few minutes, progress being watched with an image intensifier and recorded on high-quality mammography films taken every 5 minutes. Xeroradiography also produces good images; computed tomography with three-dimensional reconstruction provides even more impressive pictures.[62]

Indications

Indirect X-ray lymphography may help to differentiate between different forms of lymphoedema such as aplasia/hypoplasia or obliteration of distal lymphatics versus proximal hypoplasia or obliteration with distal distension

(*see* Chapter 7).[63,64] Its sensitivity for diagnosing lymphoedema is good (97 per cent), but it has only a moderate specificity (89 per cent).[65]

The technique has revealed pathological changes in the skin lymphatics in areas of lipodermatosclerosis caused by chronic venous insufficiency and in the vicinity of leg ulcers.[64] It has also revealed that localized lymphoedema, for example after trauma, inflammation or in morbidly obese patients,[66] is characterized by abnormal initial lymphatics in certain localized areas of skin, the large collecting lymphatics appearing normal.[51,52,64] Patients with lipoedema show a typical flame-like pattern of dye diffusion before the dye enters into the initial lymphatics, this being one of the very few pathognomonic features of this entity.[65,67] Fascinating but yet to be explained patterns may be seen after replantation surgery.[68]

Results

The contrast agent forms enlarging depots around the site of the infusion, which flows into peripheral lymph collectors. Under normal conditions, these collecting lymphatics can be followed for a mean distance of 10–30 cm.

Lymphoedema

Indirect lymphography reveals four main lymphatic patterns in lymphoedematous skin:[59]

- *Type I*: No lymphatics are opacified, but the contrast spreads in a cuff-like pattern into the adventitial spaces around the blood vessels. This appearance is often found in patients with congenital lymphoedema and is similar to the images obtained by microlymphangiography,[63] although there may also be areas of the initial lymphatic ectasis as well as aplasia.[69]
- *Type II*: A dense network of small pre-collector skin lymphatics is opacified, but only a few of the larger lymph collectors are filled (Fig. 6.9). This pattern is found mainly in patients with acquired peripheral lymphoedema obliteration (for example praecox and tarda).

- *Type III*: There is an opacification of enlarged pre-collector skin lymphatics and lymph collectors (Fig. 6.10). This pattern is usually caused by proximal obstruction or incompetent megalymphatics. Most patients with the descending form of lymphoedema caused by primary proximal obstruction have this appearance, which is also seen after infusion of the dye into areas of skin with papillomatosis cutis.[55,70]
- *Type IV*: No pre-collectors or lymph collectors are visible, but there are no cuffs around the blood vessels as there are in type 1. The significance of this pattern is unclear. It may be caused by the 'die-back' of lymphatics upstream of a severe proximal obstruction, but technical problems in patients with extremely dense and thick skin can produce a similar picture.

The retrograde filling of small skin lymphatics in any of the above groups is a sign of dermal backflow and incompetent lymphatic valves. The lymphatics of swollen

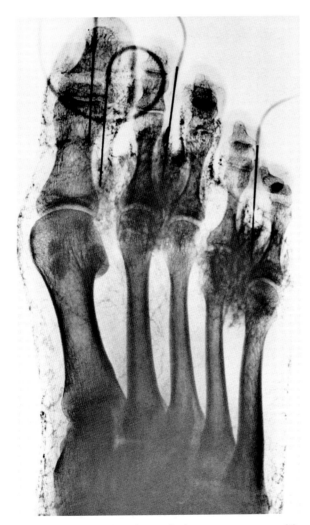

Figure 6.9 *Indirect lymphography in a young woman with congenital proximal and distal lymphoedema of one lower extremity. There are irregular dense networks of lymphatics and dermal backflow into the skin of the toes.*

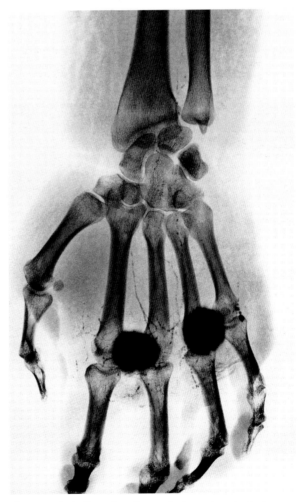

Figure 6.10 *Indirect lymphography in postmastectomy lymphoedema. After an infusion of Iotrolan into the interdigital spaces, enlarged lymph collectors fill from the two injection depots. There is also a retrograde filling of the finger and skin lymphatics (dermal backflow).*

skin are sometimes grossly abnormal when those in adjacent 'normal'-looking skin are normal or enlarged (Fig. 6.11).

Venous insufficiency

The dermal lymphatics of patients with chronic venous insufficiency may show morphological changes in abnormal lipodermatosclerotic areas of skin. The pre-collectors are often fragmented, filled by dermal backflow and surrounded by diffuse extravasation of the dye into the tissues (Fig. 6.12). The prefascial collectors are enlarged and often show increased contractility. The lymph glands in the groin may be opacified. The demonstration of wide and well-filled lymph collectors correlates with the known increase of prefascial lymph transport demonstrated by radionuclide lymphography.[51]

Injecting the contrast medium into the border of venous ulcers often fails to fill any lymphatics.

Lipoedema

Lipoedema, which is often confused with and sometimes combined with lymphoedema, shows a very characteristic and quite specific pattern. If a depot of the contrast medium is injected into the oedematous skin of a lipoedematous lower leg, a typically flame-like structure is formed (Fig. 6.13), whereas an injection into the

normal-looking skin on the dorsum of the foot of the same leg produces a normal pattern.[65,67]

Comment

Indirect lymphography is a kind of radiological 'Patent Blue' test, but with a much better resolution. A precise injection technique is a prerequisite for good results. The method has been used by those involved in scientific research but has not developed into a helpful technique

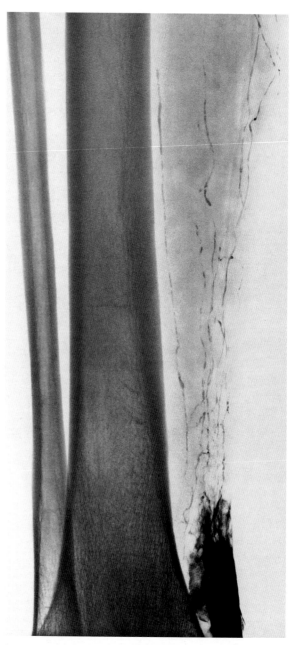

Figure 6.12 *Indirect lymphography with infusion of the contrast medium into the lipodermatosclerotic area of the medial lower leg of a patient with severe chronic venous insufficiency, showing enlarged lymph collectors with an irregular course and diffuse extravasation of the dye. After 30 minutes, inguinal lymph nodes were opacified.*

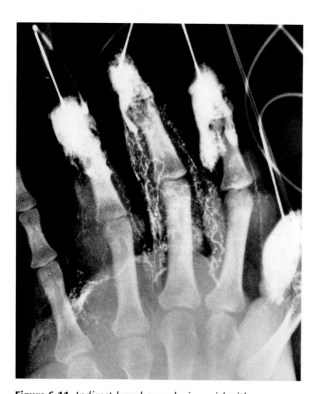

Figure 6.11 *Indirect lymphography in a girl with congenital lymphoedema of an upper limb. Although no lymphatics could be opacified after injection into the swollen parts of the fingers, dense networks of extremely enlarged lymph collectors were demonstrated after infusion of the dye into the non-swollen finger tips. Reproduced from reference 63.*

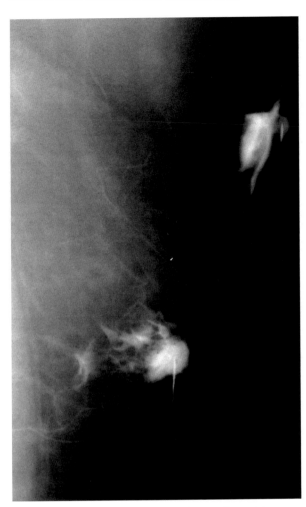

Figure 6.13 *Indirect lymphography in a patient with lipoedema. The depots of the injected contrast medium form typically flame-like structures tapering into normal lymphatics.*

for the routine clinical investigation or management of lymphoedema.

Visual lymphography

The early anatomical descriptions of the lymphatics by Aselli, Pecquet, Rudbeck and Bartholinus that led to the beautiful anatomical drawings of the whole lymphatic system by Mascagni are described in Chapter 1. These anatomists displayed the lymphatics they were dissecting by injecting them with air, milk, mercury or wax. During the middle part of the twentieth century, a number of physiologists outlined animal lymphatics with coloured dyes.[71,72] In 1933, Hudack and McMaster[73] used Patent Blue Violet to demonstrate the dermal lymphatics of their own forearms. Kinmonth, in 1952,[74] confirmed that this dye was the most effective of a large selection of vital dyes for outlining the lymphatic system of man and used it to reveal subcutaneous lymphatics large enough for direct injection.

The injection of Patent Blue Violet into the skin or subcutaneous tissues provides limited visual information about the local dermal lymphatic channels and collecting lymphatics. This vital dye, also known as Patent Blue V, is not the same as the dye commonly used for skin marking called Patent Blue. It diffuses rapidly into the lymphatics when injected into the subcutaneous tissues because it does not combine with the protein in the interstitial fluid but remains as a calcium salt with a relatively small molecular weight of 1158 Da. It is produced as a 10 per cent isotonic solution that has to be autoclaved and filtered before use. Although it rapidly enters the lymphatics, the dye is also absorbed into the bloodstream via the capillaries. It passes quickly around the body and gives the patient's skin a bluish-green colour (which can be confused with cyanosis) before being excreted by the kidneys, turning the urine blue-green but returning the patient's colour to normal. The local discoloration at the site of the injection may take several weeks to disappear.

A number of other dyes have been tried,[75,76] but all have now disappeared from use. Kinmonth[77] recommended that the maximum dose of Patent Blue Violet be 2.5 mL 10 per cent solution. We have used this dose for bipedal lymphography for 40 years, approximately 1 mL per foot, divided into four aliquots (one in each web space), without any serious complications except for the small number of patients reported by Kinmonth[77] who developed an allergy to the dye.

To visualize the dermal lymphatics, 0.2–0.5 mL Patent Blue Violet is injected in small quantities into the dermis. In normal skin, thin blue-green channels are soon seen spreading mainly proximally up the limb (Fig. 6.14a). In oedematous limbs, whatever the cause of the oedema, a fine network of dermal lymphatic capillaries appears spreading out in all directions from the point of injection (Fig. 6.14b), but this is most obvious and of maximum size when the oedema is lymphatic in origin. Kinmonth[77] felt that a failure of the dye to spread into a network of small channels indicated dermal lymphatic absence or obliteration and coincidentally implied that the skin was unsuitable for use as a skin graft donor site for a Charles operation.

The dye spreads widely throughout the skin, sometimes as far up as the thigh, if the main collecting lymphatics are absent, obliterated or incompetent (Fig. 6.14c). The finding of a greater than normal spread of the dye in the dermal lymphatic plexus (dermal blackflow) of a clinically 'normal' contralateral limb is of considerable prognostic significance because this indicates the presence of occult lymphatic disease, provided other causes of oedema such as venous obstruction have been excluded.

Visual lymphography is a very crude, non-quantifiable method of assessing the dermal lymphatics and is rarely used on its own. The Patent Blue Violet is nowadays usually injected into the subcutaneous tissues, from where it rapidly enters the subcutaneous collecting lymphatics,

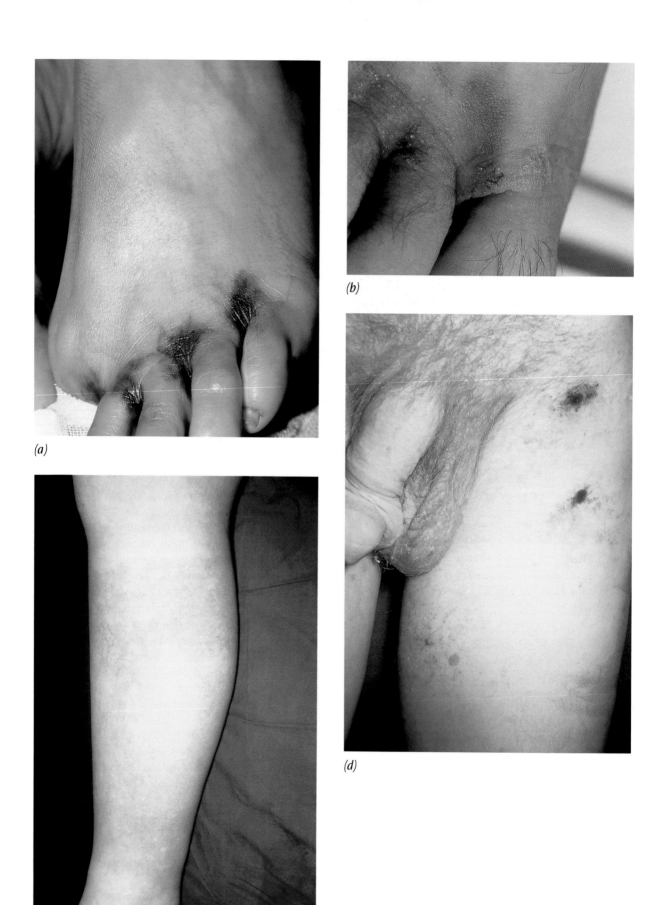

(a)

(b)

(c)

(d)

Figure 6.14 Continued on facing page.

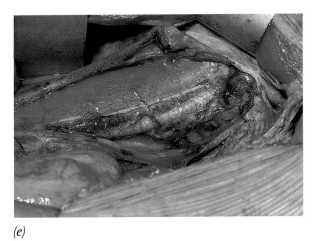
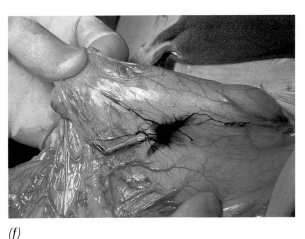

(e)   *(f)*

Figure 6.14 *Visual lymphography. (a) Many faint blue lymphatics appearing on the dorsum of a normal, non-swollen foot following the injection of Patent Blue Violet into the web spaces. (b) Patent Blue Violet spreading diffusely into the skin of the foot and into a number of lymph vesicles at the base of the toes of a patient who had megalymphatics with reflux. The vesicles often leaked clear lymph. (c) The spread of Patent Blue Violet throughout the limb following web space injections in a patient with proximal and distal obliteration. The blue edge across the leg just below the patella corresponds to the site at which sterile towels had been placed around the leg. (d) Injections of Patent Blue Violet just below the groin given to aid the visualization of the pelvic lymphatics. This patient had megalymphatics and reflux. Some of the dye has diffused out into the dermal lymphatics and into one vesicle on the inner side of the thigh. (e) Iliac megalymphatics filled by injecting Patent Blue Violet into the subcutaneous tissues of the thigh as shown in (d). Without this form of visualization, a thorough ligation of these lymphatics would be almost impossible. (f) Patent Blue Violet, injected just beneath the serosal layer of the intestine, filling lymphatics on the surface of the bowel and in the mesentery.*

as well as the dermal plexus, making them easy to expose and cannulate for radiographic lymphography.

Sites of application

Lower limb

Injections of 0.1 mL 10 per cent Patent Blue Violet into the web spaces between each toe can be painful so this is usually carried out under general anaesthesia as a prelude to X-ray lymphography (see below). The web spaces are plentifully supplied with lymphatics, and a gentle massage of the foot and toes quickly spreads the dye up into the collecting lymphatics on the dorsum of the foot. Additional injections can be made deep into the sole of the foot to display the deep lymphatics in the posterior compartment of the leg, although we rarely find this necessary. Care must be taken to avoid rubbing or dropping the dye on the skin of the dorsum of the foot and producing stains that look like subcutaneous lymphatics. After each injection, the barrel of the syringe should be pulled back as the needle is withdrawn to ensure that dye does not drip onto the patient's foot. Gloves should be worn to avoid staining the injector's fingers green, which can last for days. In obese patients, the lymphatic channels, although filled with dye, may not become visible until the skin is incised and retracted, but in a non-obese individual with normal lymphatics on the dorsum of the foot, the vessels are easy to see (Fig. 6.14a). The appearance of reticulated patches of dye in the dermis, which Kinmonth called 'dermal backflow',[77]

indicates the presence of local lymphatic obstruction or incompetence.

Pelvis

The same technique of interdigital injection of Patent Blue Violet assisted by foot elevation and massage will eventually outline the lymph nodes and lymphatics of the inguinal and pelvic regions. Additional and better filling of the pelvic lymphatics may be obtained if further injections of dye are given into the subcutaneous tissues of the thigh or even into the inquinal lymph glands, especially if there is distal lymphatic obliteration (Fig. 6.14d and e).

Upper limb and axilla

The Patent Blue Violet should be injected into the web spaces between the fingers. It can be administered deep into the palm of the hand, although we rarely inject here. If the distal limb lymphatics are obliterated, further proximal subcutaneous injections may be required along the course of the lymphatic channels on the medial side of the upper arm and lateral aspect of the axilla.

Neck

The lymphatics and lymph nodes of the supraclavicular region and posterior triangle of the neck are best visualized by injecting Patent Blue Violet into the web spaces of the hand as described above. The deep cervical lymphatics and lymph glands are seen to best effect after subcutaneous injections over the mastoid process. The thoracic duct may take up dye injected into the hand or arm, but a better method of outlining the thoracic duct is to feed the patient a large quantity of milk, fat or cream. In practice, a surgeon familiar with the anatomy of the supraclavicular fossa can usually find the thoracic duct at its termination in the jugular–subclavian vein angle without these special techniques.

Viscera

Subserosal injections of vital dyes have been used to visualize the gastric lymph glands in patients undergoing a gastrectomy for carcinoma in order to improve the efficacy of nodal excisions.[75] Patent Blue Violet can be injected under the serosa of any part of the intestine. Gentle massage then outlines the draining lymphatics (Fig. 6.14f). These lymphatics can then be cannulated for radiographic contrast lymphography. This technique is useful before performing an enteromesenteric bridge procedure (see below).

Other sites

The lymphatics of the spermatic cord (testis), liver, kidney and thyroid have all been delineated using appropriate direct injections of Patent Blue Violet in the local vicinity.

Sentinel gland biopsy

Sentinel lymph gland biopsy has recently become a popular staging technique for carcinoma of the breast and malignant melanoma.[78,79] The sentinel lymph gland is the first gland along the drainage pathway of a tumour. If Patent Blue Violet is injected into the subcutaneous tissues close to a tumour, the sentinel gland will turn green, or if an isotope is injected show a raised level of radioactivity, thus allowing the gland to be seen or detected with a scintilation counter and removed. These techniques are being used in an attempt to provide important prognostic and therapeutic information about tumour spread in patients with clinically localized disease and to avoid the morbidity associated with prophylactic block dissection, radiotherapy and chemotherapy.

Radiological (X-ray) lymphography

This is the investigation that produces an X-ray anatomical image of the lymphatics and lymph glands. It is achieved by injecting a radio-opaque material into a lymphatic that has been surgically exposed and visualized by the injection of Patent Blue Violet into the nearby tissues. The technique is correctly called a lymphogram, but the term 'lymphography' is more often used. The image obtained is a lymphograph – subdivided into lymphangiograph and lymphadenograph when the images are of lymphatics and lymph glands respectively.

Technique

Patients with swollen legs should, if possible, be admitted to hospital at least 24 hours before the investigation for bed rest, leg elevation and the application of a pneumatic compression device to reduce foot swelling and make it easier to find and dissect out a subcutaneous lymphatic in the foot.

Anaesthesia

Although it is usually easy to perform a lymphogram under local anaesthesia as an out-patient procedure when the foot is only mildly swollen and the lymphatics are normal, the procedure can be difficult and prolonged in grossly swollen limbs with abnormal or partially obliterated distal lymphatics. We thus prefer to admit our patients with lymphoedema to hospital for 24 hours and perform the lymphogram under general anaesthesia in the operating room using an operating microscope to examine, dissect and cannulate the lymphatics. This considerably increases the chance of a successful cannulation of even the most hypoplastic lymphatics. General anaesthesia has the advantage of keeping patients (and their lymphatics) still during the cannulation and subsequent injection of contrast medium. Even small movements during the injection can dislodge the needle and destroy what is sometimes the only lymphatic available for injection. Local, spinal and epidural anaesthetics are possible alternatives, but as a difficult cannulation and infusion can take between 2 and 4 hours, epidural anaesthesia is the only really credible alternative.

Instrumentation

A standard set of microsurgical instruments must be available. These should include a number of watchmaker-style forceps with fine jewelled points, sharp-pointed cross-action microsurgical scissors of different lengths, some stronger non-tooth cannulating forceps and some fine-toothed forceps to tease off the surrounding fat. A Castroviejo-style needleholder is used for the cannulation, which must be rachetless to avoid the jerking movements caused by releasing the ratchet that might damage the lymphatic during and after cannulation; other types of rachetless microneedle-holders or strong non-tooth forceps can be used.

The set should contain a number of skin hooks of differing dimensions with thread tails (small hooks that can be fixed to the patient's skin with adhesive strips being very useful) and some small self-retaining screw-apart-type or spring-apart eyelid skin retractors to hold the skin incision apart during the dissection. A fine no. 15 blade scalpel, Gillies forceps, fine curved artery forceps and suture scissors are required for opening and closing the wound. A diamond knife or microscalpel may be helpful during the dissection of the lymphatic, but a no. 15 or 17 blade is usually sufficient. Standard coagulating or bipolar diathermy must also be available.

X-ray table, apparatus and radiographer

For a lower limb lymphogram, we place a full-length radiolucent cassette tunnel on the operating table, which allows full-size radiographic cassettes to be placed beneath any part of the body from the toes to the neck. A standard portable X-ray machine can then be centred above the cassette to X-ray the contrast-filled lymphatics, bones and soft tissues. An alternative strategy is to use a mobile C-arm and image intensifier through a radiolucent operating table. This, however, produces small films that can be more difficult to interpret. An experienced theatre radiographer who has obtained lymphographs before is a major advantage. Radiographs should be taken of the abdomen and chest in the recovery room to visualize all the pelvic and abdominal lymphatics and the thoracic duct.

Preparation and position

The patient is placed supine on the radiolucent operating table or full-length cassette (Fig. 6.15). The legs are held up off the operating table by an assistant so that the skin of the feet and ankles can be sterilized with coloured alcoholic chlorhexidine. The operating table is covered with sterile drapes, and the limbs are allowed to rest back on top of them. Further drapes are then placed over the limbs to limit the exposure to the toes and dorsal surface of the feet and ankles. Towel clips should not be used as these appear on the radiographs. It is better if the over-drapes are stuck to the legs with an adhesive such as mastosol.

Good lengths of 1 inch wide sterile bandage are then looped round the big toes and passed to an operating room assistant who loops them around a convenient metal bar beneath the operating table and ties them so that the feet

and great toes are held in plantar flexion. This has the advantage of holding the feet still and the dorsum of the foot horizontal, thus providing a relatively flat surface on which to dissect out the lymphatic. We do not place the patient in the Trendelenberg position as we have not found that this appreciably reduces haemorrhage. Sterile Patent Blue Violet can be injected into the web spaces at this stage, but this will delay the procedure while the dye is massaged into the feet. An earlier injection immediately after the induction of anaesthesia is preferable.

Incision

The incision should be placed transversely across the mid-dorsum of the foot over any blue lymphatic streaks that are visible (Fig. 6.16). The length of the incision varies with the size of the limb and the number and distribution of visible lymphatics beneath the incision.

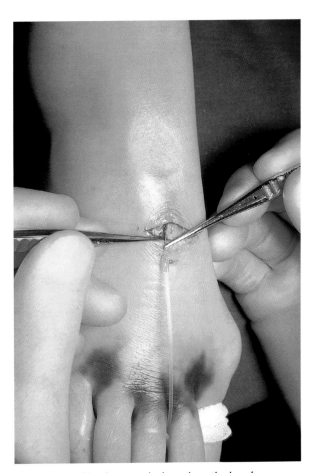

Figure 6.16 *This photograph shows how the bandages around the great toes hold the feet plantar flexed, giving good access to the transverse incision that has been made on the dorsum of the foot. A lymphatic has been dissected out and is being cannulated. The forceps in the operator's left hand are keeping the lymphatic taught while the needle is being introduced with the right hand. The distal skin hook that we usually use to hold the wound apart has been temporarily removed.*

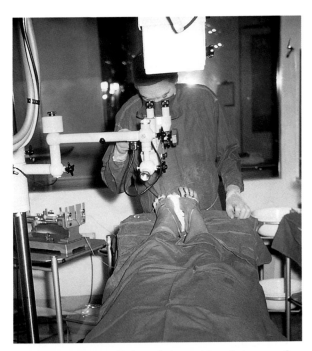

Figure 6.15 *An overall view of the position that we use for X-ray lymphography, showing the position of the operating table, the feet, the dissecting microscope, the pump and the instrument trolley.*

It is helpful to see at least two channels passing upwards in the wound so that, if the initial cannulation fails, another lymphatic is instantly accessible. A fairly long transverse incision is unavoidable if the lymphatics are clearly abnormal, thin or faint, but if the patient has had an isotope lymphoscintigram that has shown little or no uptake in the lymphatic system and no blue streaks are seen, it is not worthwhile extending the initial incision. Conversely if the lymphoscintigram has shown good uptake in the inguinal lymph glands, lymphatics should be present in the foot and the exploration should proceed. A longitudinal incision over a single lymphatic limits access to that lymphatic and prevents lateral exploration for other vessels. The shorter the incision, however, the better the cosmetic result.

An operating microscope, which should be set up and tested before the skin has been prepared, is then moved into position. The microscope should be focused on the centre of the incision and adjusted to its lowest power of magnification. The rest of the procedure should be carried out viewing through the microscope. Gentle shallow strokes of the no. 15 scalpel blade are used to deepen the incision. The incision is opened with lateral pressure from the flat surface of the blade and by pulling or pushing the wound apart with a dry swab. All this should be carried out under careful microscopic inspection to ensure that careless sharp dissection at too deep a level does not divide any exposed lymphatics, which usually lie a short distance below the dermis. Once the full thickness of the skin has been incised, it pulls apart more easily, a process that can be encouraged by traction with skin hooks or a small self-retaining retractor. Skin hooks held to the skin with adhesive strips are far less intrusive than a self-retaining retractor.

Any bleeding that is encountered must be carefully controlled by diathermy through fine forceps applied directly to the bleeding points. A small amount of blood can seriously impede vision. Bipolar diathermy may be preferred to limit the volume of tissue coagulated.

Dissection

When one or two green lymphatics have been observed running across the base of the incision, further sharp dissection is used to isolate them from their fatty surrounds. The no. 15 blade or diamond scalpel can be pointed upwards towards the microscope and its point used to cut fat and fibrous tissue away from the upper surface of the lymphatic. Once the upper surface of the lymphatic has been cleared, microscissors and fine dissecting forceps are used to pull or cut the adherent fat from the sides of the lymphatic. It is important to clear completely three surfaces of the lymphatic for about 5–6 mm to make the subsequent cannulation easy and to ensure that the needle tip can be seen within the lymph channel, which is usually covered by a fine capillary plexus visible through the dissecting microscope.

Needles and tubing

Once the lymphatic has been dissected out, the cannulating needle and its attached tubing is connected to a 10 mL syringe filled with Ultrafluid Lipiodol. The original St Thomas'/McCarthy needles that were commercially produced are no longer available so we now use a microsclerotherapy needle attached to 1 mm diameter extension tubing. Rutt devised a microsurgical needle for lymphangiograms in children, but this is rarely used today.

Contrast medium

The introduction of Lipiodol by Brunn and Engeset in 1956[80] made contrast lymphangiography a possibility. Lipiodol is an oil-soluble contrast medium, made from poppy seed, containing 35 per cent iodine. Its great advantage over water-soluble contrast media is its retention within the lymphatics and lymph glands. Water-soluble media diffuse out through the walls of the lymphatics into the subcutaneous tissues, giving poor visualization of the lymphatics and lymph glands. Lipiodol is unfortunately an extremely viscous material. This slows the speed of injection and makes the use of a mechanical injector essential.

Injection pump

We use the University of Lund pump, which is robust, dependable, reliable and versatile (Fig. 6.17),[81] although more modern slow infusion devices are commercially available. The Lund injector has an electrical motor that turns a central worm-threaded rod. This drives a metal collar forward along two smooth metal rods that prevent it rotating. The collar has three right-angle, adjustable, metal, L-shaped drivers that can be adjusted to make contact with the plungers of up to three syringes. Syringes filled with 10 mL Lipiodol are placed in front of the metal drivers in troughs and advanced up to a deeply notched vertical metal plate through which their nozzles can protrude. Before cannulation, the Lipiodol is flushed into the extension tube up to a point 5–10 cm from the needle.

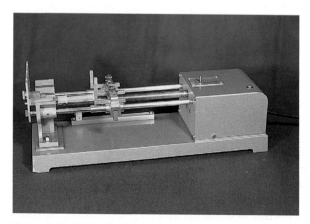

Figure 6.17 *University of Lund pump with one syringe in its central trough.*

Some air must be left in the last 5–10 cm of the tubing so that the operator can confirm that the Lipiodol is moving along the tube into the lymphatic when the pump is first turned on.

Cannulation

Once the lymphatic has been dissected from its coverings, an assistant places a curved haemostat across the foot, parallel to the wound and 3–5 cm above the incision, and presses down to obstruct the lymphatic. The foot distal to the incision is then massaged to drive the lymph and Patent Blue Violet up from the foot and distend the lymphatic. This makes cannulation easier. We have not needed to use topically applied papaverine or saline to relax spasm as the lymphatics always appear to dilate in response to these simple mechanical measures of obstruction and distal massage.

The cannulating needle and its attached tubing must be carefully positioned so that they lie without tension along the line of the lymphatic, flat on the dorsum of the foot at the correct level for puncture and cannulation. A single half-hitch of the tubing around an appropriate toe, pulled tense but not tight, fixes the tubing and prevents inadvertent dislodgment if the injector is moved. Further fixation of the tubing to the dorsum of the foot can be achieved by the application of a single 6 mm adhesive strip. The tubing should be fixed to prevent dislodgement of the needle before cannulation as attempts at fixation after cannulation can result in such movement, but there should be enough slack to allow the needle to be held and manipulated.

Once everything is in place and the lymphatic has been distended, the magnification on the microscope is increased. The needle is picked up, backhand, in a pair of Castroviejo's needle-holders without a rachet, in the dominant hand. Other cannulating forceps can be used, and any microneedle holder without a rachet will suffice perfectly well. The needle must be grasped bevel upwards and may be bent upwards at its mid-point if the lymphatic is deep and there is a large skin overhang. The surgeon's hands should rest comfortably on the opposite foot or operating table for stability, and a pair of strong non-tooth forceps is held in the non-dominant hand. With the surgeon watching carefully through the microscope, the lymphatic is stabilized and pulled taught and straight with the forceps in the non-dominant hand while the needle-holders are used to gently puncture the lymphatic with the needle, and thread the needle a few millimetres into its lumen. The initial resistance to puncture is quite marked but once the lumen has been entered, which can be confirmed by seeing dye run back into the transparent extension tubing, the resistance to feeding the needle along the lymphatic is minimal. It is important to watch the whole process carefully through the operating microscope to ensure that the needle does not pass straight through the anterior and posterior walls

of the lymphatic and lie behind its posterior surface as it is advanced.

Once the needle has been safely located in and threaded up the lymphatic, the assistant removes the obstructing haemostat and the pump is turned on. The lymphatic always collapses and sticks to the needle so it is rarely necessary to tie a ligature around the needle to hold it in the lymphatic and prevent contrast leakage provided a suitable length, i.e. about 2–5 mm, has been dissected and cannulated.

Being right-handed, we prefer to cannulate the right foot first, siting the operating microscope and infusion pump on the patient's left – the surgeon's right. The instrument nurse assists from the right. This allows the radiographer access from the patient's right to place the films beneath the limbs and bring in the portable X-ray machine or image intensifier with C-arm when the instrument trolley is moved out of the way. We feel that there is a lower risk of displacing the needle in the right foot while dissecting the lymphatics of the left foot rather than vice versa. Kinmonth and Rutt[77] designed a Perspex frame to sit over the originally cannulated foot to prevent dislodgment, but this is not necessary and can reduce access to the second side. Vigilance and attention are the best method of avoiding dislodgment. The order of cannulation can be reversed if the surgeon is left-handed, if cannulation is expected to be easy and if there is major lymphatic pathology in the left leg.

The ease or difficulty of the cannulation can often be predicted by a visual lymphogram (see above). Three, four or five blue-green streaks passing up the dorsum of the foot indicate that lymphangiography should be successful, whereas gross dermal backflow indicates that it may be difficult to find a lymphatic for cannulation and that, even if this is successful, the contrast may not pass up the whole length of the limb to the groin.

The start of the infusion of Lipiodol should be carefully watched through the operating microscope to ensure that the needle does not become dislodged and that contrast (seen as fatty droplets) does not leak out excessively around the puncture site. Fatty droplets will occasionally be seen coming out through a puncture in the lymphatic inadvertently caused during the process of threading up the needle. This will stop if the needle is advanced beyond the leakage point. Advancement is easy when the lymphatic is full of oil.

The machine has 10 speeds of delivery. After cannulation, we usually start at speed 7 and increase to speed 5 or 6 (which delivers about 1 mL Lipiodol into the lymphatic every 8 minutes); the fastest speeds deliver 1 mL every 4–5 minutes. The needle will be blown back out of the lymphatic if the infusion is started at too fast a rate, for example 5 or 6 on the Lund injector, or if the needle has not been threaded far enough up the lymphatic.

When the infusion is proceeding satisfactorily, the lower leg should be screened or a plain radiograph taken to check that the contrast medium is filling the lymphatics between the ankle and the knee. Alternatively, if the surgeon is convinced that the needle is correctly positioned, the opposite limb can be cannulated before starting to take plain radiographs of both lower limbs. We prefer to take large-dimension plain radiographs of the legs as these can demonstrate all the afferent lymphatic channels between the ankle and the groin on two radiographs. An image intensifier with spot films as a permanent record is a less acceptable alternative.

Once 1–2 mL Lipiodol have been injected and the lymphatics filled up to the groin on both sides, the rate of infusion can be increased to 6 or 7 on the Lund pump provided there is no suggestion of a proximal obstruction. A rapid infusion in the presence of blocked proximal lymphatics can cause needle dislodgement and extravasation. Repeat radiographs are taken every 5–10 minutes until the contrast has reached the level of the sacroiliac joints on both sides. No more than 7.5 mL Lipiodol should be injected into each limb unless there is considerable extravasation or leakage around the needle. Exceding the maximum dose of 7.5 mL per limb carries the risk of causing oil pneumonitis (see p. 132).

Failed exploration or cannulation

Persistence, patience and meticulous dissection are the keys to avoiding inadvertent damage to the lymphatic caused by hurried or careless deep incisions and unnecessary handling with forceps. Such an approach will increase the chances of obtaining a successful lymphogram. When no lymphatics can be found in the deep dermis, the incision should be gently deepened towards the synovial coverings of the extensor tendons. A green coloration in these deep tissues suggests that lymphatics may be present, and gentle sharp dissection with the scalpel and pointed microscissors, as described above, should expose the vessel.

The failed cannulation of a lymphatic of an abnormal limb should not deter exploration of the 'normal' side as useful information on its lymphatic drainage and the proximal pathways through the para-aortic nodes, cisterna chyli and thoracic duct should be obtained. The chance of the successful cannulation of a single abnormal lymphatic in a severely lymphoedematous limb is probably better at the beginning of an operating list than at the end. Colourless microvessels that have not taken up the Patent Blue Violet can sometimes be seen and cannulated, but these rarely extend for any distance up the leg. Occasionally, the lymphatics, although filled with dye, are so small, thin walled and tortuous that they cannot be cannulated.

On rare occasions, no vessels can be found after prolonged and careful dissection for more than an hour. Such circumstances suggest severe distal hypoplasia or even possibly true congenital lymphatic aplasia. There are two possibilities at this stage: the procedure can be abandoned, with or without biopsy of the skin and

subcutaneous tissues for immunohistochemistry (see Chapter 6), or a further transverse incision can be made in the groin and a dye-filled lymphatic, or more often a lymph node, isolated and injected with a low flow of Lipiodol (speeds 10 to 8 with the Lund injector). This has the potential to outline the proximal lymphatic channels even when there is atrophy or disappearance of the distal vessels. The incision for this approach is made parallel to and 2 cm below the inguinal ligament, unless an obviously large lymph gland is palpable, when the incision should be centred over it. In obese individuals, the lymphangiogram needle and tubing can be brought into the wound through a separate stab incision below the main wound to make the angle of cannulation easier. Groin and pelvic radiographs should be obtained after 10–15 minutes of infusion to check the passage of contrast up the lymphatics.

When the para-aortic nodes have been adequately filled with Lipiodol, the needle is removed, and a small wedge or Tru-cut biopsy of the lymph gland is taken. The gland should not be excised as this may exacerbate the lymphoedema.

Thoracic duct visualization

When the iliac and lumbar lymphatics have been filled with Lipiodol, elevation and massage of the medial side of the legs from distal to proximal along the course of the lymphatics will drive the contrast medium up into the thoracic duct of normal individuals and of patients with lymphoedema in whom there is no gross proximal or distal obstruction. Radiographs of the upper abdomen and chest should be taken 1 and 2 hours after the massage.

It is important to demonstrate the thoracic duct if an enteromesenteric bridge bypass is being considered or if there is evidence of chylothorax, chylous ascites or any form of reflux, in which abnormalities of the thoracic duct are common. Noradrenaline (norepinephrine) solution 10 mL 1:200 000 strength injected around the termination of the thoracic duct in the supraclavicular fossa improves the visualization of the duct's middle and lower sections,[82] but we rarely use this technique.

Other sites of injection

The dorsum of the foot is by far the most used site for injecting a radio-opaque contrast medium and has already been described in detail. The other sites that may be used are described briefly below.

Ankle

Patent Blue Violet may be injected subcutaneously in front of and behind the ankle on both its medial and lateral aspects. Deeper injections can be placed around the origin of the short saphenous vein to outline the lymphatics of the popliteal fossa and the medial inguinal lymph glands. Deep lymphatics within the posterior tibial vascular bundle occasionally outline with dye and can be explored and cannulated.

Inguinal region

Exploration of this area has already been described above. This approach is most often used when the no lymphatics are found in the foot, the cannulation of abnormal lymphatics has failed or the Lipiodol has only passed a short distance up the leg. It is unusual to have to use a groin injection to outline proximal megalymphatics because they usually fill well from a foot injection.

An additional uptake of Patent Blue Violet by the inguinal lymph glands can be achieved by deep injections into the side of the foot, by subcutaneous injections over the course of the long saphenous vein at the level of the knee, and by four or five subcutaneous injections in the thigh about 10 cm below the groin. Local massage, limb elevation and passive joint movements are used to drive the dye up the lymphatics to the groin. This form of visual lymphography, filling the iliac and inguinal lymphatics with dye, is an important precursor to the ligation of incompetent iliac and lumbar lymphatics (see Chapter 16).

The groin lymphatics are exposed through a transverse incision placed 2 cm below and parallel with the inguinal ligament. Contrast is injected directly into any visible lymphatics using the techniques described above; if this is not possible, the needle is inserted directly into a lymph gland.

Spermatic cord

There are very few indications for spermatic cord lymphography. In the 1970s, Kinmonth and McBrien[83] studied the testicular lymphatics of patients with hydroceles (see p. 229) and found them to be defective. There was also period when testicular lymphography was used to detect the spread of testicular cancer to the para-aortic lymph glands,[84] but the advent of CT and magnetic resonance imaging (MRI) has made this technique largely obsolete. The technique is as follows. Patent Blue Violet is injected into the tunica albuginea, which has been exposed through a small incision on the scrotum. The spermatic cord is then exposed via a separate inguinal incision and a lymphatic lying within the internal spermatic fascia, alongside the blood vessels, cannulated and injected.

Cervical region

The patient should be placed on an X-ray table in a full lateral position with the head supported on a head ring. Patent Blue Violet is injected at several points in the subcutaneous tissues over the upper part of the mastoid process. An incision is made over the tip of the mastoid process or just below the angle of the jaw, and the operating microscope is used to define and dissect out a suitable lymphatic, which is then cannulated. The infusion should be at a slow rate (8 or 9 with the Lund pump). Adequate

filling is usually achieved with 2–3 mL Lipiodol.[85] Lymphatics on the floor of the mouth may also be cannulated following submucosal injections of dye.

Upper limb and axilla

The patient is placed supine on a radiolucent table with the arm supported on a side-table. Patent Blue Violet is injected into the web spaces between the fingers, and additional booster injections can be made over the course of the arm lymphatics (see p. 37). An incision is made on the dorsum of the hand mid-way between the heads of the metacarpals and the wrist joint. The technique of cannulation is the same as that described for the lower limb – careful dissection and cannulation using the operating microscope. When detailed images of the axillary nodes are required, a more proximal injection can be made into a lymphatic in the antecubital fossa, but we have rarely found this to be necessary. Infusions of Lipiodol in the upper limb need to be slower to avoid extravasation from rupture of the more fragile arm lymphatics (e.g. Lund pump speed 8 or 9). Only 2–3mL contrast is required to fill all the arm lymphatics and axillary and supraclavicular lymph glands.

Mesentery

Mesenteric lymphangiography is used to investigate the feasibility of the enteromesenteric bridge bypass operation[86] and to investigate patients with chylous ascites and protein-losing enteropathy.

A loop of intestine is brought out onto the surface of the abdomen through a laparotomy wound and 0.5 mL Patent Blue Violet injected beneath the serosa. This is quickly taken up by the mesenteric lymphatics, which can easily be dissected out and cannulated using an operating microscope. Cannulation is helped by fixing the lymphatic by underrunning it with a heavy suture; a large artery forcep is then hung on the end of the suture to stretch the lymphatic out. The bowel is also stabilized by this manoeuvre. Radiographs can be taken through the operating table if it is radiolucent or by placing sterile films directly behind the intestine. Lipiodol 1 mL injected very slowly is usually sufficient to outline all the lymphatics of the mesentery and will often also outline the cisterna chyli and thoracic duct. The anaesthetist should be asked to stop respiratory movements when the radiographs are taken.

Completion procedures

Radiographs should be taken in the theatre until the Lipiodol injection is complete (7.5 mL to each leg, i.e. 15 mL maximum). By this stage, contrast should have reached the sacroiliac joints on both sides unless the distal lymphatics are completely obliterated or there is a proximal lymph gland obstruction. Kinmonth[77] felt that a figure of 35 minutes should be taken as the upper limit of 'normal' for the satisfactory transit of Lipiodol to this site in patients with normal lymphatics at infusion speeds of 7 with the Lund injector. We do not place great credence on transit times but ensure that the contrast has reached this level by taking an appropriate series of pelvic and abdominal radiographs.

Once the infusion has been completed and the final abdominal radiograph taken, the needle is pulled out of the lymphatic (which can be sent for biopsy or culture) and the skin wound sutured with interrupted non-absorbable stitches or a subcuticular stitch. The patient is then sent to the recovery room where further radio-graphs are taken of the abdomen and thoracic duct over the next few hours (see above). The staff in the recovery room should be warned that the blue-green appearance of the patient is a consequence of the Patent Blue Violet rather than cyanosis, although it must of course be remembered that patients can also become cyanotic. The patient is returned to the ward when fully awake.

The following day, further radiographs are taken of the pelvis, abdomen and chest to display the filling patterns of the lymph glands in these regions. These 24 hour lymphadenographs complete the examination. Patients are allowed home after the findings have been discussed with them and a plan for their future management has been formulated. Postoperative pain control rarely needs more than a simple oral non-steroidal analgesic. Non-absorbable skin sutures should be removed one week later.

Complications

The following complications are rare and mostly avoidable.

Allergy to Patent Blue Violet

Blue, itching wheals and facial swelling have been reported in 15 patients out of 16000 investigations.[87] Kinmonth[77] recorded six cases at St Thomas' Hospital, but we have not seen a single case in recent years, perhaps because we use a filter when we draw up the Patent Blue Violet. The allergy rate is also minimized by using less than the maximum recommended dose of 2.5 mL. Should an allergic reaction occur, the patient should be given antihistamines or, if the symptoms are severe, cortisone and subcutaneous adrenaline (epinephrine).

Allergy to Lipiodol

Patients with an iodine sensitivity may develop an urticarial rash (Fig. 6.18). We have never seen the more severe reactions such as facial swelling, bronchial constriction and circulatory collapse. Such reactions should be treated with antihistamines, intravenous steroids and subcutaneous adrenaline, depending upon their severity.

Exacerbation of the lymphoedema

Many have suggested that lymphography may make lymphoedema worse because, they claim, Lipiodol inflames and blocks the lymphatics. We have never seen this and do not consider it a risk of, or contraindication to, the procedure.

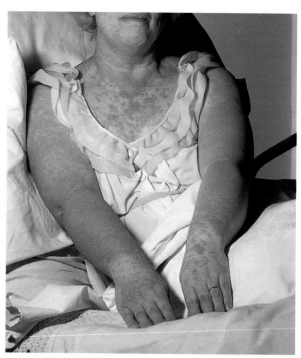

Figure 6.18 *A red urticarial rash that developed the day after a lymphogram, probably an allergic reaction to Lipiodol.*

Wound infection and cellulitis

This is extremely rare and we do not routinely prescribe prophylactic antibiotics.

Deep vein thrombosis and pulmonary embolism

We are unaware of any such cases occurring in our own practice or that of others and do not routinely prescribe prophylactic anticoagulation.

Oil pneumonitis

If an excessive amount of Lipiodol is injected into the lymphatic system, it passes via the thoracic duct into the great veins, through the right side of the heart and into the lungs via the pulmonary artery. Here the oily contrast medium is trapped in the pulmonary capillaries and behaves like a mild diffuse form of 'fat embolism'. This may cause a ventilation–perfusion mismatch and can occasionally cause severe respiratory embarrassment, particularly in patients with clinically significant pre-existing lung disease.

Although animal experiments carried out in 1964[88] suggested that doses of less than 0.3 mL/kg body weight of Lipiodol were safe, and by inference that in man up to 20 mL Lipiodol would be unlikely to cause problems, we advise that a total dose of 12–15 mL should never be exceeded. Caution, and smaller amounts, should be used when performing a lymphogram in patients with severe respiratory disease, pleural effusions or cardiac failure, as well as in young children. Patients with megalymphatics require larger doses of Lipiodol to fill their lymphatics, but the volume of contrast given to these patients must be carefully monitored.

Patients with lymphovenous shunts are another group at high risk. If an obvious 'caviar sign' (*see* p. 134) is seen on an early radiograph, it is wise to limit or terminate the injection. A mistaken injection of the Lipiodol directly into a small vein in the belief that it is a lymphatic is another potential hazard for the inexperienced lymphographer but should be detected by the first-check radiograph.

The diagnosis of pulmonary Lipiodol embolism is made when minute globules of oil scattered through the lungs can be seen on a chest radiograph (Fig. 6.19). The patient's oxygen saturation monitoring should then be carefully monitored. There is no specific treatment. Heparin and steroids may be given, more in hope than proven expectation. Oxygen should be administered through a face mask, and chest physiotherapy started at once. Antibiotics probably do no harm and may prevent secondary bacterial pneumonitis. Severe problems may require a period of artificial ventilation, but we have never seen a patient who has required this. The Lipiodol eventually breaks down and is cleared from the lungs, probably by monocytes.

Cerebral oil embolism

This has only been recorded in patients who have had radiotherapy to their lung fields, for example for lymphoma,[89,90] which presumably, by reducing the filtering efficiency of the pulmonary capillaries, allows the Lipiodol to enter the systemic circulation and the cerebral arteries. In such patients, the risk should be minimized by limiting the volume of Lipiodol injected.

Extravasation of Lipiodol

The extravasation of Lipiodol into the subcutaneous tissues does not cause any problems. Extravasation was a source of complications when radioactive material and BCG vaccine were injected into the lymphatics as a method of treatment; subcutaneous tissue radionecrosis and tuberculomata were occasionally seen after this type of infusion.

Indications for radiological (X-ray) lymphography

It may appear strange to discuss the indications for X-ray lymphography after describing in detail a technique that is now regarded by many authorities as obsolete as a consequence of the evolution of isotope lymphography (see above). In our opinion, however, there are still clear-cut circumstances when contrast lymphography remains of value.

First, radio-isotope lymphography is now the investigation of first choice for screening patients considered on clinical grounds to have lymphoedema. Most patients benefit psychologically from having their diagnosis confirmed by this investigation, but isotope lymphography can

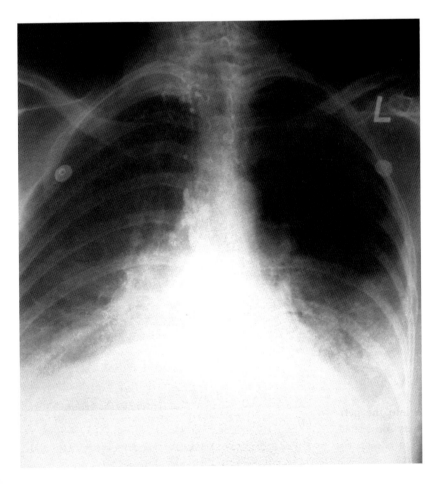

Figure 6.19 *Pulmonary Lipiodol embolism. A chest X-ray showing small droplets of oil throughout the lung fields. This patient had a cough and mild breathlessness for 2 days.*

produce both false-negative and false-positive results,[91] even though its sensitivity and specificity are quite good. Some patients who have clinical lymphoedema have a 'normal' lymphoscintigram. Many of these patients benefit both psychologically and therapeutically from having their diagnosis objectively confirmed or refuted, so we still offer X-ray lymphography to patients in this category.

Second, patients with chylous ascites, chylothorax or any other clinical signs of lymphatic reflux (e.g. skin vesicles, chyluria or chylorrhoea) should have an X-ray lymphogram performed to establish the nature and extent of the lymphatic abnormality and define any potential and actual sites of leakage (*see* Chapters 12 and 16).

Another group of patients who should undergo contrast lymphography are those being considered for a lymphovenous shunt or an enteromesenteric bridge bypass operation for a proximal obstruction indicated by the lymphoscintigram and the clinical findings of a grossly swollen limb with foot sparing (*see* Chapter 10). Some patients request the investigation to ensure that they are not candidates for such an operation.

Finally, some patients with late-onset lymphoedema who are considered to have a potential secondary cause for their lymphoedema may be diagnosed by finding a filling defect in a lymph gland on radiological lymphography even when the CT and MRI scans are normal. When a gland with a filling defect or gross enlargement has to be biopsied, a lymphogram can be a helpful guide to the surgeon and prevent the operation exacerbating the oedema through the removal of too many glands or an enlarged but normal gland.

Although the number of radiological lymphograms carried out at St Thomas' has dropped from more than 100 to fewer than 10 per year since we introduced lymphoscintigraphy, we still find it an essential investigation when choosing the correct management for a small group of carefully selected patients.

Normal lymphographic appearances

The normal cadaveric and radiological anatomy of the peripheral and central lymphatics has been fully described in Chapter 2.

Unusual lymphography appearances caused by technical errors

Extravasation

A normal subcutaneous lymphatic filled with Lipiodol is approximately 1 mm in diameter and has a smooth outline. A lymphatic may rupture if the Lipiodol is injected into it too quickly. Lipiodol spreading into the perilymphatic tissues gives the lymphatic an irregular, dilated, ragged-edged appearance (Fig. 6.20). If this is seen, the rate of injection must be reduced.

Intravenous injections

When Lipiodol is mistakenly injected into the bloodstream via a small vein, the oil breaks up into droplets and produces an X-ray appearance known as the 'caviar sign' (Fig. 6.21). Before the oil has fragmented, the vessel just looks larger than normal, but the injection should be stopped if later films show that the oil has broken up into droplets or that the oil has left the vessel within minutes. The site of the injection should then be examined and the needle removed and inserted into a lymphatic.

The appearance of the 'caviar sign' in the proximal parts of the limb or pelvis indicates the presence of a rare primary lymphovenous shunt (Fig. 6.22).[92] These shunts occasionally allow sufficient oil to pass through them to cause serious oil embolism.

Perivenous injections

If the lymphogram needle is inserted in the adventitia of a small vein, the Lipiodol spreads over the surface of the

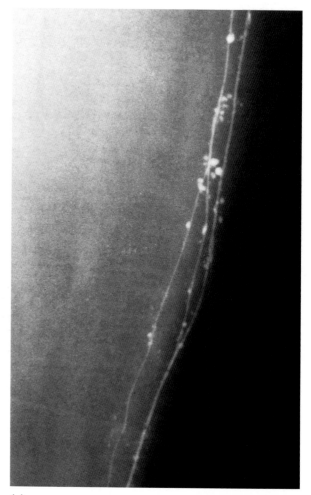

(a)

Figure 6.20 *Extravasation. (a) Lipiodol just beginning to extravasate. It is still in droplet form.*

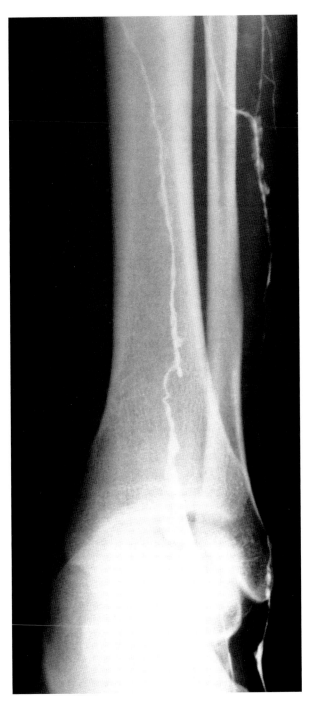

Figure 6.20b *Lipiodol extravasating around a lymphatic, giving it a fluffy, dilated appearance.*

vein (Fig. 6.23). The divisions and branches of the vein make it easy to distinguish this artefact.

Gaps in the contrast

The steady injection of Lipiodol invariably produces a continuous column of oil filling the whole length of the lymphatic. Breaks may appear in this column if the rate of injection rate is slow or intermittent, or if the needle has

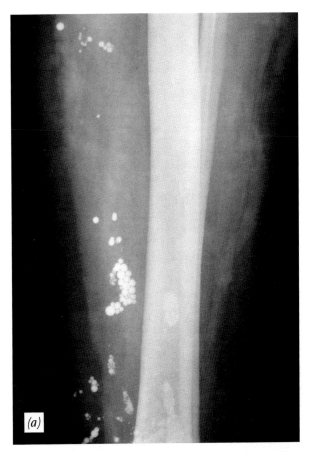

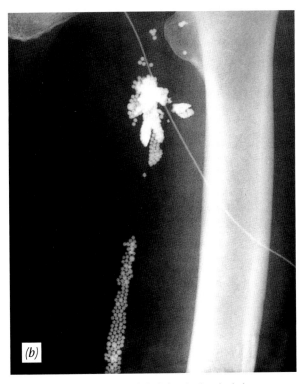

Figure 6.21 *Intravenous Lipiodol – the 'caviar' sign. (a) Lipiodol in the veins of the lower leg. (b) Lipiodol filling the superficial and common femoral veins. The valve cusps are clearly visible.*

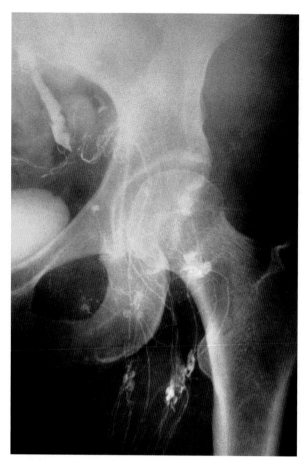

Figure 6.22 *A naturally occuring lymphovenous fistula in the pelvis. The lymphatics in the leg are normal. The Lipiodol has entered and opacified the left internal iliac vein via a lymphovenous shunt. The oil in the vein has not yet broken up into droplets.*

become displaced. Air bubbles can also enter the lymphatic (Fig. 6.24), causing localized segments of non-filling. Major segments of non-filling may occasionally be caused by vessel spasm.

Radiological lymphographic appearances of lymphoedema

Kinmonth *et al.*'s original (1957) classification of primary lymphoedema[93] was based on the lymphographic patterns that he had encountered and observed in more than one thousand lymphograms of patients with lymphoedema. This classification has now been modified to take account of other factors, for example genetic abnormalities (*see* Chapter 5). The different lymphographic appearances are briefly reviewed here but are also discussed in the chapters dealing with each of the individual presentations. It is important to correlate these appearances with the classification and aetiology of lymphoedema presented in Chapters 5 and 7.

Aplasia

There is of course no X-ray lymphographic appearance of aplasia or complete subcutaneous lymphatic obliteration because there are no lymphatics to cannulate.

Distal hypoplasia/peripheral obliteration

The presence of just one or two lymphatics in the lower limb and fewer than five entering the inguinal lymph glands is diagnostic of hypoplasia or partial distal obliteration (Fig. 6.25). This is the most frequent finding in patients with mild distal lymphoedema (60 per cent), most of whom are adolescent females (*see* Chapter 11). More severe forms completely obliterate the main superficial collecting lymphatics, the Lipiodol filling only a fine capillary plexus (Fig. 6.26) and perhaps some normal deep lymphatics. Kinmonth *et al.*[93] called these appearances 'lymphatic hypoplasia', but it is not clear what mechanism – genetic or aquired – is responsible for their development. It is to be hoped that the genetic advances now being made (*see* Chapter 5) will clarify our understanding of their aetiology.

Proximal and distal hypoplasia/obliteration

In the majority of cases with distal hypoplasia/obliteration described above, the proximal lymphatic pathways above the groin are normal, but in patients with severe whole-limb lymphoedema the lymphograph may reveal that both the proximal and the distal pathways are absent (*see* Fig. 6.25, right leg). This may be the result of long-standing proximal obstruction causing a progressive descending obliteration, a 'distal die-back' (*see* Chapter 13), or extensive hypoplasia of the pelvic lymphatics similar to that seen in the limb. As with distal hypoplasia/obliteration, we do not know the primary genetic or pathological causes of this loss of lymphatics but suspect that, in the absence of a family history or known genetic abnormality, most of these patients have an acquired obliteration following a proximal obstruction in their iliac lymph glands (see below).

Proximal obstruction

This abnormality is diagnosed when the distal lymphatic channels in the limb are normal or slightly dilated and tortuous, and the Lipiodol does not pass up beyond the inguinal or iliac lymph glands (Fig. 6.27). This appearance is often associated with severe fibrotic changes in the proximal lymph nodes.[94] Prolonged obstruction may eventually lead to distal lymphatic obliteration (die-back).[95] At an earlier stage, before die-back has occurred, these patients are suitable candidates for an enteromesenteric bypass procedure (*see* Chapter 11).

Congenital proximal obstruction caused by aplasia/hypoplasia of the iliac and lower lumbar lymphatics and lymph glands (Fig. 6.28) is a rare cause of neonatal lymphoedema.

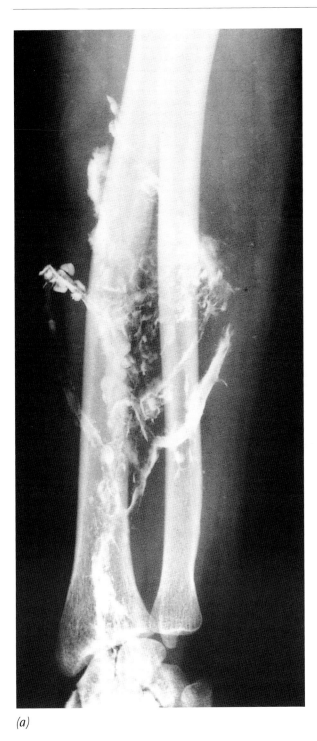

(a)

Figure 6.23 *Perivenous Lipiodol. (a) In this patient, the Lipiodol was accidentally injected beneath the adventitia of a small vein that had been mistaken for a lymphatic. The veins are outlined and recognizable as veins from their branching pattern.*

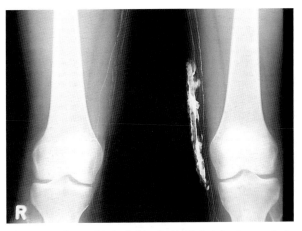

Figure 6.23b *In this individual, the Lipiodol extravasated from a lymphatic into the adventitia of the adjacent long saphenous vein.*

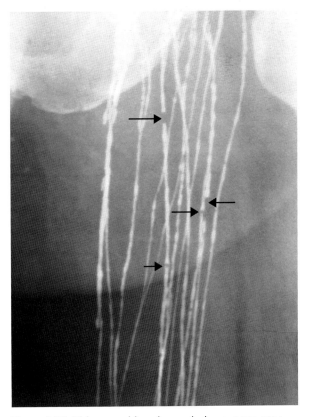

Figure 6.24 *This normal lymphograph shows many gaps (arrowed) in the columns of Lipiodol in the lymphatics. These may be caused by a slow injection, spasm of the vessel or air bubbles.*

Localized distal obstruction

This is much less common than proximal obstruction. The lymphatics (upstream) of the obstruction are distended, slightly dilated and often tortuous. Inverted Y appearances (Fig. 6.29a) are indicative of obstruction because it is caused by Lipiodol back-filling secondarily incompetent tributaries that have not been filled with Lipiodol from below. A fine dilated lymphatic plexus often fills within the local dermis as a consequence of local reflux (Fig. 6.29b). This is the appearance most often seen

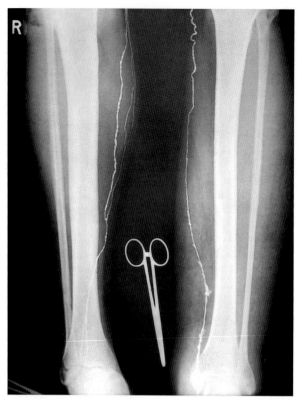 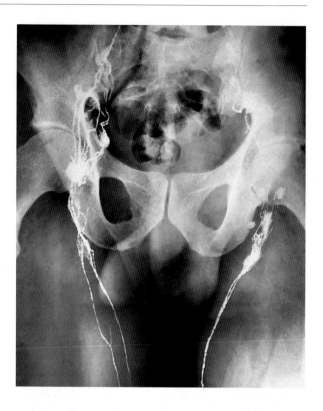

Figure 6.25 *Distal hypoplasia/obliteration. The lymphograph of this patient filled only one lymphatic between the ankle and the groin in the left leg, and two in the right leg (left panel). The lymphatics above the groin on the right-hand side are normal, whereas on the left they are poorly filled but present (right panel). This is an example of distal hypoplasia or obliteration with normal iliac (proximal) vessels. There is no evidence of proximal obstruction, but the poor filling of the iliac lymphatics on the left-hand side may be an indication of early proximal obliteration.*

below a factitious (factitial, artefactual or self-inflicted) oedema produced by a tourniquet (*see* p. 153) or following severe localized skin and subcutaneous tissue injuries.

Increased number of 'normally' sized lymphatics (Kinmonth's numerical hyperplasia)

The lymphangiogram on occasions fills many more than the normal number of lymphatics seen on the lymphograph of a normal leg, and these lymphatics are sometimes slightly wider than normal (Fig. 6.30). Kinmonth[77] found that this appearance was associated with male gender, early-onset lymphoedema, cutaneous angiomata and other associated congenital abnormalities such as distichiasis (*see* p. 104), cleft palate and cardiac defects. The lymph glands may also be increased in number, although often small, especially in the abdomen (Fig. 6.31a, p. 142), and there may be an associated abnormality of the thoracic duct (Fig. 6.31b, p. 142).

It is debatable whether this is a separate phenotypic abnormality or merely represents upstream changes produced by a genetic, partially obstructing, abnormality of the thoracic duct. As genetic abnormalities have been found in association with the lymphoedema–distichiasis syndrome, this pattern of lymphatic hyperplasia may be caused by a specific phenotype (*see* p. 104).

Megalymphatics

Large, dilated incompetent lymphatics, commonly called megalymphatics (Fig. 6.32, p. 143), are easy to recognize. They are usually unilateral and associated with the many clinical syndromes of lymphatic reflux – skin vesicles, chylous ascites, chyluria and chylothorax. Large dilated lymphatics are usually present in the pelvis, abdomen and chest as well as the limbs (*see* Chapters 12 and 16). Concomitant congenital abnormalities of the thoracic duct are common.

There may be a degree of overlap between megalymphatics and numerical hyperplasia, but it is unclear whether they have a similar aetiology (see above). Patients with megalymphatics rarely have a family history of similarly affected members or other non-lymphatic congenital abnormalities, a difference from those with numerical hyperplasia, which suggests that the two groups have a different aetiology.

Thoracic duct

Lymphographs of the thoracic duct of patients with lymphoedema may show the duct to be absent (Fig. 6.33, p. 143) or fragmented and replaced by a series of collaterals. It may, in association with lumbar and pelvic

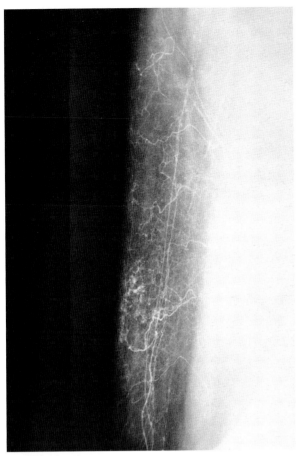

Figure 6.26 *The main collecting vessels in this leg were completely obliterated from just above mid-calf level. The Lipiodol has filled the smaller subdermal and dermal pre-collectors.*

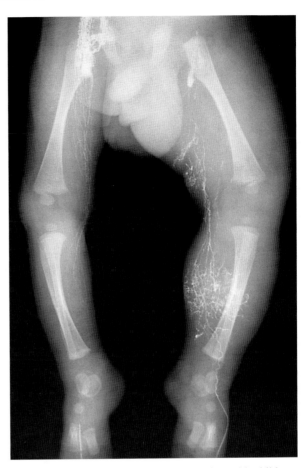

Figure 6.28 *Congenital proximal obstruction. This child presented soon after birth with lymphoedema of the leg on the right. The lymphograph shows dilated tortuous lymphatics in the leg and no lymphatics or lymph glands above the groin.*

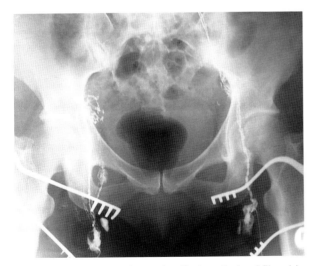

Figure 6.27 *Proximal obstruction (by lymph gland fibrosis). The lymphatics in the limbs of this patient were present, albeit reduced in number, but the Lipiodol did not ascend beyond the groin. When further injections were given into the inguinal lymph glands, the lymphangiograph revealed almost complete obliteration of the pelvic lymphatics and a few small lymph glands.*

megalymphatic changes, be grossly dilated and incompetent (*see* Chapters 12 and 16).

Summary

The four main lymphographic appearances associated with lymphoedema are summarized in Fig. 6.34, p.144. Their recognition is important for diagnosis and clinical management, but they may no longer be the best way of separating the different phenotypes that exist (*see* Chapter 5).

Comment

Contrast radiological lymphography is no longer part of the routine investigation of patients with lymphoedema. It is, however, still helpful in certain circumstances, and it is essential that those who deal with lymphatic problems are fully acquainted with the technique, normal appearances and abnormalities and artefacts described in this chapter. Further information is provided in individual sections throughout the book.

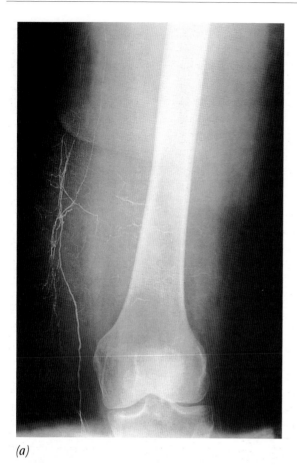

(a)

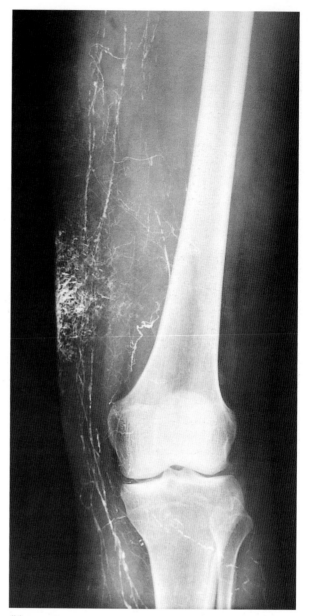

(b)

Figure 6.29 *Factitious (factitial, artefactual or self-inflicted) distal obstruction. (a) The soft tissues are indented at the site at which the patient tied a tourniquet. The lymphatics below this level show some retrograde flow and the inverted-Y appearance (see text). (b) The lymphograph of a similar patient showing extensive retrograde flow into the dermal lymphatic plexus below the level of obstruction. The lymphatics above the level of the tourniquet are not entirely normal because the level at which the tourniquet was applied varied.*

Place of contrast lymphography in the diagnosis of secondary lymphoedema

Most secondary lymphoedemas are caused by obstruction within or destruction of the lymph glands at the root of a limb. The lymphographic signs of lymphatic obstruction are upstream dilatation, tortuosity and 'hair-pin' bends, and collateral filling. The cause of the obstruction, such as filling defects seen within enlarged lymph glands or the complete non-filling or absence of the glands, may be visible.

Extensive malignant disease

Lymphomata rarely produce lymphoedema, but when they do, they are recognized by generalized nodal enlargement associated with a diffuse reticular pattern and scattered filling defects (Fig. 6.35, p. 145).

Extensive malignant infiltration by secondary malignant disease may prevent any Lipiodol entering a lymph gland. In the past, this was detected by surgical biopsy, but it can now be demonstrated by CT, MRI and positron emission tomography. These tests, followed by the guided needle biopsy of any enlarged lymph glands, have replaced lymphography in patients suspected on clinical grounds to have a secondary lymphoedema. A malignant cause of lymphoedema should be suspected if, on lymphography, the lymphatics remain opacified after 24 hours, if they have an unusual course and if the lymph glands are unusually dense or in unusual sites and/or have filling defects or a reticular pattern.

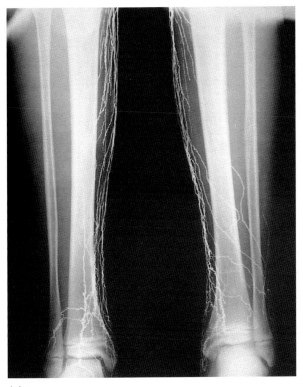

(a)

Figure 6.30 *An increased number of lymphatics. These lymphographs from a patient with distichiasis shows more than the normal number of lymphatics in the leg (a) and thigh (b) (numerical hyperplasia).*

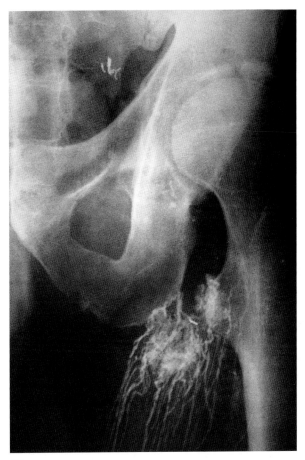

(b)

Radiation

Radiation reduces the size of normal lymph lymphatics, but their shape and pattern is usually preserved (Fig. 6.36, p.145). Excessively high doses of irradiation have to be given to normal glands before the passage of Lipiodol is impeded. This is not, however, the case if the glands contain secondary tumour, when tumour cell destruction can result in massive fibrosis and lymph gland obliteration. The lymphatics upstream of the glands have the features of obstruction or appear as an abnormal plexus of dilated collaterals.

Surgical lymph gland excision

The en bloc excision of lymph glands performed as part of the treatment of breast cancer (*see* p. 235), cervical cancer and malignant melanoma can also cause lymphoedema. Patients often receive additional adjuvant chemotherapy and radiotherapy after these procedures, and it is important, albeit quite difficult, to know whether a late onset of lymphoedema is the result of treatment or of recurrence of the tumour in the lymph glands. Lymphography is rarely used to demonstrate recurrent disease in the glands because secondary deposits need to be at least 1 cm in diameter to be detected on a lymphadenograph and the sensitivity of lymphadenography

in this respect is low, but patients with swollen legs following a Wertheim's hysterectomy are occasionally considered for an enteromesenteric bridge operation providing recurrence can be excluded and X-ray lymphography demonstrates a proximal occlusion with retained distal channels (Fig. 6.37, p.145).

Filarial disease

There are no specific lymphangiographic appearances associated with filariasis other than those that occur upstream of an obstruction, i.e. dilatation, tortuosity and collateral filling (*see* Chapter 15). The inguinal lymph glands are usually enlarged and may show patchy infiltration. The lumbar lymphatics are often large, tortuous and incompetent. The lumbar lymph glands are poorly filled, and there is frequently an associated abnormality of the thoracic duct.

Other infections and inflammations may produce the non-specific changes of distal lymphatic obstruction and lymph gland enlargement. Filling defects are unusual.

Comment

Lymphography no longer has a major role in determining the cause of secondary lymphoedema. When, however, it is difficult to know whether a patient has a primary

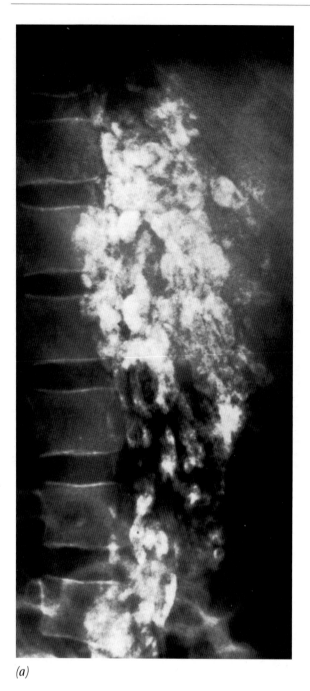

(a)

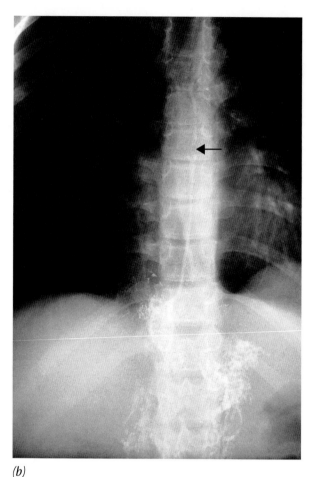

(b)

Figure 6.31 *(a) Lateral abdominal lymphograph of a patient with an increased number of lymphatics in the leg and other congenital malformations, showing a large mass of hyperplastic lumbar lymph glands. (b) The abnomal, partially obstructed thoracic duct (arrowed), with collateral vessels running along the right 11th rib, of the same patient.*

or secondary cause for the lymphoedema, and when the cross-section or radiological tests such as CT and MRI are inconclusive or unhelpful, lymphography can still be of value.

NUCLEAR MAGNETIC RESONANCE IMAGING

MRI produces excellent soft tissue images and can distinguish between fat and water, a common clinical conundrum in the differential diagnosis of lymphoedema. MRI can demonstrate a number of characteristic features of

lymphoedema (Fig. 6.38, p. 146):[96]

- a thickened skin;
- a honeycomb or 'loofah sponge' reticular pattern in the swollen subcutis;
- lakes of free fluid surrounded by fibrosis in the subcutis;
- dilated lymphatic channels related to either lymph reflux or lymphangiomata (intravenous contrast being needed to distinguish these from blood vessels).

MRI scanning can be particularly useful for diagnosing lymphoedema in infants and small children in whom lymphoscintigraphy or X-ray lymphography is inappropriate.

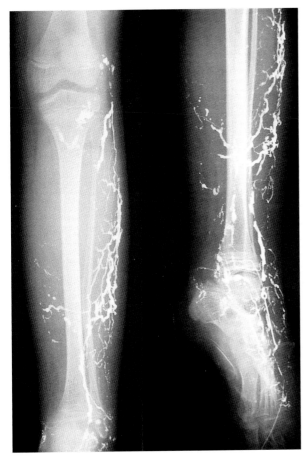

Figure 6.32 *The megalymphatics of a patient with unilateral lymphoedema and leaking vesicles on the foot.*

It is also useful for differentiating pure lymphoedema from swelling caused by expansion of the subfascial compartment following a deep vein thrombosis.[97] Lipoedema exhibits a diffuse homogenous increase in the amount of subcutaneous fat beneath a skin of normal thickness. Factors limiting the use of MRI are the size of the patient and the limb, and claustrophobia.

COMPUTED TOMOGRAPHY

CT is cheaper and more readily available than MRI but otherwise has few advantages (Fig. 6.39, p. 146). A single axial CT slice through the mid-calf has been recommended in the differential diagnosis of a swollen leg.[98] CT not only provides information on volume change through cross-sectional area views, but can also identify the compartment in which the change has occurred. Lymphoedema produces a prominent honeycomb pattern. As with MRI, CT images may reveal the features of an alternative diagnosis such as an increased cross-sectional area of the muscle compartment following venous obstruction, an increased subcutaneous fat layer in obesity and lipoedema, fluid collections between the muscle planes from the extension

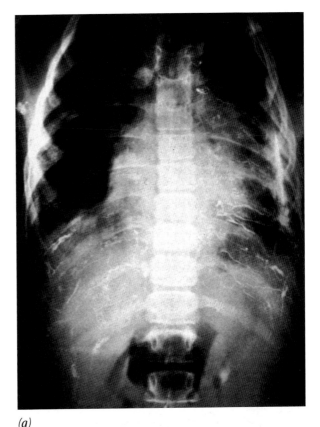

(a)

(b)

Figure 6.33 *Thoracic duct occlusion. (a) An absent or occluded thoracic duct with intercostal, paravertebral and axillary collaterals. (b) Profuse filling of the paravertebral, mediastinal and axillary glands related to the collateral pathways filled in (a).*

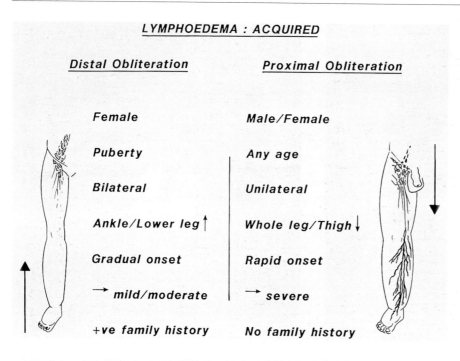

LYMPHOEDEMA : ACQUIRED

Distal Obliteration	*Proximal Obliteration*
Female	Male/Female
Puberty	Any age
Bilateral	Unilateral
Ankle/Lower leg ↑	Whole leg/Thigh ↓
Gradual onset	Rapid onset
→ mild/moderate	→ severe
+ve family history	No family history

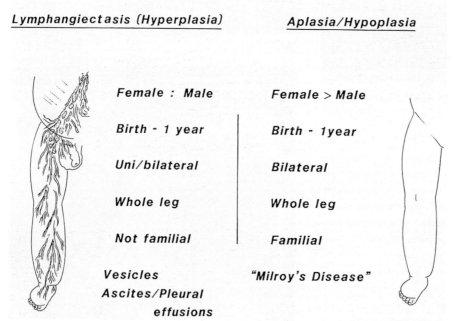

LYMPHOEDEMA : CONGENITAL

Lymphangiectasis (Hyperplasia)	*Aplasia/Hypoplasia*
Female : Male	Female > Male
Birth - 1 year	Birth - 1year
Uni/bilateral	Bilateral
Whole leg	Whole leg
Not familial	Familial
Vesicles Ascites/Pleural effusions	"Milroy's Disease"

Figure 6.34 *The four common lymphographic appearances of lymphoedema.*

or rupture of a popliteal cyst and areas of high attenuation in the muscles caused by haematomata.

ULTRASOUND

Routine ultrasound (with a 7.5 MHz transducer) can detect the thickened skin of lymphoedema and the expanded subcutaneous compartment. High-frequency ultrasound (20 MHz transducer) increases the resolution of the skin and immediate subcutis image but is limited in terms of depth. Fluid is confined to different parts of the dermis depending on the type of oedema: subepidermal in lipodermatosclerosis (seen as an echogenic band), deep dermal in heart failure and uniformly throughout the dermis in lymphoedema.[99]

BIOPSY

The histopathology of lymphoedema does not possess sufficiently specific features in itself to make tissue biopsy

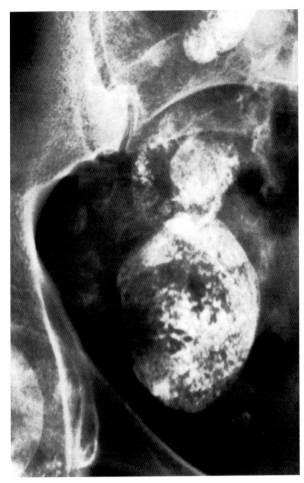

Figure 6.35 *The multiple filling defects and reticular pattern of a gland enlarged by Hodgkin's lymphoma.*

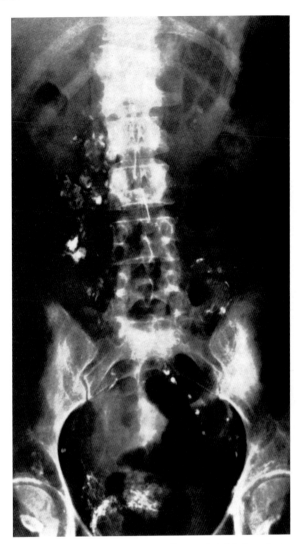

Figure 6.36 *The small dense lumbar and pelvic lymph glands that follow irradiation (in this case for lymphoma).*

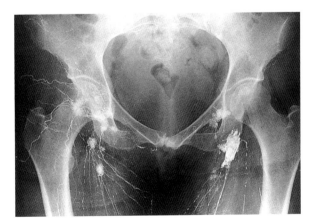

Figure 6.37 *A lymphograph of a patient with bilateral lymphoedema six years after a Wertheim's hysterectomy. No lymph glands are filled above the inguinal ligament. The lymphatics of the leg are irregular, and collateral pathways are developing. There is no evidence of recurrent carcinoma. This patient would be suitable for an enteromesenteric bridge operation.*

diagnostically useful (see Chapter 4 for details of the pathology of lymphoedema), but it can nevertheless be extremely useful on occasions for identifying the cause of lymphoedema. A lymph gland biopsy may, for example, reveal malignant deposits, or a skin biopsy may demonstrate an infiltrating and lymphophilic tumour, for example carcinoma of the breast or ovary, melanoma or malignant eccrine poroma. Similarly, a biopsy exhibiting granulomatous pathology should prompt a search for Crohn's disease or sarcoidosis. Caution should always be exercised in relation to lymph gland biopsy in patients with lymphoedema because of the risk of precipitating cellulitis, exacerbating the oedema or inducing a lymph fistula.

Ulceration is not usually a complication of lymphoedema, as it is with venous disease, unless the skin is under extreme tension from the swelling, papillomatous, hyperkeratotic or fissured. A non-healing ulcer should always be biopsied to exclude malignant change.

Classic methods to visualize lymphatics have included the injection of various materials such as colloidal carbon, vital dyes and oil, but none is a practical adjunct to biopsy in humans. Ultrastructurally, lymphatics possess certain distinguishing features, in particular open junctions and a lack of continuous basement membrane.[100] Few specific features are seen in a haematoxylin and eosin section, although a vessel with angular walls and attenuated endothelium extending some distance across the field of view would suggest a lymphatic. An elastic stain, for example acid orcein or Van Giesen, shows the elastic fibre envelope around the initial lymphatics in normal skin, but the elastic fibres tend to disappear in pathological states.[101]

ENDOTHELIAL MARKERS

There has until recently been no means of positively identifying a lymphatic vessel in a tissue section, which has seriously undermined our knowledge of the contribution of lymphatics to pathology. A number of markers are available for labelling endothelial cells, but the majority (factor VIII-related antigen, CD31 (PECAM-1), *Ulex europaeous* agglutinin-1 and EN4) stain both blood and lymph vessels.

PAL-E monoclonal antibody is the only label that is consistently negative in lymphatic vessels but positive in blood venules and small veins, the vessels most likely to be mistaken for lymphatics. Lymphatic vessels can therefore be identified only through double staining with CD31+/PAL-E−. A high activity of the enzymes 5′-nucleotidase, adenylate and guanylate cyclase has been reported specifically in lymphatic endothelial cells.[102]

New molecules have very recently been identified that allow a more precise distinction between lymphatic and blood vascular endothelium. VEGFR-3, an antibody to the receptor for the vascular endothelial growth factor-C (VEGF-C), has been shown to label lymphatic endothelium selectively in several normal tissues and certain vascular tumours. From this work, it now seems likely that Kaposi's sarcoma has lymphatic origins.[103] A hyaluronan receptor termed LYVE-1 has been shown to be restricted to lymphatic vessels in a number of normal tissues. Expression is strong in human skin and reveals a remarkably rich lymphatic network.[104]

NOTE

The sections on lymphoscintigraphy and indirect X-ray lymphography were written by Hugo Partsch, Professor of Dermatology, Department of Medicine, University of Vienna, Austria.

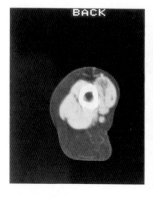

Figure 6.38 *Magnetic resonance imaging scan: longitudinal section (STIR sequence) showing bright areas of dilated lymph-filled lymphatics and interstitial tissues.*

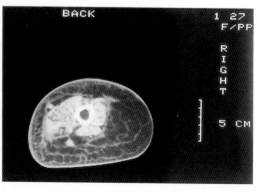

Figure 6.39 *Computed tomography cross-sectional images at thigh level in a patient with unilateral lymphoedema: normal thigh (left) compared with swollen thigh (right). There is increased skin thickness and swelling of the subcutaneous compartment with the 'honeycomb' pattern indicative of lymphoedema.*

REFERENCES

1. Stemmer R. Ein klinisches Zeichen zur Früh- und Differential-Diagnose des Lymphödems. *Vasa* 1976; **5:** 261–2.
2. Tobin MB, Lacey HJ, Meyer L, Mortimer PS. The psychological morbidity of breast cancer-related arm swelling. *Cancer* 1993; **72:** 3248–52.
3. Price EW. Podoconiosis: non-filarial elephantiasis. Oxford: Oxford University Press, 1990.
4. Casley-Smith JR, *et al.* Summary of the 10th International Congress of Lymphology working group discussions and recommendations, Adelaide, Australia. *Lymphology* 1985; **18:** 175–80.
5. Olszewski WL, *et al.* Bacteriological studies of skin tissue fluid and lymph in filarial lymphoedema. *Lymphology* 1994; **27:** 345–8.
6. Kumaraswami V. The clinical manifestations of lymphatic filariasis. In: Nutman TB ed. *Lymphatic filarasis.* London: Imperial College Press, 2000: 103–25.
7. Krywonis N, Kaye VN, Lynch PJ. Cryptococcal cellulitis in congenital lymphoedema. *International Journal of Dermatology* 1990; **29:** 41–4.
8. Stanton AWB, Badger C, Sitzia J. Non-invasive assessment of the lymphoedematous limb. *Lymphology* 2000; **33:** 122–35.
9. Bates DO, Levick JR, Mortimer PS. Starling pressures in the human arm and their alteration in postmastectomy oedema. *Journal of Physiology* 1994; **477:** 355–63.
10. Roberts CC, Stanton AWB, Pullen J, *et al.* Skin microvascular architecture and perfusion studied in human postmastectomy oedema by intravital video capillaroscopy. *International Journal of Microcirculation* 1994; **14:** 327–34.
11. Kissin MW, Della Rovere GQ, Easton D, *et al.* Risk of lymphoedema following the treatment of breast cancer. *British Journal of Surgery* 1986; **73:** 580–4.
12. Kettle JH, Rundle FF, Oddie TH. Measurement of upper limb volumes: a clinical method. *Australian and New Zealand Journal of Surgery* 1958; **27:** 263–70.
13. Kaulesar Sukul DMKS, den Hoed PT, Johannes EJ. Direct and indirect methods for the quantification of leg volume: comparison between water displacement, volumetry, the disk model method and the frustum sign model, using the correlation coefficient and the limits of agreement. *Journal of Biomedical Engineering* 1993; **5:** 477–80.
14. Stanton AWB, Northfield JW, Holroyd B, *et al.* Validation of an optoelectronic limb volumeter (Perometer®). *Lymphology* 1997; **30:** 77–97.
15. Stanton AWB, Holroyd B, Northfield JW, *et al.* Forearm blood flow measured by venous occlusion plethysmography in healthy subjects and in women with postmastectomy oedema. *Vascular Medicine* 1998; **3:** 3–8.
16. Badger C. A Study of the Efficacy of Multi-layer Bandaging and Elastic Hosiery in the Treatment of Lymphoedema and their Effects on the Swollen Limb. PhD thesis, University of London, 1997.
17. Clodius L, Deak L, Piller NB. A new instrument for the evaluation of tissue tonicity in lymphoedema. *Lymphology* 1976; **9:** 1–5.
18. Bates DO, Levick JR, Mortimer PS. Quantification of rate and depth of pitting in human edema using an electronic tonometer. *Lymphology* 1994; **27:** 159–72.
19. Roberts CC, Levick JR, Stanton AWB, *et al.* Assessment of truncal oedema following breast cancer treatment using modified Harpenden skinfold calipers. *Lymphology* 1995; **28:** 78–88.
20. Cornish BH, Bunce IH, Ward LC, *et al.* Bioelectrical impedance for monitoring the efficacy of lymphoedema treatment programmes. *Breast Cancer Research and Treatment* 1996; **38:** 169–76.
21. Proby CM, Gane JN, Joseph AE, Mortimer PS. Investigation of the swollen limb with isotope lymphography. *British Journal of Dermatology* 1990; **123:** 29–37.
22. Bollinger A, Partsch H, Wolfe JHN (eds). *The initial lymphatics.* Stuttgart: Thieme, 1985.
23. Bruna J. Computerized tomography, xeroradiography, lymphography, and xerolymphography in diagnosis of lymph stasis. In: Olszewski W ed. *Lymph stasis: pathophysiology, diagnosis and treatment.* Boca Raton: CRC Press, 1991: 412–32.
24. Cluzan R, Pecking A. Radionuclide lymphography. In: Olszewski W ed. *Lymph stasis: pathophysiology, diagnosis and treatment.* Boca Raton: CRC Press, 1991: 398–408.
25. Partsch H. Indirect lymphangiography. In: Olszewski W ed. *Lymph stasis: pathophysiology, diagnosis and treatment.* Boca Raton, FL: CRC Press, 1991: 434–42.
26. Tiedjen KU, Heimann KD, Knorz S. Radiologische Diagnostik bei Gliedmaßenschwellungen. In: Földi M, Kubik S eds. *Lehrbuch der Lymphologie.* Stuttgart: Gustav Fischer, 1999: 406–12.
27. Zum Winkel K, Sheer KE. Scintigraphic and dynamic studies of the lymphatic system with radiocolloids. *Minerva Nucl.* 1965; 390–7.
28. Baulieu F, Vaillant L, Baulieu JL, Secchi V, Barsotti J. The current role of lymphoscintigraphy in the study of lymphedema of the limbs. *Journal Maladie Vasculaire* 1990; **15:** 152–6.
29. Bourgeois P, Leduc O, Leduc A. Imaging techniques in the management and prevention of posttherapeutic upper limb edemas. *Cancer* 1998; **83:** 2805–13.
30. Cambria RA, Bender CE, Hauser MF, Gloviczki P. Lymphoscintigraphy and lymphangiography. In: Gloviczki P, Yao JST eds. *Handbook of venous disorders.* London: Chapman & Hall Medical, 1996.

31. Cambria RA, Gloviczki P, Naessend JM, Wahner HW. Noninvasive evaluation of the lymphatic system with lymphoscintigraphy: a prospective, semiquantitative analysis in 386 extremities. *Journal of Vascular Surgery* 1993; **18**: 773–82.

32. Case TC, Witte CL, Witte MH, Unger EC, Williams WH. Magnetic resonance imaging in human lymphedema: comparison with lymphangioscintigraphy. *Magnetic Resonance Imaging* 1992; **10**: 549–58.

33. Golueke PJ, Montgomery RA, Petronis JD, Minken SL, Perler BA, Williams GM. Lymphoscintigraphy to confirm the clinical diagnosis of lymphedema. *Journal of Vascular Surgery* 1989; **10**: 306–12.

34. Mandell GA, Alexander MA, Harcke HT. A multiscintigraphic approach to imaging of lymphedema and other causes of the congenitally enlarged extremity. *Seminars in Nuclear Medicine* 1993; **23**: 334–46.

35. McNeill GC, Witte MH, Witte CL, *et al.* Whole-body lymphangioscintigraphy: preferred method for initial assessment of the peripheral lymphatic system. *Radiology* 1989; **172**: 495–502.

36. Nawaz MK, Hamad MM, Abdel-Dayem HM. Lymphoscintigraphy in lymphedema of the lower limbs using 99mTc HSA. *Angiology* 1992; **43**: 147–54.

37. Richards TB, McBiles M, Collins PS. An easy method for diagnosis of lymphedema. *Annals of Vascular Surgery* 1990; **4**: 255–9.

38. Rijke AM, Croft BY, Johnson RA, de Jongste AB, Camps JA. Lymphoscintigraphy and lymphedema of the lower extremities. *Journal of Nuclear Medicine* 1990; **31**: 990–8.

39. Ter SE, Alavi A, Kim CK, Merli G. Lymphoscintigraphy: a reliable test for the diagnosis of lymphedema. *Clinical Nuclear Medicine* 1993; **18**: 646–54.

40. Witte CL, Wite MH, Unger EC, *et al.* Advances in imaging of lymph flow disorders. *Radiographics* 2000; **20**: 1697–719.

41. Bräutigam P, Földi E, Schaiper I, Krause T, Vanscheidt W, Moser E. Analysis of lymphatic drainage in various form of leg edema using two compartment lymphoscintigraphy. *Lymphology* 1998; **31**: 43–55.

42. Bräutigam P, Vanscheidt W, Földi E, Krause T, Moser E. The importance of the subfascial lymphatics in the diagnosis of lower limb edema: investigations with semiquantitative lymphoscintigraphy. *Angiology* 1993; **44**: 464–70.

43. Bull RH, Gane JN, Evans JE, Joseph AEA, Mortimer PS. Abnormal lymph drainage in patients with chronic venous leg ulcers. *Journal of the American Academy of Dermatology* 1993; **28**: 585–90.

44. Lofferer O, Mostbeck A, Partsch H. Nuklearmedizinische Diagnostik von Lymphtransportstörungen der unteren Extremitäten. *Vasa* 1972; **1**: 94–101.

45. Mortimer PS. Evaluation of lymphatic function: abnormal lymph drainage in venous disease. *International Angiology* 1995; **14(suppl. 1 to issue 3)**: 32–5.

46. Mostbeck A, Kahn P, Partsch H. Quantitative lymphography in lymphoedema. In: Bollinger A, Partsch H, Wolfe JHN eds. *The initial lymphatics.* Stuttgart: Thieme, 1985: 123–30.

47. Mostbeck A, Partsch H. Isotope lymphography – possibilities and limits in evaluation of lymph transport. *Wiener Medizinische Wochenschrift* 1999; **149**: 87–9.

48. Stewart G, Gaunt JI, Croft DN, Browse NL. Isotope lymphography: a new method of investigating the role of the lymphatics in chronic limb oedema. *British Journal of Surgery* 1985; **72**: 906–9.

49. Alex JC, Weaver DL, Fairbank JT, Rankin BS, Krag DN. Gamma-probe-guided lymph node localization in malignant melanoma. *Surgical Oncology* 1993; **2**: 303–8.

50. Krag DN, Weaver DL, Alex JC, Fairbank JT. Surgical resection and radiolocalization of the sentinel lymph node in breast cancer using a gamma probe. *Surgical Oncology* 1993; **2**: 335–9.

51. Partsch H. Assessment of abnormal lymph drainage for the diagnosis of lymphedema by isotopic lymphangiography and by indirect lymphography. *Clinical Dermatology* 1995; **13**: 445–50.

52. Partsch H. Involvement of the lymphatic system in post-thrombotic syndrome. *Wiener Medizinische Wochenschrift* 1994; **144**: 210–13.

53. Ogawa Y, Hayashi K. 99mTc-DTPA-HSA lymphoscintigraphy in lymphedema of the lower extremities: diagnostic significance of dynamic study and muscular exercise. *Kaku Igaku* 1999; **36**: 31–6.

54. Pecking AP. Evaluation by lymphoscintigraphy of the effect of a micronized flavonoid fraction (Daflon 500 mg) in the treatment of upper limb lymphedema. *International Angiology* 1995; **14**: 39–43.

55. Stöberl C, Partsch H. Congestive lymphostatic papillomatosis. *Hautarzt* 1988; **39**: 441–6.

56. Kleinhans E, Baumeister RG, Hahn D, Siada S, Bell U, Moser E. Evaluation of transport kinetics in lymphoscintigraphy: follow-up study in patients with transplanted lymphatic vessels. *European Journal of Nuclear Medicine* 1985; **10**: 349–52.

57. Gan J-L, Chang T-S, Fu K-D, *et al.* Indirect lymphography with Isovist-300 in various forms of lymphedema. *European Journal of Plastic Surgery* 1991; **14**: 109–13.

58. Gmeinwieser J, Lehner K, Golder W. Indirect lymphography: indications, technique, clinical results. *Fortschrift Geb Röntgenstrahlen Nuklearmedizin* 1988; **149**: 642–7.

59. Partsch H, Urbanek A, Wenzel-Hira BI. The dermal lymphatics in lymphoedema visualized by indirect lymphography. *British Journal of Dermatology* 1984; **110**: 431–8.

60. Partsch H. Indirect lymphography with Iotrolan. *Fortschrift Geb Röntgenstrahlen Nuklearmedizin Erganzungsband* 1989; **128:** 178–81.

61. Weissleder H. Interstitial lymphangiography: initial clinical experience with a dimeric nonionic contrast agent. *Radiology* 1989; **170:** 371–4.

62. Bruna J. Computerized tomography, xeroradiography,lymphography, and xerolymphography in diagnosis of lymph stasis. In: Olszewski W ed. *Lymph stasis: pathophysiology, diagnosis and treatment.* Boca Raton, FL: CRC Press, 1991: 412–32.

63. Partsch H, Bollinger A. Regional hypoplasia of dermal lymphatic vessels – a new variant of congenital lymphoedema. *Wiener Klinische Wochenschrift* 1986; **98:** 704–8.

64. Partsch H, Stöberl C, Urbanek A, Wenzel-Hora BI. Clinical use of indirect lymphography in different forms of leg edema. *Lymphology* 1988; **21:** 152–60.

65. Stöberl C, Partsch H, Wruhs M. Diagnostic value and criteria for evaluating indirect lymphography in lymphoedema. *Vasa* 1990; **19:** 212–17.

66. Wu D, Gibbs J, Corral D, Intengan M, Brooks JJ. Massive localized lymphedema: additional locations and association with hypothyroidism. *Human Pathology* 2000; **31:** 1162–8.

67. Weissleder H. Value of functional lymphoscintigraphy and indirect lymphangiography in lipedema syndrome. *Zeitschrift für Lymphologie* 1995; **19:** 38–41.

68. Piza-Katzer H, Partsch H, Urbanek A, *et al.* Zur Frage der Lymphgefässregeneration nach Replantation und freier mikrovaskulärer Lappenplastik. *Vasa* 1987: **16:** 60–6.

69. Pfister G, Saesseli B, Hoffmann U, Geiger M, Bollinger A. Diameters of lymphatic capillaries in patients with different forms of lymphedema. *Lymphology* 1990; **23:** 140–4.

70. Schultz-Ehrenburg U, Niederauer HH, Tiedjen KU. Stasis papillomatosis. Clinical features, etiopathogenesis and radiological findings. *Journal of Dermatological and Surgical Oncology* 1993; **19:** 440–6.

71. Homans J. Personal communications to JBK. In: Kinmonth JB ed. *The lymphatics,* 2nd edn. London: Arnold, 1982.

72. Courtice FC. Personal communications to JBK. In: Kinmonth JB ed. *The lymphatics,* 2nd edn. London: Arnold, 1982.

73. Hudack SS, McMaster PD. The lymphatic participation in human cutaneous phenomena: a study of the minute lymphatics of the living skin. *Journal of Experimental Medicine* 1933; **57:** 751–74.

74. Kinmonth JB. Lymphangiography in man. *Clinical Science* 1952; **11:** 13–20.

75. Weinberg J, Greanly EM. Identification of regional lymph nodes by means of a vital staining dye during surgery of gastric cancer. *Surgery, Gynecology and Obstetrics* 1950; **90:** 561.

76. Fitzgerald PA. Personal Communications JBK. In: Kinmonth JB ed. *The lymphatics,* 2nd edn. London: Arnold, 1982.

77. Kinmonth JB. *The lymphatics,* 2nd edn. London: Arnold, 1982.

78. Krag DN, Weaver DL, Alex JC, Fairbank JT. Surgical resection and radio localistion of the sentinel lymph node in breast cancer using a gamma probe. *Surgical Oncology* 1993; **2:** 335–40.

79. Wanebo HJ, Harpole D, Teates CD. Radionuclide lymphoscintography with technetium 99m antimony sulphide to identify lymphatic drainage of cutaneous melanoma at ambiguous sites in the head and neck and trunk. *Cancer* 1985; **55:** 1403–13.

80. Brunn S, Engeset A. Lymphadenography. A new method for the visualisation of enlarged nodes and vessels. *Acta Radiologica (Stockholm)* 1961; **45:** 389–97.

81. Clemenz S, Olin T. Apparatus for controlled infusion of saline and angiography and contrast medium in lymphography. *Acta Radiologica (Stockholm)* 1961; **55:** 109–12.

82. Cox SJ, Kinmonth JB. Lymphography of the thoracic duct. *Journal of Cardiovascular Surgery* 1975; **16:** 120–2.

83. McBrien MP, Edwards JM, Kinmonth JB. Lymphography of the testis and its adnexa in the normal and in idiopathic hydrocele. *Archives of Surgery* 1972; **104:** 819–25.

84. Chiappa S, Galli G, Barbaini S, Ravasi G, Bagliani G. La lymphographie par opératoire dans les tumeurs du testicule. *Journal de Radiol Electrol* 1963; **44:** 613.

85. Fisch U. Lymphographische Untersuchungen über das Zervikale Lymphsystem. Basle: S. Karger.

86. Kinmonth JB, Hurst PA, Edwards JM, Rutt DL. Relief of lymph obstruction by use of a bridge of mesentery and ilium. *British Journal of Surgery* 1978; **65:** 829–33.

87. Koehler PR. In: Ruttiman A ed. Progress in lymphology. Stuttgart: Georg Thieme, 1967: 323.

88. Guiney EJ, Gough MH, Kinmonth JB. Lymphography with fat soluble contrast media. *Journal of Cardiovascular Surgery* 1964; **5:** 346–54.

89. Collard M, Leroux G, Noel G, Declerq A. L'embolie cérébrale graisseuse diffuse. Complication de la lymphangiographie lipiodolée. *Journal de Radiologie, de l'Électrologie et de Médecine Nucléaire* 1969; **50:** 793.

90. Kuisk H. *Technique of lymphography.* St Louis: Green, 1971.

91. Burnand KG, McGuiness CL, Lagatolla NRF, Browse NL, El-Aradni A, Nunan T. Value of isotope lymphography in the diagnosis of lymphoedema of the leg. *British Journal of Surgery* 2002; **89:** 74–8.

92. Edwards JM, Kinmonth JB. Lymphovenous shunts in man. *British Medical Journal* 1969; **4**: 579–81.

93. Kinmonth JB, Taylor GW, Tracy GD, Marsh JD. Primary lymphoedema. *British Journal of Surgery* 1957; **45**: 1–10.

94. Kinmonth JB, Wolfe JH. Fibrosis in the lymph nodes in primary lymphoedema. *Annals of the Royal College of Surgeons of England* 1980; **62**: 344–54.

95. Wolfe JH, Fyfe NCM, Kinmonth JB. Die-back in primary lymphoedema; lymphangiographic and clinical correlations. *Lymphology* 1982; **15**: 66–9.

96. Liu N-F, Wang CG. The role of magnetic resonance imaging in the diagnosis of peripheral lymphatic disorders. *Lymphology* 1998; **31**: 119–27.

97. Duewell S. Swollen lower extremity: role of MR imaging. *Radiology* 1992; **184**: 227–31.

98. Vaughan BF. CT of swollen legs. *Clinical Radiology* 1990; **41**: 24–30.

99. Gniadecka M. Localisation of dermal oedema in lipodermatosclerosis, lymphoedema and cardiac insufficiency. *Journal of the American Academy of Dermatologists* 1996; **35**: 37–41.

100. Braverman IM. Ultrastructure and organisation of the cutaneous microvasculature in normal and pathologic states. *Journal of Investigative Dermatology* 1989; **93**: 2–9S.

101. Mortimer PS, Cherry GW, Jones RL, Barnhill RL, Ryan TJ. The importance of elastic fibres in skin lymphatics. *British Journal of Dermatology* 1983; **108**: 561–6.

102. Weber E, Lurenzoni P, Lozzi G, Sacchi G. Cytochemical differentiation between blood and lymphatic endothelium: bovine blood and lymphatic large vessels and endothelial cells in culture. *Journal of Histochemistry and Cytochemistry* 1994; **42**: 1109–15.

103. Jussila L, Valtola RO, Partanen TA, *et al.* Lymphatic endothelium and Kaposi's sarcoma spindle cells detected by antibodies against the vascular endothelial growth factor receptor-3. *Cancer Research* 1990; **58**: 1599–604.

104. Banerji S, Ni J, Wang S-X, *et al.* LYVE-1, a new homologue of the CD44 glycoprotein, is a lymph-specific receptor for hyaluronan. *Journal of Cell Biology* 1999; **144**: 789–801.

7

Aetiology and classifications of lymphoedema

Most disease classifications are based on a knowledge of the aetiology and basic pathology of the abnormality being classified. For lymphoedema, that knowledge is often sadly deficient so most of its many classifications are determined by whatever particular aspect of lymphoedema the classifier wishes to emphasize. Consequently, there are clinical, lymphographic, pathological and aetiological classifications that often overlap and confuse.

All classifications also depend upon an agreed definition of the condition being classified. Many of the earlier investigators defined lymphoedema in a manner that is now unacceptable. For example, the seminal standard textbook on peripheral vascular disease, written in 1946 by Allen, Barker and Hines,[1] which summed up the views of the angiologists of the first half of the twentieth century, subdivided all cases of chronic lymphoedema into two main categories: non-inflammatory and inflammatory. The inflammatory group was divided into primary and secondary, and included oedema caused by tissue inflammation rather than lymphatic insufficiency. Such cases are excluded by the modern definition of lymphoedema. It is therefore essential to define lymphoedema before attempting to classify it.

DEFINITION

Lymphoedema is defined as:

> the accumulation of lymph in the interstitial spaces caused by the failure of the lymph-conducting system (lymphatics and lymph glands) to accept and/or conduct lymph back to the blood circulation.

Put another way, all the conditions that cause lymphoedema interfere with the lymph-collecting and conducting system.

We do not classify oedema caused by an excessive production of interstitial fluid in the presence of a normal, functioning, lymph-conducting system as lymphoedema. We do not, for example, consider the oedema of inflammation caused by excessively leaky capillaries to be lymphoedema even though the lymph-collecting system may become overwhelmed and might be considered to have failed. Earlier workers[1] did not take this view. The oedema fluid of lymphoedema has a composition similar to that of lymph, in particular a high protein content.[2–4]

A comprehensive classification based on aetiology could be produced if we knew why the lymph-conducting system failed, but in many cases that knowledge is incomplete or completely absent. Although, for example, it is possible to demonstrate that the lymphatics of a limb are present but occluded, we rarely know whether the occlusion has been caused by an external agent or an intrinsic/genetic abnormality. Similarly, we may know the age at which a patient's lymphatic problem presented but often do not know whether it was acquired as a result of an external agent such as a bacterial infection or an intrinsic genetic deficiency that had not made itself manifest until adult life (*see* Chapter 5). These questions will one day be answered; until then, we must use the different classifications as guides for investigation, treatment and clinical audit and as stimulants of further research.

CLASSIFICATIONS OF LYMPHOEDEMA

Every case of lymphoedema should first be assigned to one of two categories: secondary or primary (also often called intrinsic, idiopathic, unknown or spontaneous). All possible secondary causes should be excluded before considering a diagnosis of primary lymphoedema because many of the causes of secondary lymphoedema require treatment in their own right, treatment that often also relieves the lymphoedema.

Secondary lymphoedema is lymphoedema caused by events, abnormalities or disease processes that have arisen outside the tissues of the lymph-conducting system. There is usually no difficulty in identifying secondary lymphoedema even when the underlying disease process is difficult to define, but it is important to remember that the lymphocytes and germinal follicles of the lymph glands do not function as part of the lymph-conducting system, even though they are intimately related to it, so lymphoedema caused by, for example, a lymphomatous proliferation of the lymphocytes within the lymph glands is secondary rather than primary lymphoedema.

Primary lymphoedema is caused by a failure of the lymph-conducting system (the lymphatics and the lymph-conducting spaces within the lymph glands) caused by disease or abnormalities of the components of that system.

Classification of secondary lymphoedema

Secondary lymphoedema is much more common than primary lymphoedema and is further classified according to its cause. The events, abnormalities and diseases that do not arise directly from the components of the lymph-conducting system that may cause secondary lymphoedema are legion (Table 7.1) but can usually be assigned to one of the following seven broad categories:

1 Infection
2 Trauma and tissue damage
3 Malignant disease
4 Inflammation
5 Factitious (factitial, artefactual or self-inflicted)
6 Immobility and dependency
7 Venous disease.

Infection

Although confined to certain geographical areas, *filariasis* (*see* Chapter 15) is by far the most common cause of secondary lymphoedema worldwide. Filariasis is endemic in the Far East, West and East Africa, the northern parts of South America and the Caribbean and should be excluded by complement fixation tests and midnight blood smears on any patient from these areas who presents with a swollen limb.

All causes of chronic lymphadenitis, such as *tuberculosis*, *toxoplasmosis* and *lymphogranuloma venereum*, and repeated episodes of *acute cellulitis*, *lymphangitis* and *lymphadenitis* cause a progressive fibrosis within the affected lymph glands that gradually obstructs the passage of lymph flow through the gland and ultimately causes lymphoedema.

Patients with primary lymphoedema who develop severe cellulitis and lymphangitis as a complication of their lymphoedema frequently experience an increase in the swelling of their limb, which, although usually transient, can be permanent. Lymphatics may also be permanently blocked by a single episode of acute lymphangitis, and if this happens in an area drained by a relatively

Table 7.1 *Some causes of secondary lymphoedema*

Infection
  Filariasis
  Tuberculosis
  Toxoplasmosis
  Non-specific cellulitis and lymphadenitis
Trauma
  Surgical lymphadenectomy
  Radiotherapy
  Varicose vein operations
  Vein harvesting
  Degloving injuries
  Burns
Malignant disease
  Secondary deposits in lymph glands
  Infiltrative carcinoma
  Lymphoma in lymph glands
  Kaposi's sarcoma
Inflammation
  Podoconiosis
  Rheumatoid disease
  Dermatitis
  Psoriasis
  Pretibial myxoedema
  Granulomatous disease
    Orofacial granulomatosis
    Sarcoid
Factitious
  Tourniquet application
  Hysteria
Immobility and dependency
  Dependency syndrome
  Paralysis
  Hysterical paralysis
Venous disease
  Post-thrombotic syndrome
  Venous ulceration
Intravenous drug abuse causing venous thrombosis
  and subcutaneous abscesses

small number of lymphatics – such as the scrotum – lymphoedema may develop.

Trauma and tissue damage

Lymph gland excision

Lymph gland excision is recognized to be one of the most common causes of secondary lymphoedema. Block dissection of the regional lymph glands of patients with malignant tumours has for many years been an accepted technique for enhancing survival and providing important prognostic information. This has led to a high incidence of lymphoedema of the arm after mastectomy, especially when combined with radiotherapy, and lymphoedema of the leg after block dissection of the inguinal glands. The swelling can develop many years after the original surgery, at a time when tumour recurrence is a possibility so must be carefully excluded.

Other tumours treated by block dissection that may cause secondary lymphoedema include malignant melanoma, carcinoma of the cervix, carcinoma of the ovary and body of the uterus, teratoma of the testis and carcinoma of the prostate, penis, scrotum or vulva.

Radiation therapy

Radiation therapy often causes lymphoedema because, although it destroys malignant cells, it also damages the normal cells in the lymph glands, causing necrosis and fibrosis, which interfere with the passage of lymph through the gland. High doses of irradiation should be avoided whenever possible and given through multiple fields to reduce the incidence of this complication. Fast neutron beam therapy appears to be particularly damaging to tissues and lymph nodes, and has consequently been largely withdrawn as a treatment modality.

The combination of *irradiation* and *lymphadenectomy* produces a very high incidence of lymphoedema, especially in the arm (*see* Chapter 13).

Surgical misadventure

The removal of a single enlarged lymph gland, inadvertently or for diagnosis in patients with a latent or subclinical primary lymphoedema, may precipitate severe swelling. In these circumstances, a Tru-cut biopsy or lymphogram should be performed rather than an excisional biopsy.

Recurrent varicose vein operations

Recurrent varicose vein operations in the groin and the removal of fatty lumps or enlarged axillary tails in the axilla can also cause secondary lymphoedema. All groin operations should be undertaken with caution and performed in a way that avoids dividing lymphatics and/or removing an excessive number of normal lymph glands.

Severe wounds

Severe wounds in the thigh, including *vein harvest incisions*, can cause lymphoedema, although this is usually mild and causes little disability. Similarly, *large* or *circumferential wounds*, *degloving injuries* and *burns* with extensive tissue loss are prone to lead to lymphoedema.

Malignant disease

The passage of lymph through the lymph glands may be obstructed by the presence of enlarging deposits of secondary carcinoma or deposits of Hodgkin's or non-Hodgkin's lymphoma. The possibility of an occult malignancy causing lymphoedema must be considered in any patient, especially those presenting with late-onset lymphoedema without any preceding history of mild leg swelling, before concluding that they have primary lymphoedema. Cancers that infiltrate through the soft tissues may occlude the main subcutaneous collecting trunks and cause lymphoedema.

Inflammation

Inflammation without infection is a feature of various conditions, many of which are autoimmune diseases. Lymphoedema may develop as a complication of *rheumatoid arthritis*, *dermatitis* and *psoriasis*. *Pretibial myxoedema* also contains a lymphoedematous element. The granulomatous diseases such as *oral–facial granulomatosis* and *sarcoidosis*, cause inflammatory changes in the skin lymphatics and lymph glands that cause lymphoedema, often of the face. Silica may reach the inguinal lymph glands through bare-foot walking and the resulting inflammatory response can cause lymphoedema – *podoconiosis*.

Factitious (artefactual or self-inflicted) lymphoedema

Every year, we see one or two patients who have deliberately applied some form of tourniquet around a limb and developed 'classical lymphoedema'. The disorder should be suspected if there is a sharp cut-off point at the upper end of the swelling (*see* Fig. 6.8). In our experience, some of these patients are using their condition as a means of escaping from social and other commitments, very few having a definable psychiatric abnormality. Objective tests invariably show anatomically normal lymphatics with local distortion where the tourniquet has been applied.

Immobility and dependency

If a limb is kept dependent and immobile, it becomes oedematous. Most of this oedema is caused by a gravitational increase in capillary pressure and filtration, but because lymph transport is affected by the lack of muscle tone and limb movement, the swelling can in part be categorized as lymphoedema. *Dependency oedema* is seen in patients confined to a wheelchair, in genuinely *paralysed limbs* and in patients with *hysterical paralysis*.

Venous disease

Oedema is a common complication of venous insufficiency. Thrombosis of the major veins and deep vein incompetence do not affect the main collecting lymphatics, but the small initial and pre-collecting lymphatics of the skin and subcutaneous tissues of the lower leg are damaged by prolonged venous hypertension, especially in areas of lipodermatosclerosis (*see* Chapter 6). Any lymphatic deficiency that develops exacerbates the underlying oedema caused by the venous hypertension.

Classification of primary lymphoedema

The many alternative titles for the term 'primary' – idiopathic, intrinsic, spontaneous and unknown – reveal that this group consists of those cases in which the problem is thought to be a primary abnormality of the lymph-conducting system but whose nature and cause is unknown. For this reason, these patients are often classified according to those features of their clinical presentation that we do know, as described below.

By age of onset

In this classification, primary lymphoedema is divided into the following categories:

- *congenital*: primary lymphoedema present at birth;
- *praecox*: primary lymphoedema that appears after birth and before 35 years of age;
- *tarda*: primary lymphoedema that appears after the age of 35 years.

Allen[5] originally divided all primary lymphoedemas into two categories – congenital and praecox – Kinmonth[6] adding the tarda group to separate out those in whom the oedema, albeit primary, was late in onset and probably of a different aetiology.

Although the term 'congenital' implies that the abnormality is present at birth, it would be wrong to assume that all cases of lymphoedema that are present at birth are caused by a genetic abnormality: although it is unlikely, the cause might have been an external agent acting via the mother, in utero, on a normal lymphatic system. The same argument applies to lymphoedema appearing after birth, even those cases which appear after the age of 35 years. Some may be caused by genetic abnormalities, others by an external agent so all may in the future be subdivisible into genetic and acquired rather than congenital and acquired.

By lymphography

Kinmonth[7,8] classified primary lymphoedema in terms of the lymphographic appearances (*see* Chapter 6):

- *Aplasia*: No collecting vessels detectable by the techniques used to obtain lymphographs.
- *Hypoplasia*: A lower than normal number of vessels opacified.
- *Numerical hyperplasia*: More than the normal number of normally sized vessels opacified.
- *Hyperplasia*: An increased number of lymphatics of greater than normal diameter opacified. As these lymphatics are dilated, tortuous and have incompetent valves, they are commonly called *megalymphatics*.

It is usually easy to allocate lymphographs to one of these categories.

The descriptive words used by Kinmonth – aplasia, hypoplasia and hyperplasia – unfortunately have common meanings far beyond those he attributed to them. In general medical terminology, 'aplasia', 'hypoplasia' and 'hyperplasia' are terms used to describe tissues or organs that have not developed at all, have developed subnormally or have overdeveloped.[9] Kinmonth's use of the first of four terms listed above to describe circumstances in which lymphatics cannot be found on the dorsum of the foot, so cannot be opacified by lymphography, suggests an unproven aetiology because there may be lymphatics in other parts of the limb.

When we began to question the significance of failing to find a collecting vessel on the dorsum of the foot, we started to explore the subcutaneous tissues higher up the limb, at the level of the knee and the middle of the thigh.[10] In the majority of patients, we found collecting vessels at these sites and were able to perform lymphangiograms. Between 1957 and 1982, 1027 lymphograms were performed at St Thomas' Hospital, London. Over this period, the incidence of lymphographic 'aplasia', if defined by finding no lymphatics in any part of the limb as opposed to finding none in the dorsum of the foot, dropped from 15 to 0 per cent. When defined by finding lymphatics in any part of the limb, the incidence of lymphographic 'hypoplasia' (a reduced number of lymphatics opacified) increased from 61 to 90 per cent.[11] Over the same period, the mean incidence of lymphographic 'hyperplasia' did not change, varying between 6 and 24 per cent with a mean incidence of 11.7 per cent.[11]

Lymphatics are an essential component of the mechanism that controls the quantity and nature of the interstitial fluid (*see* Chapter 3). Their complete absence may be incompatible with life so a failure to find lymphatics large enough to inject in the subcutaneous tissues must not be interpreted as meaning a complete absence of lymphatics. In fact, when subcutaneous collecting lymphatics are difficult to find, the intradermal lymphatics revealed by an intradermal injection of Patent Blue Violet are always increased in size and number (*see* Chapter 6).

In 1967, Kaindl et al.[12] suggested alternative descriptive terms as substitutes for the term 'hyperplasia', based on the histological appearance of the lymphatics. His classification subdivided lymphoedema into hypoplasia and aplasia, lymphangiopathia obliterans, ectasia, Milroy's disease and lymphangitis. This classification has not been generally adopted as it combines, in a confusing manner, clinical, radiological and pathological features.

In 1970, Craig[13] produced another classification based upon a small number (40) of lymphograms. He combined hyperplasia and megalymphatics under the term 'lymphangiectasia' and suggested a new cause of lymphoedema – 'leaky lymphatics' (lymphatica porosa) – based upon the lymphographic finding of extravasation of contrast medium through the vessel wall. Most of his lymphograms were unfortunately performed with a water-soluble contrast medium so the extravasation he observed was almost certainly an artefact caused by the normal diffusion of the contrast medium through the lymphatic wall (*see* Chapter 6).

'Lymphatica porosa' is in fact a term that was originally used by Buocone and Young in 1965[14] to describe the fluffy perilymphatic appearance of contrast medium outside the lymphatics that is produced when they are injected with a water-soluble, low molecular weight contrast medium or with Lipiodol at an excessively high pressure. There is to date no proof that this appearance indicates a pathological level of lymphatic wall permeability or that 'leaky' lymphatics cause lymphoedema.

By known abnormality

The preceding review of the classifications of lymph-oedema that were in use in the early 1980s reveals the confusion caused by ignorance of the cause of many cases of primary lymphoedema. The past 25 years have seen a steady, albeit small, increase in understanding so that more is known more about the role of genetic abnormalities and the development of acquired lymph vessel obliteration. In 1985, we published a new classification of lymphoedema,[15] which, although based upon the known detectable abnormalities, did not imply any unproven, causative mechanisms. There are three groups of patients with primary lymphoedema for which we know the pathological abnormality and the way it causes lymphoedema, those with:

1 lymphoedema caused by aplasia, obstruction or incompetence of the thoracic duct and cisterna chyli, many instances of which are probably genetically determined;
2 lymphoedema caused by aplasia or valvular incompetence of the collecting ducts in the limbs, most cases probably being genetically determined;
3 lymphoedema caused by a fibrosis of unknown aetiology in the hilum of the lymph nodes.

The remainder, which constitute the majority, are the lymphoedemas in which lymphography reveals a reduced number of lymphatics. Most patients who have this abnormality, present at birth or within the first 15 years of life (Allen's congenital and praecox groups). A few may have a true genetic aplasia or hyperplasia, but the majority, particularly those whose oedema appears at a later age, often have histological evidence of 'thrombosed' or obliterated lymphatics so we can reasonably assume that they have an acquired condition rather than a true genetically determined aplasia or hypoplasia. Believing that these patients have an acquired condition, we suggest that this group be described as having 'lymphangio-obliterative lymphoedema' while acknowledging that we do not know the trigger for the obliteration or the mechanism by which it occurs.

When the proximal vessels are involved, it is impossible to determine whether they have become occluded secondary to lymph node fibrosis or independently. Whatever the mechanism, there are likely to be secondary changes, such as dilatation and tortuosity, in the lymphatics distal to the obstruction. Many of the vessels below an obstruction gradually become obliterated.[16–18]

In 1985, the St Thomas' classification of the lymphatic abnormalities that cause lymphoedema was as follows:[15]

A. Congenital
1 Congenital aplasia or hypoplasia of the peripheral lymphatics (the lymphographic abnormality and/or oedema usually presenting at/or within 2 years of birth)
2 Congenital abnormalities of the abdominal or thoracic lymph trunks

3 Congenital valvular incompetence (always associated with megalymphatics and often with chylous reflux)
B. Acquired
4 Intraluminal or intramural lymphangio-obstructive oedema
   a) Distal: acquired obliteration of the limb's distal lymphatics, cause unknown
   b) Proximal: acquired obliteration of the lymphatics in the proximal part of a limb, usually associated with distal dilatation, cause unknown.
   c) Combined: acquired obliteration of all the lymphatics of a limb
5 Obstruction of the lymph-conducting pathways in the lymph glands by hilar fibrosis. This may cause the changes classified above as lymphangio-obstructive oedema; i.e. types 4 and 5 often co-exist.

Acquired distal valvular incompetance may follow any form of obstruction.

We have now altered the classification by changing the word 'congenital' to 'genetic' because the latter has a more specific meaning, and the term 'lymphangio-obstructive' to 'lymphangio-obliterative' because this more accurately indicates the underlying pathology.

Current St Thomas' classification of the lymphatic abnormalities that cause lymphoedema

Genetically determined abnormalities
1 *Aplasia, malformations and valvular incompetence of the central lymphatic ducts*, namely the cisterna chyli and thoracic duct
2 *Aplasia, hypoplasia or dilatation and valvular incompetence of the collecting ducts in the subcutaneous tissues of the limbs and trunk.* This group includes the familial conditions – Milroy's, Meige's and lymphoedema/distichiasis syndromes (*see* Chapter 5) – and the congenital but sporadic lymphoedemas associated with other congenital abnormalities (Box 7.1).

Box 7.1 *Clinical syndromes associated with primary lymphoedema*

Distichiasis (familial)
Klippel–Trenaunay syndrome
Mixed lymphatic and vascular deformities
Maffuci's syndrome
Lymphangiomatosis
Neurofibromatosis
Proteus syndrome
Turner's syndrome
Noonan's syndrome
Amniotic bands
Yellow nail syndrome

Acquired abnormalities
1 *Lymphangio-obliterative lymphoedema*
   a) Distal
   b) Proximal
   c) Combined
2 *Intralymph gland (hilar) fibrosis.* This is probably the same process as lymphangio-obliterative oedema beginning in the lymph-conducting parts of the lymph gland rather than in the lymphatics.

It is clear that this classification does not fit well with those based on age of onset or lymphography because, although genetically determined abnormalities may be present at birth, their clinical presentation may be delayed until early childhood, adolescence or adult life. The time of onset does not indicate the true aetiology of the disease. We no longer use Kinmonth's solely descriptive lympho-graphic classification because it is usually possible to make a functional as well as an anatomical diagnosis, such as distal or proximal lympho-obliterative lymphoedema, or valvular incompetence with reflux, from the lymph-angiograph. The truly genetically determined aplasias/hypoplasias can be separated from the acquired obliterations when these patients present at or soon after birth and have a definite family history.

This leaves one group of lymphoedemas whose cause, genetic or acquired, cannot be surmised from lympho-angiography – the group of patients whose lymphoan-giographs reveal more than the usual number of normally sized lymphatics (Kinmonth's numerical hyperplasia). Is this a true abnormality, or an appearance produced by the unusual hydrodynamics that exist during the injection of Lipiodol, or a very early sign of proximal obstruction caused by early lymph gland fibrosis? Further studies are needed to resolve this question. The authors' opinions are divided: Professor Burnand thinks this is probably a true genetically determined abnormality (although how it produces lymphoedema is not clear), whereas Professor Browse thinks it is more likely to be a very early sign of proximal obstruction, which would explain how it causes lymphoedema.

Of one thing we can be quite certain, by the time the second edition of this book has been written, this classification will have been significantly altered to take account of new knowledge, especially that which is steadily appearing in the field of genetics.

REFERENCES

1. Allen E, Barker NW, Hines EA. *Peripheral vascular diseases*. Philadelphia: Saunders, 1946.
2. Taylor GW, Kinmonth JB, Dangerfield WG. Protein content of oedema fluid in lymphoedema. *British Medical Journal* 1958; **2:** 1159–60.
3. Courtice FC. The transfer of proteins and lipids from plasma to lymph in the leg of the normal and hypercholesterolaemic rabbit. *Journal of Physiology* 1961; **155:** 456–69.
4. Szabo G, Gerzely S, Magyar ZS. Immunoelectrophoretic analysis of the lymph. *Experientia* 1963; **29:** 98–9.
5. Allen EV. Lymphoedema of the extremities. Classification, aetiology and differential diagnosis: a study of 300 cases. *Archives of Internal Medicine* 1934; **54:** 606–24.
6. Kinmonth JB, Taylor GW, Marsh JD. Primary lymphoedema. *British Journal of Surgery* 1957; **45:** 1–5.
7. Kinmonth JB. Primary lymphoedema: classification and other studies based on oleo-lymphography and clinical features. *Journal of Cardiovascular Surgery (Torino)* Special number for the XVII Congress of the European Society of Cardiovascular Surgeons 1969; 65–77.
8. Kinmonth JB. *The lymphatics*, 2nd edn. London: Arnold, 1982.
9. Skinner HA. *The origin of medical terms*. London: Baillière Tindall & Cox, 1949.
10. Kinmonth JB. Lymphography 1977. A review of some technical points. *Lymphology* 1977; **10:** 102–6.
11. Browse NL. The diagnosis and management of primary lymphoedema. *Journal of Vascular Surgery* 1986; **3:** 181–4.
12. Kaindl F, Mannheimer E, Pfleger L, Thurner B. Histology of lymphangiopathies. In: Ruttiman A ed. *Progress in lymphology*. Stuttgart: Georg Thieme Verlag, 1967: 15–17.
13. Craig O. Radiology of lymphatic disorders. *British Journal of Hospital Medicine* 1970; **3:** 276–82.
14. Buocone E, Young JR. Lymphangiographic evaluation of lymphoedema and lymphatic flow. *Roentgenology* 1965; **95:** 751–65.
15. Browse NL, Stewart G. Lymphoedema: pathophysiology and classification. *Journal of Cardiovascular Surgery (Torino)* 1985; **26:** 91–106.
16. Danese C, Howard JM. Post-mastectomy lymphoedema. *Surgery, Obstetrics and Gynecology* 1965; **120:** 797–802.
17. Jackson RJA. A study of the lymphatics of the lower limbs in the normal state and after inguinal lymphadenectomy. *Journal of Obstetrics and Gynecology of the British Commonwealth* 1966; **73:** 71–87.
18. Fyfe NCM, Wolfe JHN, Kinmonth JB. 'Die-back' in primary lymphoedema: lymphographic and clinical correlations. *Lymphology* 1982; **15:** 66–9.

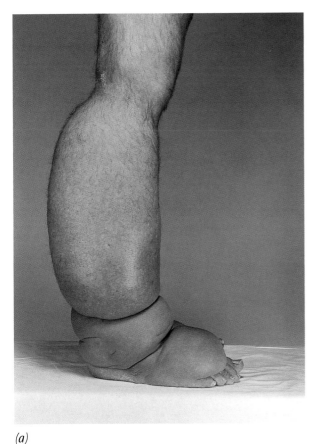

(a)

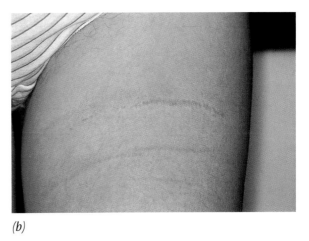

(b)

Figure 8.6 *Factitious (factitial, artefactual or self-inflicted) oedema. (a) This patient was producing lymphoedema in his lower leg by tying a tight narrow bandage just below his knee beneath a below-knee elastic stocking. The rest of his right leg was normal. True lymphoedema does not stop abruptly, the transition from lymphoedematous tissues to normal tissues always being gradual. (b) This young woman presented with a swollen leg. Careful examination revealed the superficial scars on her thigh where she had been applying a tourniquet.*

subcutaneous tissues are swollen and thickened. Both legs are affected. The symptoms are worse in the winter, and there is often a family history of this problem. Although the swelling leads to the misdiagnosis of lymphoedema, the seasonal variation of the symptoms, the localized discoloration of the skin and the absence of oedema in the feet usually make it easy to refute a diagnosis of lymphoedema.

LIPOEDEMA

Lipoedema (lipidosis, lipohypertrophy; Fig. 8.7) is a common but infrequently recognized condition causing bilateral enlargement of the legs in women.[10] It is frequently misdiagnosed as lymphoedema. In its later stages, some true chronic oedema can supervene, the so-called lipoedema–lymphoedema syndrome. The profusion of synonymous terms used in the literature, including adipositas spongiosa, massive obesity of the legs, painful fat syndrome and lipodystrophy, testify to the poor understanding of the condition.

Lipoedema results from the excessive subcutaneous deposition of fat in the lower limbs between the ankle and waist, and to a lesser extent in the upper limbs from the wrist to the shoulder. The condition is distinct from morbid obesity even though the two frequently co-exist. Dieting tends to result in a loss of fat from non-lipoedema

areas, for example the face, neck and chest, with little effect on the lipoedema, whereas weight gain preferentially affects the lipoedema sites, particularly the thighs and hips. Although it has been described in males, it is a condition almost exclusively affecting females. The onset is usually at puberty, when the sufferer becomes conscious of fat legs or shapeless ankles. The cause is not known, but genetic factors are probable as it is not unusual to find a positive family history. Pubertal onset suggests hormonal influences, as does later onset with pregnancy.

The distribution of the swelling in the legs is characteristic, giving rise to a bracelet effect around the ankle with inverse shouldering immediately above and an increased gaiter girth. Unlike lymphoedema, lipoedema exhibits remarkable symmetry. The feet are typically spared unless or until lymphoedema co-exists. The skin in lipoedema remains soft with a 'mattress' contour (cellulite) caused by expansion of the subcutaneous fat lobules with tethering of the skin from the interlobular septa that connect the skin and fascia. Cellulite can be part of lipoedema, but the conditions are distinct. The tissues are tender and bruise easily. Spontaneous pain or allodynia (pain from an innocuous stimulus) may be also a feature. Sufferers complain of fluid retention in that the swelling can fluctuate with heat, standing or the menstrual cycle, yet pitting is *absent* and lymphoscintigraphy reveals relatively normal function within the main

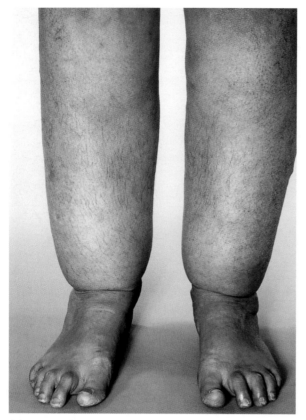

(a)

Figure 8.7 *Lipoedema. (a) Lipoedema in the lower limb characteristically presents as swelling of the lower third of the leg, above the malleoli, with no swelling of the feet. The fat areas are often tender and bruise easily but do not pit on pressure. The lymphatics are normal. (b) Gross generalized lipoedema tends to collect in the thighs and around the hips and buttocks, but not in the face and upper torso. When this strange redisposition of fat from the upper to the lower half of the body occurs gradually, it is called lipodystrophy progressiva.*

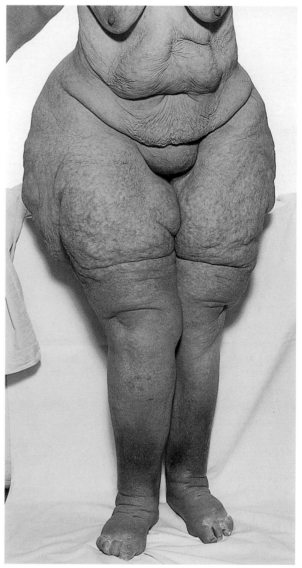

(b)

lymphatic routes following a standard web space injection of isotopic tracer into the foot.[11]

Indirect lymphography has shown extremely distended pre-lymphatic spaces within the affected subcutis compared with those of normal controls (*see* Chapter 6).[12] This finding would support the hypothesis of oedema formation localized to the lipoedematous tissues (rather than the limb generally) and arising from low tissue compliance. The 'flabby' nature of the affected tissues would also explain the occurrence of superficial varicosities despite normal venous function.[11]

PRETIBIAL MYXOEDEMA

Pretibial myxoedema (Fig. 8.8) may cause limb swelling indistinguishable from that of lymphoedema. Studies have demonstrated impaired initial lymphatic function possibly

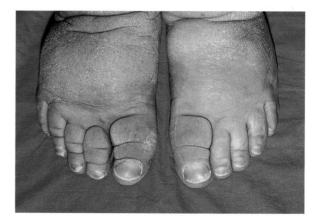

Figure 8.8 *Pre-tibial myxoedema extending into the feet. This example shows the typical thickening and roughening of the skin, which usually appears first in the pre-tibial skin but often spreads down into the feet. A skin biopsy showed a heavy deposition of mucopolysaccharides.*

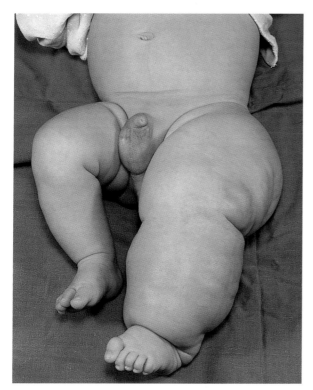

Figure 8.9 *The swelling of this infant's limb was caused by plexiform neurofibromatosis. The lymphatics were normal.*

related to the tissue deposition of mucopolysaccharide.[13] The swelling may increase when the thyrotoxicosis is treated.

INFLAMMATORY SKIN DISEASE

Inflammatory skin diseases such as eczema, psoriasis and cellulitis can provoke marked oedema because of the increased vascular permeability causing an extravasation of protein and fluid and the increased blood flow associated with the vasodilatation.

PLEXIFORM NEUROFIBROMATOSIS

This uncommon diffuse subcutaneous variety of neurofibromatosis (Fig. 8.9) presents as a soft subcutaneous tissue swelling that, when it affects a foot or covers part of the face, looks like lymphoedema. Palpation reveals that it has a distinct edge and does not pit. Biopsy is the only method of confirming the diagnosis.

GIGANTISM

The congenital overgrowth of a limb or part of a limb (Fig. 8.10) in the presence of normal arteries, veins and

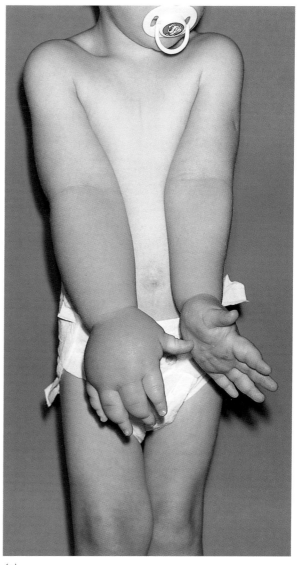

(a)

Figure 8.10 *Gigantism. The soft enlargement of an otherwise healthy looking limb or digit is often misdiagnosed as lymphoedema. (a) Local gigantism, in this patient simple partial hemihypertrophy, may be associated with congenital lymphoedema.*

lymphatics is called gigantism. Because the hypertrophy of the soft tissues makes the limb look swollen, the swelling is often misdiagnosed as lymphoedema. These limbs or digits are often deformed, something that does not occur with lymphoedema. The fact that the arteries and veins are normal can usually be ascertained by clinical examination, but it may be necessary to perform a lymphoscintigram to confirm that the lymphatics are normal.

The very many other conditions that may cause a limb to swell are listed in Box 8.1. A description of their clinical features, diagnosis and treatment is beyond the scope of this book but can be found in many other medical textbooks.

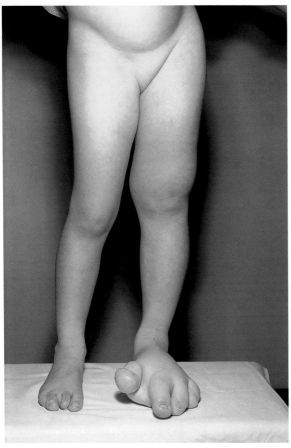

(b)

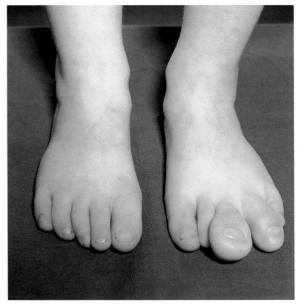

(c)

Figure 8.10b,c *(b) The lymphatics in this child's shortened leg with an overgrown oedematous foot were normal. The oedema was thought to be caused by the lack of a proper gait and poor muscle activity. (c) Gigantism of the third and fourth toes of an otherwise normal left limb (Proteus syndrome may look similar). Lymphoedema of a single digit is invariably caused by a constricting band at its base. This young girl had a large abdominal lymphangioma but normal limb lymphatics.*

REFERENCES

1. Browse NL, Burnand KG, Irvine AT, Wilson NM. *Diseases of the veins*. London: Arnold, 1999.
2. Klippel M, Trenaunay P. Du noevus variqueux osteo-hypertrophique. *Archives of General Medicine (Paris)* 1900; **185:** 641–8.
3. Parkes Weber F. Angioma formation in connection with hypertrophy of limbs and hemi-hypertrophy. *British Journal of Dermatology* 1907; **19:** 231–8.
4. Alavi S, Chakrapani A, Kher A, Bharucha BA. The proteus syndrome. *Journal of Postgraduate Medicine* 1993; **39:** 219–21.
5. Carleton A, Elkington JStC, Greenfield JG, Robb-Smith AH. Maffucci's syndrome (dyschondroplasia with haemangiomata). *Quarterly Journal of Medicine* 1942; **11:** 203–9.
6. Ouvry PA, Guenneguez H. Lymphatic complications from variceal surgery. *Phlébologie* 1993; **46:** 563–8.
7. Hannequin P, Clement C, Liehn JC, Eurard P, Nicaise H, Valeyre J. Superficial and deep lymphoscintigraphic findings before and after femoro-popliteal bypass. *European Journal of Nuclear Medicine* 1988; **14:** 141–6.
8. Reading G. Secretan's syndrome. Hard edema of the dorsum of the hand. *Plastic and Reconstructive Surgery* 1980; **65:** 182–7.
9. Schwartzman RJ. New treatments for reflex sympathetic dystrophy. *New England Journal of Medicine* 2000; **343:** 654–6.
10. Wold LE, Hines EA, Allen EV. Lipoedema of the legs. *Annals of Internal Medicine* 1949; **34:** 1243–50.
11. Harwood CA, Bull RH, Evans J, Mortimer PS. Lymphatic and venous function in lipoedema. *British Journal of Dermatology* 1996; **134:** 1–6.
12. Partsch H, Stoberl C, Urbanek A, Wenzel-Hura BI. Clinical use of indirect lymphography in different forms of leg oedema. *Lymphology* 1988; **21:** 152–60.
13. Bull RH, Coburn PR, Mortimer PS. Pretibial myxoedema: a manifestation of lymphoedema. *Lancet* 1993; **341:** 403–4.

Principles of medical and physical treatment

WITH A CONTRIBUTION FROM THOMAS O'DONNELL

Lymphoedema represents an irreversible failure of the lymphatic system so treatment can only aim to control rather than to cure. One of the problems with lymphoedema is the lack of sensitive investigations to give information about a failing system before an irreversible situation arises. Our inability to identify reduced vessel contractility, early valvular incompetence, vessel fibrosis and obliteration seriously undermines the opportunity for early corrective treatment. Once swelling has been established, the associated changes in the tissues make it difficult to return to them to normal. Unlike all other oedemas, which are solely fluid, lymphoedema possesses a 'solid' component caused by the accumulation of protein, lipid, cells, debris and eventually fibrous tissue.

The management of lymphoedema varies greatly around the world. Drug therapy is disappointing and should not be the first line of treatment. In developed countries, the emphasis is more on physical forms of therapy, mainly massage and external compression, whereas in less-developed and hot countries, surgery is often the mainstay of treatment.

PHYSICAL THERAPY

The basic objective of physical therapy is to enhance whatever lymph drainage capacity remains by applying the physiological principles that make lymph flow in normal circumstances. Unlike the situation with blood flow, lymph has no central heart pumping the lymph around the body. There are many small peripheral lymph 'hearts' (the lymphangions or contractile segments between the valves of the lymphatic collectors), but these respond only to the supply of lymph to them from the initial lymphatics.

Initial lymphatic function is essentially a passive process dependent upon local changes in tissue pressure arising from skeletal muscle activity, arterial pulsation and other massaging influences. Without exercise and movement, lymph flow therefore falls to a very low level. Physical therapy attempts to mimic these physiological mechanisms by encouraging exercise and compression. Compression not only enhances the effect of skeletal muscle activity, but at the same time helps to control lymph formation (capillary filtration). Manual massage (manual lymphatic drainage therapy) seeks to enhance initial lymphatic function and direct drainage into collateral lymph pathways, particularly at sites where compression cannot be applied, i.e. midline sites such as the trunk, head and neck.

Principal forms of physical therapy

Physical therapy comprises exercise and movement, compression, massage and skin care.

Exercise and movement

It is probable, but by no means certain, that lymphatic contractility (intrinsic pumping) fails in lymphoedema. If so, extrinsic pumping must be made to play a far greater role. Stimulating lymph flow in lymphoedema should be considered to be similar to external cardiac massage.[1] Pressure is required to expel lymph from a segment of lymph vessel, but an equal period of relaxation is required to permit refilling.

Isotonic exercises (muscle contraction with muscle shortening followed by rest) are therefore ideal, whereas isometric exercise (sustained contraction with no muscle shortening) is undesirable. Patients often comment that walking improves leg swelling yet carrying a suitcase will promote swelling in the arm. Overexertion and excessive static exercise are counterproductive because they increase blood flow and consequently capillary filtration. If active exercise is not possible, for example because of paralysis caused by spina bifida, passive exercise is better than nothing.

Compression

In theory, *non-elastic* external support rather than elastic compression should be used.[2] The former resists the outward expansion of the tissues during muscle contraction but does not generate much inward pressure on the skin during muscle relaxation. This results in high pressure during muscle contraction and low pressure (to allow lymphatic refilling) at rest. Conversely, elastic compression provides little resistance to muscle expansion because elastic bandages and hosiery stretch and apply a sustained pressure at rest as the elastic recoils, thus preventing the collecting lymphatics refilling. The principles are similar to those underlying the 'non-stretch' versus 'stretch' bandage arguments advanced for leg ulcer treatment.

It is in practice not possible to provide true non-stretch external support hosiery because a certain amount of elasticity is necessary for the garment to conform and to be taken on and off. For the purposes of this discussion, we will thus use the term 'compression' broadly to refer to the use of whatever form of bandage or elastic hosiery the clinician considers appropriate.

Massage therapy, manual lymphatic drainage and simple lymphatic massage

Exercise and compression will passively move lymph proximally along a limb towards the adjoining quadrant of the trunk. Although this quadrant will also be a site of compromised lymph drainage, the opportunity for the lymph to escape to normally draining lymphatic basins is higher here than from the limb itself. Consequently, less oedema is usually present in the trunk, although significant swelling can be present. Indeed, compression of the limb can push fluid into the trunk, with, for example, unfortunate consequences for the genitalia. Although an exercise such as swimming can improve oedema of the trunk, there is generally no satisfactory treatment except massage.

Manual lymphatic drainage is a specific form of lymphatic massage performed by trained therapists that is designed to direct lymph away from congested lymph-oedematous areas through collateral routes on the trunk to normally draining lymphatic basins. Simple lymphatic massage is a copy of manual lymphatic massage performed by the patients themselves, their partners or their carers.

Skin care

The skin undergoes significant changes in lymphoedema, becoming thicker and harder with increased scaling (hyperkeratosis), warty changes and papillomatosis, which contributes to morbidity through its appearance, reduced compliance and an increased tendency to infection. The skin acts as an important collateral route for lymph drainage in lymphoedema. Skin with reduced compliance is stiffer and likely to compromise lymph flow even further. This makes it more likely to suffer damage as stiff skin will not withstand pressure and shearing forces so easily. Hyperkeratosis tends to harbour greater populations of micro-organisms so the risk of both fungal and bacterial infections is increased.

Elevation

Elevation (gravity) will enhance the rate of lymph flow to the root of the limb only while the lymphatics are full. Once the lymphatics have collapsed, which is likely after a short period of elevation, there is no reason to believe that elevation per se will enhance the rate of lymph flow; indeed, it may well do the opposite. What it does do is reduce venous pressure and consequently capillary filtration. By reducing lymph production, lymph drainage can play 'catch-up', and this is probably the main reason why elevation to some extent reduces swelling in lymphoedema. Overall, elevation has a much slower impact on lymphoedema than it does on other forms of chronic oedema in which excessive filtration is the predominant factor. Extreme elevation, for example by suspending a lymphoedematous arm in a sling attached to a drip stand, has no long-term benefit once the high elevation has been discontinued, whereas the regular, daily comfortable positioning of the limb at heart level or above during rest and sleep is a help.

The practice of physical treatment

Physical treatment aims to reduce or delay the progression of swelling, restore limb shape, improve skin quality and prevent infection. The best results are obtained with care delivered by a multidisciplinary team, ideally from a dedicated lymphoedema clinic. Success depends not only on the ability to deliver all the components of care (exercise, compression, manual lymphatic drainage and skin care), but also on the skill of the therapist and the time, resources and funding to provide it. Physical therapy is simple and safe, but it is time consuming and can use resources indefinitely.

Enabling patients to understand their condition and know what they should and should not do for themselves is central to care; only then can a high level of motivation and compliance with treatment be generated. Successful treatment should result in controlled lymphoedema and an independent patient able to self-manage with minimal intervention from health professionals. A healthy lifestyle with regular exercise, good weight control and a positive attitude to self-treatment works wonders. So often the patients with lymphoedema who do badly are overweight and sedentary and do not comply with treatment.

Skin care

Emollients, because they soothe, smooth and hydrate the skin, are first-line treatments in the management of most skin conditions, lymphoedema being no exception. Grease or oil, for example a 50 per cent liquid/50 per cent white soft paraffin mixture, is best but is cosmetically unacceptable in the daytime and may ruin hosiery. Water-soluble ointments containing macrogols which can be washed off (e.g. Diprobase) are better. When skin scale (hyperkeratosis) is excessive, salicylic acid ointment in increasing strengths (2–5 per cent) can be used.

For deep cracks and crevices where bacteria readily flourish, regular washing followed by an antiseptic drying agent, for example eosin, brilliant green or magenta paint (or betadine paint if the traditional coloured paints are unavailable or unacceptable), is essential. For extensive smelly, suppurating or weeping eczematous skin, 0.01 per cent potassium permanganate solution is advised as a soak. Topical steroids may be necessary for the treatment of eczema/dermatitis, which can both contribute to and result from lymphoedema, but care is required because of the increased risk of infection.

Decongestive lymphatic therapy (combined decongestive therapy)

In developed countries, the ideal approach is an intensive course of treatment comprising manual lymphatic drainage, multilayer bandaging and exercise followed by maintenance treatment using elastic hosiery, exercise and simple lymphatic massage or occasional courses of manual lymphatic drainage.[3] This combination of treatments, known as decongestive lymphatic therapy, combined decongestive therapy or complex physical therapy, is designed to reduce limb volume and restore limb shape as much as possible.

Manual lymphatic drainage followed by multilayer bandaging and then exercises is administered daily for approximately 3 weeks. Thereafter, off-the-shelf or made-to-measure hosiery is fitted and the maintenance phase begins. Severe lymphoedema with oedematous limbs too large or irregularly shaped to fit hosiery requires very intensive treatment. Mild lymphoedema should not need intensive treatment and can enter the maintenance phase directly unless the condition of the skin precludes the use of hosiery.

Combination therapy using manual lymphatic drainage, multilayer bandaging and exercise has been shown to be effective in an open study.[4] This study also identified a reduction in the incidence of cellulitis as a result of treatment.

Manual lymphatic drainage

Manual lymphatic drainage involves the use of specific hand movements in contact with skin without the use of oils. Rubbing or friction is discouraged. The first stage of manual lymphatic drainage stimulates lymph drainage within the normal, contralateral quadrant of the trunk; in the case of right-sided breast cancer-related lymphoedema, for example, massage begins on the left side, encouraging drainage to the left side of the neck and axilla. It is hoped that this will create a 'suction' effect, drawing lymph across the midline watershed from the compromised lymphatic basin to the normally draining basin.

The second stage involves massage within the congested trunk to 'push' the lymph (gently) along skin and subcutaneous collateral routes into the normal basin. The final stage attempts to move the lymphoedema within the arm, forearm and finally the hand towards the emptied vessels at the root of the limb and on the opposite side. Manual lymphatic drainage relies on good preparatory work in 'clearing the way ahead' so that lymph is more likely to flow from filled to empty vessels.

Massage, in accordance with the principles of manual lymphatic drainage, was first advocated by the surgeon Von Winiwarter in 1892,[5] and a number of schools have refined the practice.[6]

Manual lymphatic drainage has been shown to have a number of physiological effects. These include an increase in the contraction rate of the lymphatics,[7] increased reabsorption of protein into the lymphatics,[8] reduced microlymphatic hypertension[9] and improved collateral lymph drainage across the lymphatic territories of the skin.[10]

A number of studies have compared manual lymphatic drainage with various forms of compression. In 1984, Zanolla et al.,[11] using limb circumference and subjective assessment of mood to measure change, found no difference between patients receiving manual lymphatic drainage and those having massage and pneumatic compression, but the authors commented that the significance of their results was limited by the small number and the lack of standardization of methods. Another similar study found no significant benefit when manual lymphatic drainage was added to a standard compression regimen.[12]

Two randomized controlled clinical trials of manual lymphatic drainage have been published. The first[13] compared manual lymphatic drainage with sequential pneumatic compression (using an inflatable sleeve), each treatment being given as the only intervention for two weeks, in 28 women with breast cancer-related lymphoedema. In this study, both treatments reduced baseline arm volume by 7–15 per cent, but there was no significant difference between the two. The second randomized controlled trial, by the same author,[14] compared the effects of compression bandaging with and without manual lymphatic drainage, again in arm swelling following curative breast cancer treatment. The group receiving manual lymphatic drainage achieved a significantly greater reduction in arm volume and pain. Those who had bandaging and manual lymphatic drainage showed a significant reduction in limb volume ($P = 0.04$) and decreased pain ($P = 0.03$) even though the manual lymphatic drainage was given only once a week.

In our own, randomized cross-over trial comparing hosiery with and without manual lymphatic drainage,[15] manual lymphatic drainage achieved:

- a significantly higher reduction in arm volume;
- a reduction in oedema within the posterior axillary fold, measured using modified Harpenden calipers;
- a reduction in skin thickness, as measured by high-resolution ultrasound.

Manual lymphatic drainage is highly popular with patients, who perceive great benefit, but it is time consuming and labour intensive.

Manual drainage is probably relatively ineffective unless combined with some form of compression and exercise. When used in conjunction with multilayer bandaging, exercises and skin care as an intensive daily treatment course, it is referred to as decongestive lymphatic therapy or combined decongestive therapy. In some circumstances, for example facial lymphoedema, it may be the only possible and realistic form of treatment. Although manual lymphatic drainage and simple lymphatic drainage are widely used, studies of their cost-effectiveness and long-term value are lacking. Patients must adhere to a strict treatment schedule and make it part of the regular routine of their daily lives, some patients finding the time constraints imposed by such a strict schedule of treatment sessions unacceptable.

Simple lymphatic massage

A simplified version of manual lymphatic drainage, often referred to as simple lymphatic massage, is commonly taught to patients and their relatives in the UK. Patients are encouraged to massage their swollen limb daily for 15–20 minutes as a long-term self-health measure.

Comment

Although both manual and simple lymphatic drainage are widely used in lymphoedema centres, there is very limited research into their overall long-term value, their effect depending more on the vigour and diligence with which they are applied than on any other factor. Several studies have evaluated the effects of the combined decongestive therapy programme[4,16,17] or examined specific components of the treatment regimen, such as bandaging and hosiery.[18]

Multilayer bandaging

Multilayer bandaging[19] is designed, through the application of several layers of non-extensible bandages, to generate high pressures during exercise and low pressures at rest by acting as a counterforce to dynamic muscle activity (Fig. 9.1). The use of padding is intended to 'iron out' large folds and improve shape. Multilayer bandaging also

reverses skin changes, stops lymphorrhoea and softens underlying fibrosis. A reduction in swelling leads to a loosening of the bandages (as there is no elasticity to take up slack) so reapplication is required every 24 hours. When using non-extensible support, as opposed to elastic compression with extensible or elastic bandages, the sub-bandage pressure is proportional to the tightness of the bandage when applied and to the number of bandage layers, the bandage width and the circumference of the limb (Laplace's law).

The efficacy of multilayer bandaging has been assessed in a randomized controlled trial.[18] In this study, which lasted 24 weeks, patients with lymphoedema (mainly of the arm and breast cancer related) were randomized to multilayer bandaging (applied daily for 18 days) followed by hosiery for the rest of the trial, or to hosiery alone throughout the trial. All the patients performed exercises, skin care and simple lymphatic massage every day. At 24 weeks, the reduction in swelling was significantly greater in the multilayer bandaging group, the benefit being maintained for at least 6 months.

Elastic hosiery

Compression garments[19] are designed to contain swelling rather than to reduce it to any great extent, although, in practice, the introduction of hosiery together with other components of treatment (massage, exercise and skin care) should improve mild and moderate lymphoedema. For good compliance, the patient should be carefully fitted, as poorly fitting garments will understandably not be tolerated, and instructed on methods of application and removal. For whole-limb swelling, a garment that encompasses as much of the root of the limb, for example hip or shoulder, is desirable. The use of more than one layer of a garment of a lower compression class is sometimes preferable to a single garment of a high compression class. Lycra cycling or Bermuda-type shorts may help to control lower truncal swelling.

Garments come in many forms, for example sleeves with and without a hand piece, pantyhose and foot gloves, expertise being required when choosing the most appropriate size and style. Off-the-shelf hosiery is quicker and cheaper to obtain, but custom-made hosiery may be necessary for limbs that remain large or misshapen even after decongestive lymphatic therapy. Hosiery needs careful maintainance if it is to last: regular washing and rotating between several pairs will extend hosiery's useful life. In general, the management of lymphoedema requires arm sleeves of compression classes 1 and 2 ($<40\,mmHg$) and leg stockings of compression classes 3 and 4 ($>40\,mmHg$), but caution is required when prescribing the latter for patients with any degree of arterial ischaemia or neuropathy.

The efficacy of hosiery on lymphoedema has not been assessed in any randomly controlled clinical trials, but the wearing of an elastic sleeve for several months by

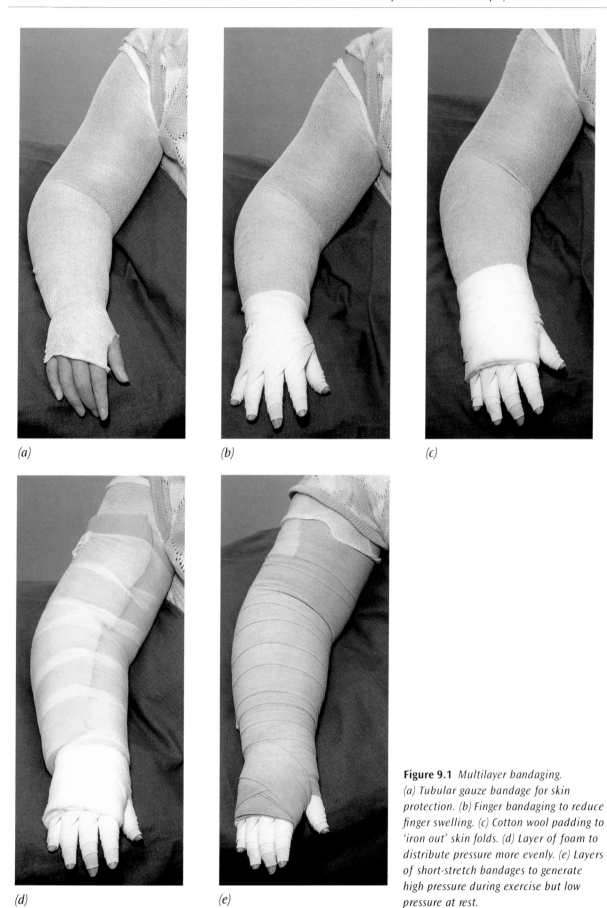

(a)

(b)

(c)

(d)

(e)

Figure 9.1 *Multilayer bandaging.*
(a) Tubular gauze bandage for skin
protection. (b) Finger bandaging to reduce
finger swelling. (c) Cotton wool padding to
'iron out' skin folds. (d) Layer of foam to
distribute pressure more evenly. (e) Layers
of short-stretch bandages to generate
high pressure during exercise but low
pressure at rest.

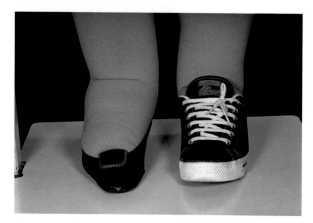

Figure 9.2 *The importance of good footwear in controlling lymphoedema. A court shoe encourages swelling of the dorsum of the foot, whereas a lace-up shoe provides additional compression to the dorsum and around the malleoli.*

women with arm oedema has been shown to reduce swelling.[20–22] The Circaid is a non-elastic, adjustable compression appliance that can be a useful adjunct to hosiery to prevent re-swelling.[23] It is essential that the effect of any form of lower limb stocking is assisted by well-fitting footwear (Fig. 9.2).

Mechanical sequential external compression

The introduction of multicompartmental sequential compression devices designed to reduce limb volume has led to an improvement in the short- and long-term outcomes of patients with lymphoedema.

Rationale

Centripetal lymph propulsion in the normal individual is determined by several factors: the intermittent elevation of interstitial tissue pressure caused by muscle contraction, the integrity of lymphatic valves that prevent the reflux of lymph during muscle relaxation, the alternating pressure gradient between the thoracic and abdominal cavities and finally intrinsic lymph vessel contraction.

The response to compression therapy using an external pump depends on the centripetal lymphatic pressure gradient it produces and the patency of any remaining collateral lymphatics. The establishment of an efficient centripetal extrinsic compression mechanism requires a multicompartment system with synchronized sequential inflation from its most distal to its most proximal cell, followed by a simultaneous total deflation in all the cells. Studies with ^{131}I-labelled albumin have shown that limb reduction is accomplished by clearance of free water and protein.[24] In contrast, Partsch *et al.*,[25] using lymphoscintigraphy, have shown that non-synchronized or single-compartment devices cause intraluminal lymphatic contents to flow in a bidirectional fashion, therefore increasing lymph reflux into the distal areas of the limb and out into the interstitium.

External compression devices

There are several commercially available external compression devices, varying in their degree of sophistication from single-cell, low-pressure, inflatable bags to the more sophisticated multicompartmental, synchronized, sequence-adjustable pressure devices.

The 20 year clinical experience of the New England Medical Center has been with the Lymphapress, one of the devices that provides sequential intermittent pneumatic compression. The Lymphapress consists of 9–12 overlapping cells along with a single-cell boot for the foot. The cells inflate sequentially from the most distal to the most proximal, this being followed by a simultaneous deflation of all cells. The complete cycle lasts 25 seconds, with a compression time of 20 seconds. These short cycles of compression allow for a significantly better tolerance to pressures up to 120–160 mmHg, although pressures should be individually adjusted for the patient's comfort.

Use of external compression devices

The use of external compression therapy is dictated by the prime therapeutic objectives of the management of lymphoedema, namely the reduction of limb volume, weight and girth, and the restoration of limb contour, in order to relieve the symptoms of heaviness, fatigue and disfigurement. The secondary objective, obtained through the reduction of limb size, is a decrease in the incidence of infection and inflammatory episodes.

In order to quantify the response to therapy, the circumference and volume of the affected limb must be accurately measured. The simplest way to measure limb girth is to use the template commonly employed for fitting elastic stockings, which requires the measurement of the circumference at nine sites on the leg and six sites on the arm. Relative and absolute limb reduction can be determined from the pre- and post-treatment values. Limb volume is determined by volume displacement.[26]

The best results are obtained by admitting the patient to hospital or to a short-stay ambulatory unit in order to ensure rest in a controlled environment for a 2–3 day period. The patient is restricted to complete bed rest with the leg elevated, and external compression therapy is initiated with the Lymphapress device over a fitted, lightweight, full-length cotton sock to absorb moisture. The inflation pressures are set so that the patient experiences a firm but tolerable sequential milking sensation. The pressures should be gradually increased to the patient's maximum tolerance, usually just above the diastolic pressure, the maximum tolerated pressures usually being between 80 and 90 mmHg. The compression pressures should not be allowed to exceed the patient's systolic blood pressure. The sleeve is removed after 6–8 hours of treatment and the limb allowed to air-dry for 1–2 hours until the next compression cycle is started. The total duration of treatment in a 24 hour period is usually 12 hours, therapy being continued for 2–3 days to obtain the optimum response. Once the period of treatment with the Lymphapress has concluded, patients are fitted with a two-way stretch elastic stocking measured at the limb's *new post-reduction girth*. Stockings must be replaced once their elasticity has been lost, usually once every 3 months.

Patients who show a partial response to therapy during their hospital admission, and those who are unable to maintain limb volume reduction with their elastic stockings, may need to continue external sequential compression in their home. Treatment for 4–6 hours each day, 3–4 times a week hours is arranged around the patient's regular work schedule, most frequently in the evening or during sleep (Fig. 9.3).

Results and outcome

A review of the New England Medical Center experience of 49 lymphoedema patients treated with the Lymphapress was published in 1992.[27] Patients were admitted to hospital for 2–3 days of twice-daily, 8 hour periods of compression at 20 seconds total inflation time and 80–90 mmHg maximum pressure, after which they were fitted with two-way stretch elastic stockings (40 mmHg compression). Antifungal agents were applied daily to the interdigital spaces and a water-soluble skin lotion over the whole of the affected limb. After the initial treatment, further maintenance sequential compression therapy

was used according to the degree and rate of fluid reaccumulation. Patients with rapid rates of reaccumulation were advised to use the Lymphapress daily at home, at the same settings as used during the initial treatment, for a minimum of 4 hours at times convenient to the patient's lifestyle, whereas those with a slower rate of oedema accumulation were treated at 4–6 month intervals in the out-patient department.

The study population consisted of 49 patients, 43 with lymphoedema of the lower limb (22 primary and 21 secondary) and 6 with secondary lymphoedema of the upper limb. Patients were seen and limb measurements obtained at 4–6 month intervals. The average follow-up time after beginning sequential compression therapy was 25 ± 4 months. The reduction in limb size was determined from the differences between the pre-treatment, immediate post-acute treatment and long-term treatment girths at nine points on the limb. Reduction to a size similar to that of the normal limb was classified as a full response, a clinically significant but less than full response being classified as a partial response and the remainder as no response. As there were only six patients with arm oedema, distributed evenly between the three groups, they have not been included in this analysis.

Twenty-six of the 43 patients with lymphoedema of the lower limb demonstrated a full response (a return to normal size), 10 a partial response and 7 no response (Fig. 9.4, Table 9.1). None of the clinical characteristics

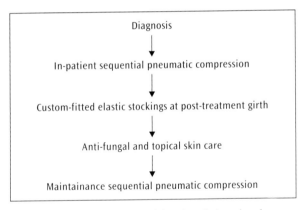

Figure 9.3 *Treatment protocol for chronic lymphoedema.*

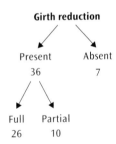

Figure 9.4 *Therapeutic response to sequential external pneumatic compression in 43 swollen lower limbs.*

Table 9.1 *Absolute reduction of lymphodematous tissue: comparison of changes in limb girths with acute compression and long-term treatment*

Level	Reduction of limb girth (cm)		
	Full responders (n = 26)	Partial responders (n = 10)	No response (n = 7)
Gluteal fold	4.28 ± 1.79	4.77 ± 2.00	3.70 ± 2.45
Upper thigh	4.20 ± 1.76	4.30 ± 1.84	4.74 ± 2.59
Lower thigh	5.10 ± 1.75	5.67 ± 1.80	4.00 ± 2.82
Knee	5.47 ± 1.43	3.25 ± 1.16	2.64 ± 1.75
Calf	6.76 ± 1.54	4.95 ± 1.58	4.54 ± 0.88
Distal calf	7.24 ± 1.98	5.83 ± 3.30	4.45 ± 3.19
Ankle	6.28 ± 1.40	4.72 ± 2.14	4.48 ± 2.80
Instep	3.64 ± 0.83	3.77 ± 1.01	3.50 ± 1.77
Metatarsophalangeal joint	1.55 ± 0.56	1.53 ± 0.53	1.45 ± 0.41

recorded, such as lymphoedema type, gender, extremity involved or amount of lymphoedematous tissue present before treatment, appeared to predict or determine the therapeutic response except for the condition of the subcutaneous tissue: those with less-fibrotic and more-compliant tissues appeared to have a better response. This study thus showed that both primary and secondary lymphoedema respond equally to a programme of external sequential compression followed by the constant use of elastic stockings, custom fitted to the post-reduction limb girth, and regular topical skin care. After this, 80 per cent of patients showed a worthwhile response in some part of their swollen limb and 60 per cent had a worthwhile response over the whole limb.

Patient instructions and self-care

Since there is a degree of local immunocompromise in a lymphoedematous extremity, preventing the development of portals of entry for bacteria that could lead to limb and/or life-threatening infection is of the utmost importance. In order to decrease the risk of acute cellulitis and inflammatory episodes, patients should be thoroughly instructed in the basic pathophysiology of lymphoedema and the self-care of their involved limbs. These instructions emphasize diligent hygiene and the avoidance of trauma. The following is a précis of the educational package given to our patients at the New England Medical Centre:

- Wash the affected limb daily with a mild antiseptic soap and inspect the limb for early signs of infection during each wash. Avoid leaving the skin moist, especially in the skin creases, by thorough but gentle drying. A hair-dryer may help, particularly in warm moist climates.
- Apply a hydrophilic skin lotion twice a day to avoid and/or remove any eczematous hyperkeratotic scaling, which can become an entry site for bacteria.
- Trim your nails regularly. Do not damage the cuticles or make them bleed.
- Avoid sandals, slippers and barefoot walking, and make sure that new shoes fit well and do not cause blisters.
- Avoid all forms of injury to the affected limb.
- Avoid strenuous exercise of a swollen lower limb, including long-distance running and contact sports. If you have a swollen arm, do not use heavy bags with over-the-shoulder carrying straps.
- Avoid tight jewellery.
- Use insect repellents and protective sun screen to prevent insect bites and sunburn.
- Avoid venepunctures and injections in the affected limb. In order to avoid such an event, we recommend wearing a 'lymphoedema alert' bracelet or necklace.
- If you want to remove hair from the swollen limb, use an electric rather than a safety razor.
- Regular normal walking while wearing your elastic stocking is helpful, but avoid walking long distances. You should refrain from sitting and standing still for long periods.

Box 9.1 *Lymphoedema support groups*

Several support groups for the lymphoedema patient have been formed. These institutions are an excellent source of patient education, and some offer monthly meetings for patients and health-care providers, as well as other related links. The groups listed below are easily accessed through their respective web sites.

National Lymphedema Network at www.lymphnet.org

Online lymphoedema support group at http://LISTSERV@ACOR.ORG

Online support group for lower extremity lymphoedema at http://lowerlimblymphedema@onelist.com

Lymphoedema Association of Australia at http://www.lymphoedema.org.au/index.htm

The International Lymphedema Guest Book at http://weezenhof.nl.eu.org/lymphedema/

American Lymphedema Institute at www.imsa.edu/~bug/alih.html

The Lymphedema Foundation by calling (in the USA) 1-800-596-7439, or (worldwide) by writing to The Lymphedema Foundation at Post Office Box 834, San Diego, California 92014-0834, USA

Lymphoedema Support Network, London, UK at www.lymphoedema.org/lsn/index.html

British Lymphology Society at www.lymphoedema.org/bls/

Lymphovenous Canada at www.lymphovenous-canada.com

Lymphatic Research Foundation at www.lymphaticresearch.org/

- Protect yourself against the development of fungal infections between the toes by applying a topical antifungal cream or spray. Soft split skin between the toes is an ideal portal of entry for bacteria. Antifungal agents should be prescribed if you develop tinea pedis.
- Well-fitting elastic stockings must be worn at all times, especially during all air and long car travel trips, to avoid recurrence or exacerbation of the oedema.
- Elevate the involved limb at night.
- Report immediately to your treating physician at the first sign of infection (redness, increased swelling, warmth and skin breakdown).
- Contact your local or national lymphoedema support group (or start one yourself) (Box 9.1).

CONTROL OF INFECTION

The lymphatics are responsible for conveying antigen via the Langerhan's cells, macrophages and lymphocytes to lymph glands. Without intact lymphatics, a primary immune response cannot develop. T-lymphocytes constantly recirculate between the central organs, blood and tissues for the purpose of immunosurveillance.[28] In lymphoedema, disturbances in lymphocyte trafficking may interfere with host defence mechanisms within the oedematous lymphatic basin, thereby predisposing to infection.

Acute inflammatory episodes, cellulitis

In lymphoedema, acute inflammatory episodes (*see* Chapter 6) may not always produce an area of clearly demarcated erythema with a migrating border, as seen in classical cellulitis and erysipelas, maybe because the inflammatory process sometimes spreads so rapidly throughout the oedematous tissues. Consequently, an acute inflammatory episode may present as a blotchy rash or just focal inflammatory spots. A not infrequent inability to isolate an offending micro-organism prompted the introduction of the term pseudo-erysipelas.[29] Acute inflammatory episodes may fail to resolve despite standard treatment with antibiotics. Recurrent acute inflammatory episodes can be a major problem that even prophylactic antibiotics sometimes fail to prevent, thus challenging infection as the sole cause.

Prevalance

Acute inflammatory episodes of the arm after curative treatment for breast cancer have been reported in 15 out of 273 patients (6 per cent) over 42 months.[30] All patients with acute inflammatory episodes had lymphoedema. The mean interval between the cancer surgery and the acute inflammatory episode was 38 months. In another series, 41 per cent of patients with post-mastectomy lymphoedema developed an acute inflammatory episode, the incidence increasing with the interval since the original cancer treatment.[31] There are also reports of acute inflammatory episodes occuring in the breast after breast irradiation. These episodes are probably related to impaired lymph drainage from the breast because breast oedema is usually present.[32]

Of more than 300 women who underwent a hysterectomy with pelvic lymphadenectomy, only nine, all of whom had received radiation therapy, developed acute inflammatory episodes in their legs.[33]

Causes

The simplistic view of acute inflammatory episodes is that stagnant lymph fluid provides an ideal medium for bacterial growth, but the reality is almost certainly more complex. The low yield of bacteria in microbiological specimens does not exclude infection, and the good response of acute inflammatory episodes to penicillin (particularly when given prophylactically) supports the view that bacteria, probably streptococci, are the cause. The isolation of non-group A streptococci in a substantial number of cases of acute inflammatory episodes associated with lymphoedema suggests that opportunistic infection as a result of a regional immunodeficiency ('regional AIDS') may be a factor. Organisms other than group A streptococci and *Staphylococcus aureus* are rarely found in classical cellulitis.[34]

Predisposing factors

It is assumed that the portal of entry for the infection causing acute inflammatory episodes is through the skin, and many patients report a direct relationship between accidental skin puncture and the onset of an acute inflammatory episode. There is also a widely held belief that breaches in the skin integrity from dermatitis, from fungal infection (tinea pedis) and at points of lymphorrhoea increase the likelihood of acute inflammatory episodes.[35] Some patients notice a direct relationship between foci of infection elsewhere, such as pharyngitis or a dental abscess, and their acute inflammatory episodes. Only a minority of patients, however, notice any precipitating factor. The majority of patients receive no warning of an impending attack other than a headache and a general feeling of malaise.

It is possible that once an infection has gained entry, it is never fully eradicated but remains quiescent with varying episodes of reactivation. This would explain why acute inflammatory episodes can relapse immediately on stopping taking antibiotics, even after 1 or 2 years of successful prophylaxis, and why they can be triggered by physical events such as excessive exercise, multilayer bandaging or even a course of manual lymphatic drainage.

Management

Acute inflammatory episodes are easily diagnosed when accompanied by constitutional upset, fever and rigors. If there is only minimal systemic upset, the distinction from other forms of inflammation, such as thrombophlebitis, deep vein thrombosis and acute lipodermatosclerosis, is not easy. The rash may be minimal and the suspicion of cellulitis based solely on the patient's 'not feeling well', on pain and on increased swelling. Diagnosis therefore often depends solely on clinical judgement. A duplex Doppler ultrasound examination is advisable to exclude deep vein thrombosis. The white cell count may or may not be elevated.

The treatment of a single acute inflammatory episode is no different from that of classical acute cellulitis, i.e. rest, elevation and antibiotics. In severe cases when there is a marked systemic upset and concern for the patient's welfare, the patient should be admitted to hospital and given intravenous antibiotics, usually benzylpenicillin. The addition of flucloxacillin may be sensible to cover against *Staphylococcus aureus* (Fig. 9.5). Penicillin may, however, fail to control severe streptococcal infection. Clindamycin has greater efficacy in experimental models

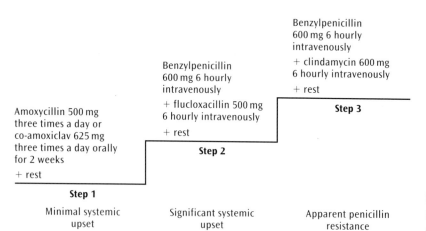

Benzylpenicillin
600 mg 6 hourly
intravenously

+ clindamycin 600 mg
6 hourly intravenously

+ rest

Step 3

Benzylpenicillin
600 mg 6 hourly
intravenously

+ flucloxacillin 500 mg
6 hourly intravenously

+ rest

Step 2

Amoxycillin 500 mg
three times a day or
co-amoxiclav 625 mg
three times a day orally
for 2 weeks

+ rest

Step 1

Minimal systemic
upset

Significant systemic
upset

Apparent penicillin
resistance

Figure 9.5 *Stepladder approach to the treatment of acute inflammatory episodes (cellulitis).*

of streptococcal infection and is recommended in addition to benzylpenicillin if there is no improvement after 48 hours' treatment, although it carries with it the risk of pseudomembranous colitis.[36] If the systemic upset is not severe, oral amoxycillin, 500 mg three times a day, or co-amoxiclav, 625 mg three times daily, for a full 2 weeks is recommended, as relapses are common. Patients allergic to penicillin may be given erythromycin, clarithromycin or a cephalosporin.

Although moderate exercise as a stimulant to lymph flow is always recommended as a treatment for lymphoedema, rest is essential and should be enforced during an acute inflammatory episode. The decision of when exercise or other components of lymphoedema treatment, for example the reapplication of compression garments, should be reintroduced, rests solely on clinical judgement.

Patients who suffer recurrent (possibly relapsing) acute inflammatory episodes require prophylactic antibiotics, although no randomized controlled trials exist proving their efficacy. Accepted practice is to give phenoxymethylpenicillin, 500–1000 mg daily, or erythromycin if penicillin allergy exists. There is one open uncontrolled prospective study of long-acting benzathine penicillin, which claims that attacks of acute inflammatory episodes were abolished in 41 out of 45 patients by giving 1 200 000 units intramuscularly every 3 weeks for 1 year.[37] Some patients continue to suffer 'breakthrough' attacks of inflammation despite prophylactic penicillin. Interestingly, the use of stronger broad-spectrum antibiotics appears to convey no additional benefit, but trial data are lacking.

There is a general belief that a reduction in oedema through physical therapy reduces the incidence of acute inflammatory episodes. In one prospective open study of 229 consecutive patients treated with manual lymphatic drainage, multilayer bandaging, exercises and skin care with a maintenance regimen of a compression garment, exercise and nocturnal bandaging, the incidence of cellulitis decreased from 1.1 attacks per patient per year to 0.65.[4] Other groups have also reported similar reductions in acute inflammatory episodes after physical therapy.[38]

Fungal infections

Lymphoedema affecting the foot and toes is invariably accompanied by tinea pedis. Although the close apposition of swollen toes, leading to skin maceration, may be the main cause, underlying immunodeficiency is also likely to contribute. In one report, all 25 individuals with recurrent 'lymphangitis' had co-existent fungal infection of their feet. Of the 15 patients whose fungal infection was eradicated, none had further acute inflammatory episodes, but the remainder, in whom the fungus persisted, continued to suffer such episodes.[35]

Acute fungal infection is best treated with a 3 month course of topical or oral terbinafine. Regular local toilet is essential. Long-term, half-strength compound benzoic acid (Whitfield's) ointment or miconazole nitrate (Daktarin) cream or powder is recommended at night as prophylaxis.

Ulceration

Unlike venous disease, lymphoedema does not commonly result in ulceration, but superficial ulceration can follow a superficial infection, and cutaneous necrosis can be caused by a blistering erysipelas or septic folliculitis. Malignant change should always be excluded by biopsy if the ulcer is long-standing or of rapid onset without an obvious cause.

The treatment of ulceration consists of local care similar to that given for venous ulcers and external compression. A period of bed rest followed by split-skin grafting may be necessary, but if the oedema is not controlled thereafter, the skin graft is likely to break down and the ulcer recur.

DRUG THERAPY (EXCLUDING ANTIBIOTICS)

Drug therapy is generally used as an adjunct to physical therapy in the management of lymphoedema.

Diuretics

Diuretics remain the most widely prescribed drug treatment for lymphoedema but incorrectly so in the majority of cases. Diuretics alone have very little effect on lymphoedema because their main action is to limit capillary filtration by reducing circulating blood volume. In fact, a marked improvement from diuretic use suggests that the predominant cause of the oedema is not lymphatic. Nevertheless, diuretics may be of value in oedemas of mixed origin through a reduction in lymph load. If diuretics have to be prescribed, a thiazide or low-dose spironolactone is to be preferred.

Benzopyrones

The benzopyrones are a group of substances comprising coumarin, hydroxyethylrutin and flavanoid derivatives such as diosmin. Trials of coumarin have produced conflicting results. The initial randomized controlled trials suggested some effect on post-mastectomy oedema, leg lymphoedema[39] and filarial lymphoedema,[40] but a subsequent study of women who developed lymphoedema after treatment for breast cancer found that coumarin did not alleviate lymphoedema and that coumarin-related hepatotoxicity occurred in 6 per cent of patients.[41]

Other trials in breast cancer-related lymphoedema using hydroxyethylrutosides have demonstrated statistically significant effects but small and clinically unimportant benefits.[42,43] Our experience with these drugs suggests that they soften the lymphoedema, particularly in the lower limb, indicating that the mode of action is predominantly vascular rather than lymphatic. Experimental studies have shown hydroxyethylrutosides to reduce capillary hydraulic permeability.[44]

Purified micronized diosmin and hesperidin (Daflon 500) has also been shown to have a small effect on breast cancer-related lymphoedema, and there are experimental studies indicating that these drugs reduce microvascular permeability in the hamster cheek pouch[45] and increase canine thoracic lymph duct pumping.[46]

NOTE

Dr Thomas F. O'Donnell and Dr Marcos F. Barnatan, MD, Department of Surgery, New England Medical Center, Boston, Massachusetts, USA, contributed the section on mechanical sequential external compression and parts of the section on manual lymphatic drainage.

REFERENCES

1. Roddie IC. Lymph transport mechanisms in peripheral lymphatics. *News in Physiological Science* 1990; **5:** 85–9.
2. Thomas S. Bandages and bandaging. *Nursing Standard* 1990; **4:** 4–6.
3. Földi E, Foedli M, Weissleder H. Conservative treatment of lymphoedema of the limbs. *Angiology* 1985; **36:** 171–80.
4. Ko DSC, Lerner R, Klose G, Cosimi AB. Effective treatment of lymphoedema of the extremities. *Archives of Surgery* 1998; **133:** 452–8.
5. Von Winiwarter A. Chirurgischen krankheiten der Haut. In: *Deutsche Chirurgie.* Stuttgart: Enke, 1892: Chapter 17.
6. Vodder E. Le drainage lymphatique, une nouvelle méthode thérapeutique. *Revue d'Hygiène individuelle Santé pour Tous.* Paris, 1936.
7. Hutzschenreuter P, Brummer H, Ebberfeld K. Experimental and clinical studies of the mechanisms of effect of manual lymph drainage therapy. *Journal of Lymphology* 1989; **13:** 62–4.
8. Leduc O, Bougeois P, Leduc A. Manual lymphatic drainage: scintigraphic demonstration of its efficacy on colloidal protein reabsorption. In: Partsch H ed. *Progress in Lymphology XI.* Excerpta Medica, 1988: 551–4.
9. Franzeck UK, Spiegel I, Fischer M, Bortzler C, Stahel HU, Bollinger A. Combined physical therapy for lymphoedema evaluated by fluorescence micro-lymphography and lymph capillary pressure measurements. *Journal of Vascular Research* 1997; **34:** 306–11.
10. Ferrandez JC, Laroche JP, Serin D, Felix-Faure C, Vinot JM. Lymphoscintigraphic aspects of the effects of manual lymphatic drainage. *Journal Maladie Vasculaire* 1996; **21:** 283–9.
11. Zanolla R, Monzeglio C, Balzarini A, Martino G. Evaluation of the results of post-mastectomy lymphoedema treatment. *Journal of Surgical Oncology* 1984; **26:** 210–13.
12. Andersen L, Hotris I, Eriandsen M, Andersen J. Treatment of breast cancer related lymphedema with and without manual lymphatic drainage. *Acta Oncologica* 2000; **39:** 399–405.
13. Johansson K, Lie E. A randomized study comparing manual lymph drainage with sequential pneumatic compression for the treatment of postoperative arm lymphedema. *Lymphology* 1998; **31:** 56–64.
14. Johansson K, Albertsson M, Ingvar C, Ekdahl C. Effects of compression bandaging with or without manual lymphatic drainage treatment in patients with postoperative arm lymphoedema. *Lymphology* 1999; **32:** 103–110.
15. Williams AF, Vadgama A, Franks P, Mortimer PS. A randomised controlled crossover study of manual lymphatic drainage therapy in women with breast cancer-related lymphoedema. *European Journal of Cancer Care* 2002; **(Dec.)**.
16. Mirolo BR, Bunce IH, Chapman M, *et al.* Psycho-social benefits of post-mastectomy lymphoedema therapy. *Cancer Nursing* 1995; **18:** 197–205.

17. Sitzia J, Sabrido L. Measurement of health related quality of life of patients receiving conservative treatment for limb oedema using the Nottingham Health Profile. *Quality of Life Research* 1997; **6**: 373–84.

18. Badger CMA, Peacock JL, Mortimer PS. A randomized controlled, parallel-group clinical trial comparing multi-layer bandaging followed by hosiery versus hosiery alone in the treatment of lymphedema of the limb. *Cancer* 2000; **88**: 2832–7.

19. Todd J. Containment in the management of lymphoedema. In: Twycross R, Jenns K, Todd J eds. *Lymphoedema.* Oxford: Radcliffe Medical Press, 2000: 165–202.

20. Swedborg I. Effects of treatment with an elastic sleeve and intermittent pneumatic compression in post-mastectomy patients with lymphoedema of the arm. *Scandinavian Journal of Rehabilitation Medicine* 1984; **16**: 35–41.

21. Zeissler RH, Rose GB, Nelson PA. Postmastectomy lymphoedema: late results of treatment in 385 patients. *Archives of Physical and Medical Rehabilitation* 1972; **53**: 159–66.

22. Bertelli G, Venturini M, Forno G, *et al.* An analysis of prognostic factors in response to conservative treatment of postmastectomy lymphedema. *Surgery, Gynecology and Obstetrics* 1992; **175**: 455–60.

23. Lund E. Exploring the use of Circaid® legging in the management of lymphoedema. *International Journal of Palliative Nursing* 2000; **6**: 383–91.

24. O'Donnell TF. Abnormal peripheral lymphatics. In: Clouse MF, Wallace S eds. *Lymphatic imaging: lymphography, computed tomography, and scintigraphy,* 2nd edn. Baltimore: Williams & Wilkins, 1985: 142–79.

25. Partsch H, Mostbeck A, Leitner G. Experimental investigations on the effect of a pressure wave massage apparatus (Lympha-Press) in lymphedema. *Phlébologie Proktologie* 1980; **80**: 124–8.

26. Raines JK, O'Donnell TF, Kalisher L, *et al.* Selection of patients with lymphedema for compression therapy. *American Journal of Surgery* 1977; **133**: 430–7.

27. Pappas CJ, O'Donnell TF. Long-term results of compression treatment for lymphedema. *Journal of Vascular Surgery* 1992; **16**: 555–64.

28. Streilen JW, Toews GB, Bergstresser PR, *et al.* Langerhans cells: functional aspects revealed by in-vivo grafting studies. *Journal of Investigative Dermatology* 1980; **75**: 17–21.

29. Edwards EA. Recurrent febrile episodes in lymphedema. *Journal of the American Medical Association* 1963; **184**: 858–62.

30. Simon MS, Cody RL. Cellulitis after axillary lymph node dissection for carcinoma of the breast. *American Journal of Medicine* 1992; **93**: 543–8.

31. Mozes M. The role of infections in post-mastectomy lymphoedema. *Surgical Annals* 1982; **14**: 73–83.

32. Hughes LL, Styblo TM, Thoms WW, *et al.* Cellulitis of the breast as a complication of breast conserving surgery and irradiation. *American Journal of Clinical Oncology* 1997; **20**: 338–41.

33. Dankert J, Bouma J. Recurrent acute leg cellulitis after hysterectomy with pelvic lymphadenectomy. *British Journal of Obstetrics and Gynaecology* 1987; **94**: 788–90.

34. Hook EW, Hooton TM, Horton CA, *et al.* Microbiologic evaluation of cutaneous cellulitis in adults. *Archives of Internal Medicine* 1986; **146**: 295–7.

35. Young JR, De Wolfe VG. Recurrent lymphangitis of the leg associated with dermatophytosis: report of 25 consecutive case. *Cleveland Clinic Quarterly* 1960; **27**: 19–24.

36. Bisno AL, Stevens DL. Streptococcal infections of skin and soft tissues. *New England Journal of Medicine* 1996; **334**: 240–5.

37. Olszewski WL. Episodic dermatolymphangioadenitis (DLA) in patients with lymphoedema of the lower extremities and benzathine penicillin administration. *Scope – On Phlebology and Lymphology* 1996; **3**: 20–4.

38. Földi E. Prevention of dermatolymphangioadenitis by combined physiotherapy of the swollen arm after treatment for breast cancer. *Lymphology* 1996; **29**: 48–9.

39. Casley-Smith JR, Morgan RG, Piller NB. Treatment of lymphedema of the arms and legs with 5,6-benzo-α-pyrone. *New England Journal of Medicine* 1993; **329**: 1158–63.

40. Casley-Smith JR, Wang CT, Casley-Smith JR, Zi Hai C. Treatment of filarial lymphoedema and elephantiasis with 5,6 benzo-α-pyrone (coumarin). *British Medical Journal* 1993; **307**: 1037–41.

41. Loprinzi CL, Kugler JW, Sloan JA, *et al.* Lack of effect of coumarin in women with lymphedema after treatment for breast cancer. *New England Journal of Medicine* 1999; **340**: 346–50.

42. Taylor HM, Rose KE, Twycross RG. A double-blind clinical trial of hydroxyethylrutosides in obstructive arm lymphoedema. *Phlebology* 1993; **8 (suppl. 1)**: 22–8.

43. Mortimer PS, Badger C, Clarke I, *et al.* A double-blind, randomised parallel-group, placebo-controlled trial of O-(β-hydroxyethyl)-rutosides in chronic arm oedema resulting from breast cancer treatment. *Phlebology* 1995; **10**: 51–5.

44. Kendall S, Towart R, Michel CC. Effects of hydroxyethylrutosides on the permeability of microvessels in the frog mesentery. *British Journal of Pharmacology* 1993; **110**: 199–206.

45. Bouskela E, Verbeuren TJ, Donyo KA. Effects of diosmin–hospieridin on increased microvascular permeability in the hamster cheek pouch. *International Journal of the Microcirculation: Clinical and Experimental* 1994; **14 (suppl.)**: 79.

46. Cotonat A, Cotonat J. Lymphangogue and pulsatile activities of Daflon 500mg on canine thoracic lymph duct. *International Angiology* 1989; **8 (suppl.)**: 15–18.

Principles of surgical treatment

WITH A CONTRIBUTION FROM PETER GLOVICZKI

The ideal surgical treatment of lymphoedema would return the lymphoedematous limb to a normal size with minimal scarring and a near-perfect cosmetic result. This is at present unachievable, the main goal of surgery being to produce a functional limb with the best cosmetic result that can be achieved. Current surgical procedures can be categorized into 'bulk-removal' operations, often called 'reducing' operations, and 'bypass' operations, which connect the normal lymphatics below an obstruction to normal lymphatics above it (lympho-lymphatic anastomosis) or to adjacent veins (lymphovenous anastomoses). These operations, their indications, aims and complications are described in this chapter, and their application to the surgical treatment of lymphoedema of particular areas is discussed in Chapters 12, 13, 14 and 16.

REDUCING OPERATIONS

Bulk-removal operations only became a reality in the twentieth century following the development of modern analgesia, anaesthesia and plastic surgical techniques. The reducing operations described in the following chapters have been fully illustrated in a colour atlas by Browse.[1]

Preoperative preparation for reducing operations

The limb is first reduced in size by bed rest, elevation and the application of external sequential pneumatic compression (*see* Chapter 9). This makes the tissues soft and lax by taking the tension out of the skin and subcutaneous fat.

We do not give our patients low-dose prophylactic subcutaneous heparin because we have had only one patient suffer a pulmonary embolus in 40 years of practise and heparin is likely to increase the incidence of postoperative haematoma. We advise our patients against surgical treatment if there is any suggestion of a deep vein abnormality or a previous deep vein thrombosis. If they insist on surgery, they should have full anticoagulation and accept all its attendant risks.

We do not give prophylactic antibiotics unless the incisions are to be made high on the medial side of the thigh close to the perineum. In such cases, we use penicillin or a broad-spectrum antibiotic. Operations on patients with septic lesions or ulcers should be delayed until the infection has been abolished or the ulcer has healed. If this cannot be achieved, the operation should be carried out with cover from the relevant antibiotic.

Because a tourniquet will be used, the blood supply to the limb should be assessed preoperatively by palpating the foot pulses or measuring the ankle/brachial pressure index with a Doppler flow meter. The operation is usually performed under general anaesthesia, although spinal or epidural anaesthetia can be used.

The swollen limb is elevated and abducted by connecting a wire from a pulley in the operating room ceiling to a Steinmann pin passed through the calcaneum and held in a sterile stirrup (Fig. 10.1). The whole limb can then be raised up 30–40 degrees and abducted at the hip by 30–40 degrees to provide easy access to both the medial and the lateral side of the whole leg up to the groin. Further

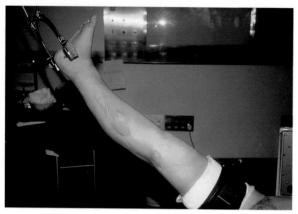

Figure 10.1 *The position of the leg that gives the best all-round access for a reducing operation. The leg has been elevated by a wire from the operating room ceiling attached to a stirrup and Steinmann's pin through the calcaneum. The skin has been prepared with povidone-iodine, exsanguinated with an Esmarch bandage and kept bloodless with a tourniquet around the top of the thigh inflated to 300 mmHg.*

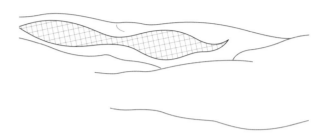

Figure 10.2 *The incision used for a Sistrunk's operation. The length of the incision above the knee depends upon the degree and extent of the swelling in the thigh. It is easier to obtain a cosmetically acceptable scar in the upper thigh and just below the groin if the incision is curved laterally, just below but parallel to the crease of the groin. The cross-hatching indicates the area of skin and subcutaneous tissue to be excised.*

access can be gained by rotating the operating table to throw the limb clear of its fellow.

The skin is prepared with an antiseptic solution (Hibitane or Betadine). A tourniquet, sterile or unsterile as the situation demands, is fixed around the upper thigh just below the groin crease. A sterile Esmarch bandage is wound tightly around the prepared limb from the foot up to the thigh to exsanguinate the tissues. The tourniquet is then inflated to 300 mmHg and the Esmarch bandage removed. The time of tourniquet inflation is recorded. The duration of tourniquet ischaemia *must not exceed 2 hours*. The incision lines are then marked out on the skin.

Sistrunk's reducing operation

This was the first attempt to reduce the bulk of the subcutaneous tissue.[2] The procedure entails the excision of a long wedge of skin and subcutaneous tissue from the limb to reduce its diameter. It is used today to reduce the diameter of the thigh as an adjunct to the Homans' or Charles's below-knee reduction (*see* pp. 181 and 184).

A long 'melon slice' wedge of skin and subcutaneous tissue is excised down to the deep fascia of a width that will allow primary apposition and suture of the skin edges (Fig. 10.2). The skin edges are not undercut and must be apposable without skin grafting. Large veins, including the long saphenous vein, should be divided between haemostats, and all smaller potential bleeding points leaking blood ligated with 2/0 polyglactin (Vicryl). *Diathermy coagulation must not be used on a cold ischaemic limb*. The tourniquet is then released and final haemostasis achieved by further ligatures and coagulating diathermy.

The upper part of the vertical thigh wound can, after removing the tourniquet, be extended and curved laterally, parallel to the groin crease (Fig. 10.2), to produce a better cosmetic result. Careful haemostasis before and after removal of the tourniquet reduces blood loss and the need for transfusion as well as the risk of postoperative haematoma formation. The wound is then carefully closed with interrupted nylon sutures and/or staples over suction drainage. External compression is applied over Jelonet dressings, gauze, cotton wool and compression bandages. The patient is nursed with the leg elevated. A self-retaining urethral catheter may be inserted to measure urine flow and avoid postoperative retention of urine.

Analgesia, limb elevation and bed rest are required for 3–5 days, after which the wound can be inspected and the suction drains removed. The sutures or staples are left in place for 10–12 days, but the patient may start to walk, with the compression bandages in place, after the initial inspection. Most patients can be discharged home 10–15 days after this operation, with strict instructions to use their compression bandages until new elastic stockings have been measured and fitted at the first follow-up appointment 6 weeks later. It is very important to use the compression bandages to maintain the limb at its postoperative reduced size until new stockings are fitted.

The results of a Sistrunk's type of reduction have never been scientifically assessed, but, as they are usually combined with a Homans' or Charles's reduction of the calf, our clinical impression is that they reshape the thigh in line with the reduction of the lower leg and improve the overall final appearance, although we clearly recognize that this opinion is based on the subjective opinion of the operating surgeon and usually the patient (*see* Chapter 11). The limb is reduced in diameter by the width of the strip of skin that is excised. The medial and/or lateral scars partially fix the skin to the deeper tissues, thus preventing the oedema re-accumulating in this area. The operation can be performed on both sides of the thigh. The muscles and deep tissues must be preserved. The results are less satisfactory if there is subfascial oedema.

Homans' reducing operation

John Homans improved on Sistrunk's operation by elevating skin flaps and removing subcutaneous fat beyond the area of skin excision before suturing the flaps over the exposed deep fascia or muscle.[3] The length and thickness of the flaps is critical: excessive undermining of the skin can cause ischaemic necrosis of the edge of the flaps, a cosmetically disastrous complication.

Medial side reduction

The flaps are marked out with an indelible pen (Fig. 10.3). The longitudinal (vertical) incision should lie 1–2 cm behind the posterior border of the tibia. Horizontal lines for the circumferential darts may be made 7–10 cm below the knee joint and, if required, just above the medial malleolus, but these incisions may be made at a later stage. The incision may pass below and behind the ankle and up into the thigh, sometimes to join up with a thigh Sistrunk's procedure (see Fig. 10.2).

The skin is raised from the subcutaneous lymphoedematous fat using sharp dissection and skin hooks, leaving the minimum amount of fat on the deep surface of the first 3–4 cm of the flaps. The flaps are then gradually thickened until, when the dissection reaches the midline of the leg anteriorly and posteriorly, it reaches the deep fascia (Fig. 10.4). The flaps should not extend beyond the anterior and posterior meridians of the limb.

The subcutaneous tissue is then removed from beneath the flaps by dissecting beneath it on the surface of the deep fascia (Fig. 10.5). Haemostasis is achieved by ligating or underrunning all the divided veins, such as the long and short saphenous veins and perforating vessels, with 2/0 Vicryl. The skin flaps are then pulled together, and any excess skin is excised (Fig. 10.6). There will also be excess skin in a longitudinal direction because of the loss of subcutaneous fat; this is corrected by excising triangular darts from both sides of the incision approximately 5–10 cm below the knee and, if necessary, 2–3 cm above the ankle. Circumferential darts below the knee heal well and do not spoil the shape of the limb. Darts just above the ankle can leave scars that interfere with footwear.

When adequate haemostasis has been achieved and the flap lengths have been adjusted, the tourniquet is released and complete haemotasis achieved with further ligatures, sutures and diathermy. Releasing the tourniquet sometimes affects the position and tension of the skin, especially at the level of the knee, and it may be necessary to trim the flaps again to make them fit snugly together without undue tension (Fig. 10.7a). The circumferential darts in the flaps should be sewn together before closing the longitudinal wound. Suction drains

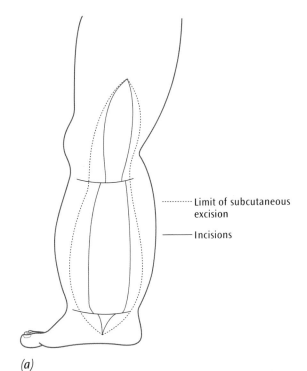

(a)

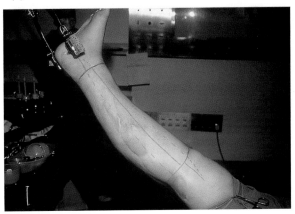

(b)

Figure 10.3 (a) Incision lines for a Homans' operation. (b) Incision lines marked on the leg before performing a Homans' operation. The dotted lines indicate the probable area of skin to be excised. The continuous line marks the line of the initial excision used to start raising the skin flaps. It is safer to decide upon the precise amount of skin to be excised after raising the skin flaps. This leg was grossly swollen but has been reduced before the operation by 5 days of elevation and compression.

Limit of subcutaneous excision
Incisions

are placed beneath the flaps. The skin is closed with interrupted nylon sutures or staples (Fig. 10.7b). Whenever possible, the junctions of the darts and flaps should be sewn together in a way that avoids four corners meeting (Fig. 10.8).

The wound and patient are managed as described above for the Sistrunk operation, taking care to inspect the junctions between the darts and the longitudinal suture line as these corners are the areas most likely to become

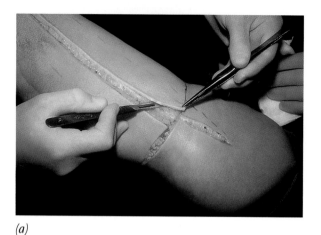

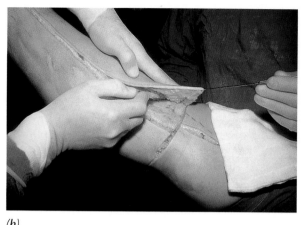

(a)   *(b)*

Figure 10.4 *Raising the skin flaps. The flaps should be only skin thick at their edge (a) but become gradually thicker towards the anterior and posterior midlines (b).*

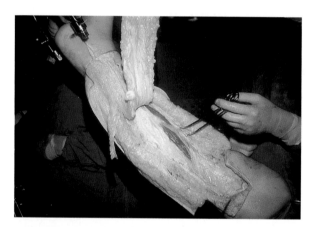

Figure 10.5 *The subcutaneous tissue being removed down to the deep fascia. Note that the communicating arteries and veins are being clipped and ligated. The skin flaps have been turned back and are at this stage slightly thicker than they should be. At this point, much of their fat can be removed by gently squeezing the fat globules out of the tissues, a procedure not unlike liposuction.*

ischaemic. The sutures are removed, the patient then being mobilized and usually discharged 10–15 days later.

Complications of the Sistrunk's and Homans' operations

Haematoma

Haematomata can be avoided by careful haemostasis, good drainage and adequate external compression. Large haematomata should be evacuated under anaesthesia. The sutures should be removed, all the clot cleared out and the wound resutured over suction drains.

Skin necrosis

Excessive undermining and tension on the wound edges can cause skin necrosis, which may require a further operation to excise the dead skin and sometimes to carry out

skin grafting. Skin necrosis is made worse by the presence of a large haematoma.

Infection

Infection can be a problem if either haematomata or ischaemia occur. Infection is more likely if there is preoperative ulceration or if the skin is thickened and infected. Preoperative preparation with antiseptic baths, and even prophylactic antibiotics, is appropriate if a heavy growth of a single organism is cultured.

Deep vein thrombosis and pulmonary embolus

These are rare complications: we are only aware of one case in our 40 years of clinical practise. We do not routinely give prophylactic anticoagulants to patients undergoing a reducing operation because we had several problems with haematoma formation when this approach was introduced. A control trial to test our clinical impressions is never likely to be performed.

A reducing operation performed, mistakenly, on a swollen post-thrombotic limb is highly likely to be complicated by deep vein thrombosis and pulmonary embolism so care should be taken to exclude deep vein disease before advising a reducing operation.

Keloid scars

These are common, particularly in black races and especially around the knee, and may necessitate re-excision with local triamcinolone infiltration.

Recurrence of the lymphoedema

This is inevitable. All patients must be told that they may need further operations 5–10 years after the first. The improvement tends to diminish because the unexcised tissue becomes more oedematous. Computed tomography scanning or magnetic resonance imaging can show the site and extent of the swollen subcutaneous tissues and determine, especially in recurrent cases, whether surgery might be successful.

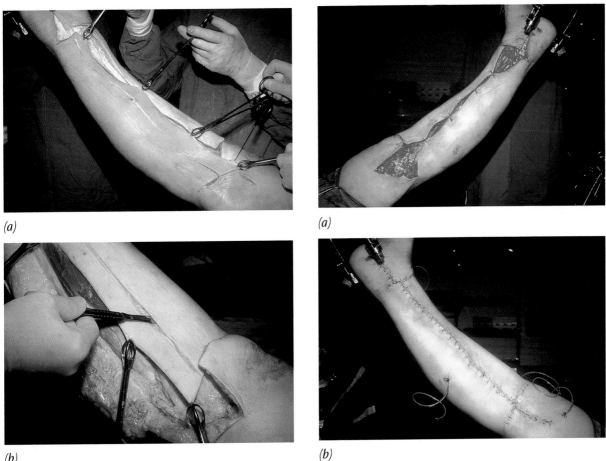

(a)

(a)

(b)

(b)

Figure 10.7 (a) After deflating the tourniquet and obtaining complete haemostasis, the tension in the skin flaps should be tested by placing a series of stitches to hold them in place. At this stage, suction drains should be placed beneath the flaps. (b) The completed suture line.

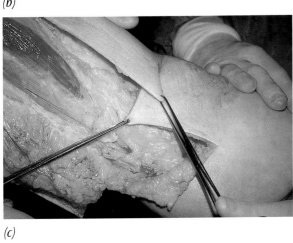

(c)

Figure 10.6 (a) The skin flaps are pulled together to see whether they will, when sutured together, be taut but not over-stretched. (b) The flaps often need to be revised at this stage. (c) The skin flaps should also be stretched lengthwise and the excess skin excised to form circumferential darts.

Figure 10.8 (a) Corner mattress stitches. These hold two corners against the opposing flap in a way that does not disturb the blood supply at the corners of the skin. (b) Whenever possible, having four corners come together at one point should be avoided; two corners against a straight edge of skin are much more likely to heal well.

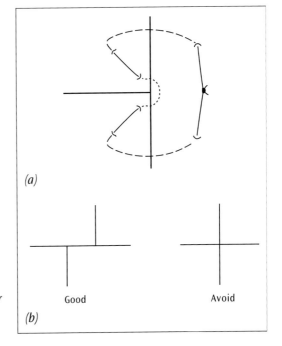

(a)

Good   Avoid

(b)

Mortality

The mortality in our practice is effectively zero. Our only case of pulmonary embolism did not die.

Lateral side reduction

A lateral below-knee Homans' operation can be performed 6 months after the medial side of the limb has been reduced. The lateral-side operation is only performed first when the lateral side of the thigh or the dorsum of the foot is especially swollen. The limb can be suspended as previously described, or the patient can be placed in the full lateral position with the affected limb uppermost, the trunk being held in this position with a pommel against the chest and a belt across the haunches.

After marking out the flaps, the limb is exsanguinated, the flaps are raised and the subcutaneous tissues are excised. Release of the tourniquet and careful haemostasis are again followed by skin closure over Redivac drains. The use of a dart just above the ankle is optional. The longitudinal incision can be carried down over the lateral side dorsum of the foot to allow excision of the swollen subcutaneous fat overlying the extensor tendons. The incision can also be carried up on to the thigh, and flaps can be raised here or, more commonly, a modified Sistrunk performed. Care must be taken not to go through the deep fascia over the neck of the fibula as the common peroneal nerve lies beneath it just below the neck of the fibula.

Thompson's buried dermis flap operation

Although this operation is rarely performed, it is described here for completeness and historical interest.[4] The theory underlying it was that if the cut edges of the dermal lymphatics were fixed underneath the deep fascia, they would link up with the deep lymphatics and form a new pathway for lymph drainage. We stopped using this operation because we could not show, with the lymphography, that superficial-to-deep anastomoses developed and because, when re-exploring some of the limbs that had undergone this operation, we found that the deep flap had necrosed and become a thin fibrous sheet.

The preparation and positioning of the patient and the incision lines on the skin are the same as those described above for a medial Homans' operation. An electric dermatome is used to remove a 5 cm wide, 0.1 mm thick layer of the epidermis and dermis (split-skin graft thickness) along the whole length of the proposed posterior flap. As this becomes the 'buried' flap, it is important to take off all the hair follicles and remove a reasonable width of skin in order to avoid burying undenuded skin when suturing the wound.

The incisions and flaps that are raised are identical to those of the Homans' operation. After excising the subcutaneous fat, the deep fascia is incised between the anterior border of the calf muscles and the posterior border of the deep flexor muscles behind the tibia. The tourniquet is released and haemostasis achieved. The posterior flap is trimmed appropriately and sutured deep to the deep fascia in the intermuscular groove between the deep flexors and the calf muscles with fine non-absorbable nylon sutures. The anterior flap is then brought over the top of the denuded flap, trimmed as required, upper and lower darts being cut if necessary, and sutured to the denuded skin with interrupted sutures.

Complications

The exposed area of denuded skin sometimes becomes hyperkeratotic. Pilonidal sinuses and sebaceous collections may develop from the buried skin flap if too much epidermis is left on the buried portion. If this flap becomes necrotic in the early postoperative period, it may cause pain and suppurate.

Charles's reducing operation

This is an effective radical operation for the reduction of massive swelling of the calf and foot, especially when the skin is in poor condition.[5] The operation produces a thin lower leg, but the appearance of the split-skin grafts is sometimes irregular and unsightly.

The limb is prepared by admitting the patient to hospital for several days before surgery for bed rest, limb elevation, daily antiseptic baths and external pneumatic compression. Prophylactic antibiotics may be given if there is a heavy growth of organisms cultured from the skin, especially if they are anaerobes. The operation is performed under general anaesthetic and the limb suspended from the operating room ceiling by the technique described above.

The area to be excised is marked out. It is important not to extend the excision of the skin over the ankle or above the knee, but the medial and lateral incisions at the side of the knee can be extended up on to the thigh to allow either a medial and lateral Homans' or Sistrunk's type of excision. It is better to stop the excision above the ankle, but if the dorsum of the foot is very swollen the excision can be extended to include all the superficial tissues over the extensor tendons (Fig. 10.9). The patient's skin and subcutaneous tissues beyond the upper and lower ends of the excised area should be tapered to form a smooth transition between the graft and the normal skin, avoiding a 'pantaloon effect' at the knee (see Fig. 11.2a).

The limb is exsanguinated and a tourniquet inflated around the thigh to 300 mmHg. All the skin and subcutaneous tissue of the lower leg between the knee and the ankle is removed down to the deep fascia. It is important to leave as little fat on the deep fascia as possible because residual nodules of subcutaneous fat may swell up and cause 'bosses' beneath the skin grafts. Some surgeons excise the deep fascia; we do not do this because haemostasis is more difficult if the underlying muscle is damaged, and

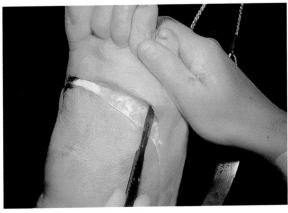 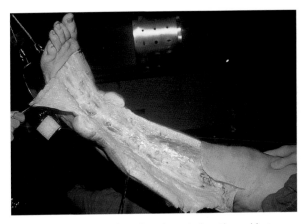

Figure 10.9 *When the swelling on the dorsum of the foot is excessive, the excision can be taken down below the ankle to include the dorsum of the foot.*

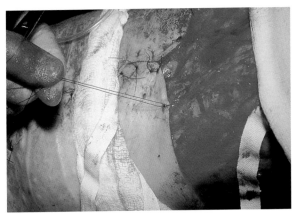 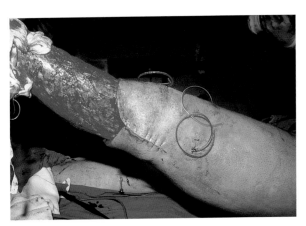

Figure 10.10 *After fashioning the flaps immediately below the knee, the skin edge must be sewn down to the deep fascia to prevent the development of a 'pantaloon' effect (see Fig. 11.2a).*

the periosteum of the tibia and the common peroneal nerve are more likely to be damaged. The long and short saphenous veins, with their accompanying saphenous and sural nerves, are excised. All the veins and visible vessels must be ligated or underrun with 2/0 Vicryl sutures.

The upper anterior flap must be carefully raised towards the knee to preserve, if possible, the infragenicular branch of the saphenous nerve, to ensure that there is enough skin to cover the tibial tuberosity (for kneeling) and to avoid a big step-down to the skin graft that is to be placed on the deep fascia. The posterior flap must not be cut too short as it tends to retract. For comfort when walking, there must be normal skin at and below the level of the posterior skin crease of the knee joint. Similar care must be taken at the ankle when undermining the skin, thinning off the subcutaneous fat and cutting the circumferential darts to bring the edge of the skin down on to the deep fascia.

The tourniquet may have to be let down and removed to allow further skin preparation and incision up to the level of the groin. In such cicumstances, all the potential visible bleeding points must be carefully ligated before the tourniquet is released, to avoid excessive blood loss, and haemostasis meticulously completed after its release.

The lateral incisions on the thigh and the ankle are sutured, and then the skin of the anterior and posterior flaps below the knee and above the ankle or around the dorsum of the foot carefully sutured to the deep fascia with 4/0 polydioxone sutures in order to produce a smooth, tapering appearance (Fig. 10.10).

Once the extent of the 'raw' area of exposed deep fascia or muscle can be assessed, an appropriate amount of skin is harvested to cover the defect. An electric dermatome is used to take partial-thickness skin strips. The preferred donor site is the opposite 'normal' thigh, but, if the condition is bilateral, ipsilateral thigh skin may be taken from the anterior and posterior surface between any thigh incisions. The excised skin is never used as a donor source because it is invariably abnormal and thickened. Skin may be taken from the abdomen and torso, but there is usually enough healthy donor skin on the thigh. The split-skin grafts are *not meshed* as this produces an unsightly 'string vest' appearance.

The grafts are stretched out, deep surface uppermost, on strips of tulle gras until an adequate quantity has been obtained. The grafts and the tulle gras are then applied directly onto the denuded deep fascia or muscle and fixed

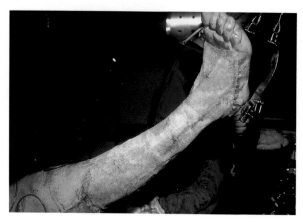

Figure 10.11 *The skin grafts in place, covered with tulle gras, ready for the next layer of wool and bandage.*

in place with sutures or staples (Fig. 10.11). Small pieces of skin are fixed to fill the gaps between the large sheets. The whole of the deep fascia and muscle must be carefully covered. Excess split skin is stored in a refrigerator for later use on any areas of slippage or graft failure. The grafted area is then covered with another layer of tulle gras, dressing gauze, wool and a crêpe bandage. The donor sites are covered with transparent adhesive plastic (Opsite) dressings.

The limb is elevated and the patient kept in bed until the grafted areas have been inspected on the fifth postoperative day. The stored skin may be applied at this stage if there are any patches of graft that have not taken. If no further skin grafts have to be applied, the limb is then exposed during the day and mobilization begun. The sutures or staples can be removed after 7–10 days. It may be necessary to obtain further pieces of split skin to cover areas where the grafts are not adherent. This is rare if careful attention to detail is taken at the time of the first operation. It is best to wait 7–10 days before applying new grafts. Most patients can be discharged home 2–3 weeks after their operation. Tulle gras and bandages should be used while there are unhealed or discharging areas, but the bandages can be discarded once full healing has occurred. At least 6 months should be allowed to elapse before surgery on the opposite limb is considered.

Foot reductions

Massive foot swelling can be treated by excising the skin and subcutaneous tissue on the dorsum of the foot down to the extensor tendons. The remaining skin needs to be undermined, thinned and sutured to the deep fascia before a split-skin graft is applied and fixed over the bare central area. Whenever possible, the skin over the front of the ankle should be left intact to prevent contractures and fixity, which reduce ankle movement. It is often better to carry out a standard sub-cutaneous reduction through a longitudinal incision on the dorsum of the foot.

'Tidy-up' re-do surgery

Patients who have had a Charles's reduction often require further small procedures to tidy up disfiguring areas at the ankle or foot that were not fully corrected by the initial surgery. This can be combined with the shaving off of any papillomata or keloid scars that have developed in the postoperative period. Additional skin grafts can be applied to any resulting raw areas at the same time.

Postoperative complications

The following complications can be encountered (*see also* Chapter 11):

- *Haematoma formation and 'graft loss'*. These are preventable by meticulous haemostasis and the avoidance of heparin.
- *Flap necrosis*. It is important to avoid any long and potentially poorly vascularized flaps.
- *Condylomata formation*. This can be avoided by taking off all the subcutaneous fat.
- *Ulceration* at sites where the graft has failed. Ulcers require currettage and re-grafting.
- *Foot oedema*. This is a fairly common complication and should be discussed with the patient before the operation. It may require an additional foot reduction (see above).
- *Papillomata and hyperkeratosis*, especially on the toes. This is unfortunately quite a common long-term complication. Papillomata are treated by shaving them off with a skin-grafting knife and either allowing the raw area to epithelialize spontaneously or applying split-skin grafts. Amputation of the toes provides a radical solution in some patients whose toes are severely affected.

Results

The long-term results of the reducing operations are discussed in Chapter 11, p. 212.

LIPOSUCTION

Liposuction was introduced by plastic surgeons in the 1980s as a method of removing subcutaneous fat.[6] As the effect of removing subcutaneous fat from a limb is to reduce the limb's overall size, it was not surprising that those caring for patients with large lymphoedematous limbs should investigate the effect of liposuction on such limbs,[7–11] even though there was no logical reason for so doing because the swelling of a lymphoedematous limb is caused not by fat alone but by lymph and fat as well as, after many years, fibrosis between the fat lobules and thickening of the skin. Therefore although subcutaneous suction will permanently remove a small proportion of the fat, it will only remove the oedema fluid temporarily;

unless there is an excess of fat, liposuction can therefore have only a minor effect on limb size. Furthermore, the trauma of the suction technique might well damage any functioning subcutaneous collecting lymphatics.

In spite of these theoretical objections, we, like others[7–11] and in conjunction with our plastic surgical colleagues, tried out the effect of liposuction on a small group of patients with primary lymphoedema of the lower limb. The procedure appeared to have no long-term benefit. There was an initial reduction in size produced by sucking out the oedema fluid and a little fat, but the swelling soon recurred unless it was restrained by the continuous use of good-quality compression. The overall effect appeared to us to be no better than the effect of elastic compression, massage and elevation alone. Because of these disappointing results and the doubtful theoretical basis of the technique when applied to lymphoedema of the leg, we did not conduct a full clinical trial.

In contrast, the results of the use of liposuction combined with compression therapy for breast cancer-related lymphoedema of the arm have been much more encouraging and have been the subject of a series of clinical studies by Brorson.[12] None of these studies compared the long-term effect of liposuction alone against compression alone or against compression and liposuction combined. The reason for this is clear: it was soon appreciated that the initial effect of liposuction was, although significant, short lived, the oedema rapidly returning if the arm were not compressed.

Brorson's first study,[13] on 28 women with fatty as well as oedematous arms, showed that the initial fat/fluid aspiration reduced the mean arm volume, measured 2 weeks after operation, from 1800 to 550 mL, a reduction that, provided high-quality compression was then applied, was maintained and actually improved during the ensuing months until, at the end of a year, the arm regained its normal size (see Fig. 13.8).[13,14] Brorson and colleagues have since shown that this degree of reduction can be maintained for 5 years.[15] The effect of combining suction and subsequent compression was better than the mean reduction in volume from 1700 to 1350 mL produced by compression alone,[14] although this reduction also improved over the 12 months that followed its initiation.

There are two reasons for the significant effect of liposuction on the arm. First is the observation that there is a reduced skin blood flow in lymphoedematous arms, which may stimulate the growth of adipose tissue.[16–19] Consequently, lymphoedematous arms are literally fatter than normal so liposuction has proportionally a much greater effect.[20] Second, the degree of fibrosis induced by lymphoedema in the arm appears to be less than that which develops in the leg, a feature that makes sucking out the fat far easier.

We do not know whether liposuction damages the subcutaneous collecting lymphatics, but Brorson and colleagues have shown that it does not worsen the already

reduced clearance of lymph from the skin,[21] and for some unexplained reason it also appears to increase the skin blood flow.[21]

Liposuction followed by a vigorous lymphoedema clinic regimen of compression hosiery, massage and elevation is therefore a worthwhile treatment for lymphoedema of the arm[22] but of little value for lymphoedema of the leg. In legs in which leg swelling is caused primarily by excess fat but there is perhaps a minor degree of lymphoedema (the so-called lipoedema–lymphoedema syndrome), liposuction is effective.

BYPASS OPERATIONS

In 1912, Kondoleon hoped that he was achieving a lymphatic bypass by excising a window in the deep fascia that would allow the lymphatics in the skin to reconnect with the deep lymphatics.[23] The method failed, presumably because fascial defects heal over and there was no stimulus to encourage the two sets of lymphatics to join together.

Handley, in 1908, inserted silk threads in the subcutaneous tissue of patients with lymphoedema, which he hoped would act as 'wicks' to carry lymph past sites of obstruction.[24] This technique failed too as the threads were rapidly walled off by fibrosis and scarring. In the 1960s, Kinmonth tried implanting fine tubes of nylon and polyethylene in experimental animals, but when these were removed, they were found to be walled off and blocked with old clotted lymph or blood within their lumen.[25]

In 1935, Sir Harold Gillies developed a 'skin bridge'.[26] This consisted of a long pedicle graft of healthy skin and subcutaneous tissue moved in stages from the upper limb to the lower limb, where it was placed as an inlay graft from the upper thigh to above the umbilicus. It was hoped that this would form connections between the leg lymphatics and the lymphatics that drained to the axillae, bypassing occluded iliac and aortic channels. Although Gillies, Fraser and Kinmonth reported a few good individual clinical results, the operation fell out of favour because the results were unpredictable and the staged operations required such a prolonged stay in hospital. When Kinmonth used visual lymphography to see whether there were lymphatic connections between the dermal lymphatics of the skin of the leg and the pedicle, he found that the Patent Blue Violet failed to cross through the scar at the leg–pedicle junction.

Thompson developed the buried dermis flap operation (see above) in 1962 in an to attempt to stimulate the development of connections between the dermal and deep subfascial lymphatics of the limb.[4] In our experience, however, the buried skin flap and its lymphatics rarely survived; even when they did, we never found evidence of superficial to deep lymphatic connections.

In 1966 and 1968, Nielubowicz and Olszewski described an operation in which a lymph gland was transected and anastomosed to the side of a vein (*see* Fig. 10.18b, p. 193).[27,28] They claimed that this allowed lymph to drain directly into the bloodstream below the level of any obstruction through the transected channels in the gland. The capsule of the gland was anastomosed to an opening in the vein, care being taken not to damage any adjacent collateral vessels. These authors originally reported favourable results in patients with lymphatic obstruction in the proximal lymph glands caused by secondary malignant disease, but Kinmonth was unable to obtain satisfactory results in patients with proximal obstructive primary lymphoedema.[25] One of Kinmonth's patients developed a deep vein thrombosis postoperatively. A lymphographic study performed on eight patients who had undergone this procedure failed to demonstrate evidence of persisting lymphovenous communications.[29]

Kinmonth suggested that a modification of the Nielubowicz procedure, in which the contents of the lymph node were shelled out before the capsule was anastomosed to the vein, might improve the results, but we are unaware that this has been subjected to any formal evaluation. The probable cause of the failure of this operation is the growth of vascular endothelium across the cut surface of the lymph gland, which the low intermittent flow of lymph from the leg fails to prevent.

The greater omentum has also been used as a potential lymphatic bridge between obstructed lymphatics and the base of the limb and the pre-aortic coeliac lymph glands.[30,31] Kinmonth achieved disappointing results in two patients on whom this procedure was attempted. He attributed this to the paucity of lymphatics in the omentum, as demonstrated by visual lymphography. As even Goldsmith's results were very inconsistent – only half of his 22 operations being considered successful – this procedure has never gained acceptance.

The natural extension of these procedures was the direct anastomosis of lymphatics to veins, at first using implantation techniques[32] and subsequently microvascular anastomosis.[33] This approach is discussed in detail on p. 192.

Enteromesenteric bridge bypass operation

The use of a mesenteric pedicle to bypass a lymphatic obstruction was first reported by Pugnaire in 1968.[34] He brought down a flap of mesentery and ileum beneath the inguinal ligament into the subcutaneous tissues of the thigh in patients with lymphoedema. Pugnaire claimed encouraging results, but these were unfortunately not confirmed by lymphography. John Kinmonth independently developed a similar concept at St Thomas' Hospital, London. Impressed by the richness of the intestinal lymphatics when studying patients with protein-losing enteropathy, he developed a technique which, by

placing the submucosal lymphatics of an isolated length of small bowel over the cut surface of lymph glands below an iliac gland obstruction, encouraged lympho-lymphatic connections to develop that would bypass the obstruction.

After preliminary laboratory experiments had demonstrated that the mucosa could be stripped off the luminal surface of the small bowel without damaging the submucosal lymphatics, Kinmonth performed a series of experiments on the pig in which an isolated, opened, 5 cm length of terminal ileum that had had its mucosa stripped off was sutured over a partially divided and opened lymph gland, the gland's efferent lymphatics having been clipped and divided to mimic downstream obstruction. The gland's afferent lymphatics were carefully preserved (Fig. 10.12). The development of connections between the lymph sinuses of the gland and the submucosal plexus and mesenteric lymphatics was confirmed 1 month later by contrast lymphography and injection studies.[35] An animal in whom the mucosa was left intact failed to form any lymphatic connections and developed a mucocele at the site of anastomosis.

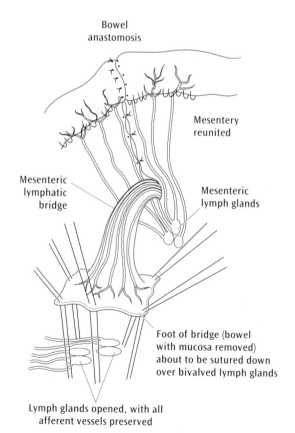

Figure 10.12 *A diagrammatic representation of the principles of the enteromesenteric bridge operation showing a pedicle of a segment of opened small bowel, denuded of its mucosa, being sutured down over opened lymph glands.*

Encouraged by these experimental successes, Kinmonth and colleagues carried out a number of bypasses on a selected group of patients. It rapidly became apparent that only patients with normal downstream lymphatics, i.e. pre-aortic glands, cisterna chyli and thoracic duct, benefited from the procedure. Four of the 8 patients in Kinmonth's early report obtained significant benefit and developed lymphographically proven lympho-lymphatic anastomoses.[36] Others, who were, with hindsight, incorrectly selected, did not improve.

The indications and procedure of this technique have now been refined, and this operation is an established treatment option at St Thomas'. Patients are first considered as possible candidates if they have whole-leg oedema with relative sparing of the foot, a clinical indication of the presence of a proximal lymphatic obstruction. An isotope lymphogram is then performed to confirm that there is no onward passage of the isotope beyond the inguinal and distal iliac glands. A bipedal X-ray lymphogram is then carried out to confirm that there are normal afferent lymphatic pathways up to the groin and a proximal ilio-inguinal obstruction (Fig. 10.13). The injection of Lipiodol into the unaffected, contralateral limb is essential to confirm the presence of normal upper abdominal glands, a normal cisterna chyli and a normal thoracic duct.

The limb must be of sufficient size to justify major abdominal surgery with bowel anastomoses but not so huge that distal changes, for example lymphatic die-back, make success unlikely. The patient must understand the risks, potential benefits and unpredictability of the procedure and must accept the chance (30–40 per cent) of failure. A prolonged delay in proceeding to operation should be avoided as persistent proximal gland obstruction may, over a number of years, lead to the disappearance of the afferent lymphatics.

Technique

Patients are admitted to hospital 1 or 2 days before their operation for bed rest, elevation of the affected limb and external pneumatic compression. They should be generally fit for surgery without any contraindications to laparotomy such as a frozen pelvis or previous radiotherapy. Subcutaneous low molecular weight heparin, for example tinzaparin, is given as there is no contraindication to thromboembolism prophylaxis in patients having this procedure, in contrast to those undergoing limb reduction surgery.

The patient is given a general anaesthetic and placed supine on the operating table with the lower limbs abducted on a vein board. Patent Blue Violet (1 mL per limb) is injected subcutaneously into the web spaces of the foot. The skin of the abdomen and groin is shaved and the skin prepared with chlorhexidine or Betadine. Drapes are placed to expose both the affected groin and the abdomen. If the preoperative lymphograph shows that the occlusion is high and the distal iliac glands are filling, the abdomen is opened through a lower midline incision to expose and confirm the presence of distal iliac glands coloured with the Patent Blue Violet. When the obstruction is lower, the Lipiodol reaching only the inguinal glands, the initial incision is made in the groin, below the inguinal ligament, centred just 1 cm medial to the femoral pulse. The incision must have a vertical component but can be placed slightly obliquely.

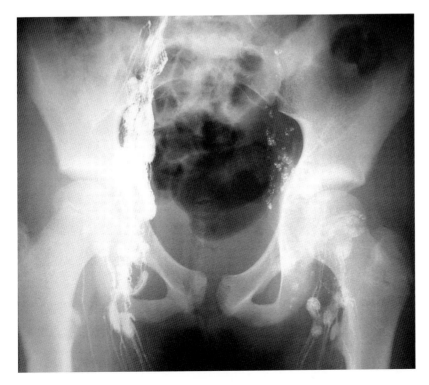

Figure 10.13 *A lymphograph taken 6 hours after the pedal injection of Lipiodol showing the Lipiodol stopping at the left inguinal lymph glands because the left iliac lymphatics and glands are fibrotic and obliterated.*

The incision is deepened into the subcutaneous fat by blunt dissection until the long saphenous vein is seen passing up to its termination in the femoral vein. Blue staining lymph glands should be visible within the subcutaneous fat around the saphenous and femoral vein. They can sometimes be quite large when they are obstructed. The glands can be quite superficial and it is important not to destroy their afferent channels when clearing fat from their inferior margins. One, two or even three glands should be identified and their upper surface partially cleared of connective tissue before leaving the groin and opening the abdomen to construct the entero-mesenteric bridge. The procedure is the same for exposing the iliac lymph glands, which can usually be seen and felt lying on the surface of the iliac vessels.

The abdomen is opened through a lower midline incision, although a paramedian or rectus-splitting incision on the relevant side may be equally appropriate. A transverse lower abdominal incision may be used to provide access, but dividing and lengthening a short small bowel mesentery may prove difficult through this approach.

A laparotomy is performed. The iliac, aortic and mesenteric lymph nodes should all be inspected and palpated. A 7–10 cm length of that part of the terminal ileum that has the longest mesentery is then selected and marked; this segment should have a good blood supply and its mesentery must be long enough to allow it to reach down to the groin. This can be roughly tested by pulling the loop down outside the abdomen towards the groin wound. In an obese patient with a thick, fatty mesentery, the Patent Blue Violet can be injected beneath the serosa to outline the lacteals and lymph glands. They must not be damaged while the mesentery is being divided.

The anterior and posterior peritoneal layers of the mesentery are divided in a vertical direction, from the anti-mesenteric border of the bowel towards the root of the mesentery, taking care to preserve an appropriate arcade of blood vessels with a broad base because the lymphatics (lacteals) do not form arcades but run directly from the bowel to the mesenteric glands. The mesenteric vessels beneath the divided peritoneum are then carefully ligated and divided (Fig. 10.14a). Transillumination with a bright light and vessel ligation in continuity with a fine suture material may aid this process. Enough mesentery, with its contained blood vessels, should be divided to allow the isolated segment of bowel to lie in front or behind the re-anastomosed small bowel without the pedicle being constricted. It is usually better to anastomose the small bowel behind the pedicle as the pedicle usually needs to lie in the front of the abdomen to reach the inguinal ligament. The bowel is divided at both ends of the isolated segment between intestinal clamps and then anastomosed end to end with one or two layers of 2/0 or 3/0 polyglactin (Vicryl) sutures to re-establish bowel continuity (Fig. 10.14b).

The clamps on the isolated segment of bowel are removed and the bowel irrigated and cleaned with

Hibitane. Any ischaemic or crushed portions are excised. The bowel is then opened along its anti-mesenteric border with a diathermy point. The mucosal surface is again thoroughly wiped clean of any residual attached contents with Hibitane-soaked swabs. A solution of 1:200 000 adrenaline (epinephrine) in saline or plain isotonic saline is then injected beneath the mucosa to elevate and aid its separation from the submucosa (Fig. 10.15). The edge of the mucosa is then separated from the submucosa by sharp scalpel dissection. Once a plane has been developed, most of the mucosa can be removed by wiping it off the submucosa with a small dry swab (Fig. 10.16). Sharp dissection is needed only where the mucosa adheres to underlying Peyer's patches. It is important to clean off *all* the mucosa to prevent the development of a mucocele or abscess.

The exposed submucosal surface of the bowel is then ready to be brought into apposition with one or more of the opened, bivalved inguinal or iliac lymph glands and sutured to their exposed inner surfaces. This is simple if there are suitable iliac glands, but a tunnel has to be made beneath the inguinal ligament if the inguinal glands have

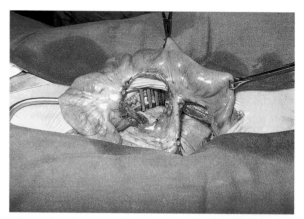

(a)

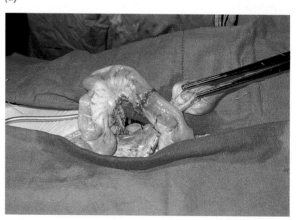

(b)

Figure 10.14 *(a) Preparation of the mesoenteric bridge by careful division of the vessels on either side of the lacteals in the mesentery. (b) Anastomosis of the bowel, and testing the length of the pedicle to ensure that it will reach the groin.*

to be reached. The tunnel beneath the inguinal ligament is created with forceps and finger dissection medial to the external iliac/femoral vein, and the bowel is pulled into the groin with forceps passed up from below. The mesentery will often have to be stretched to reach down to this level. Horizontal incisions in the peritoneum of its anterior and posterior surface may allow it to stretch to the required length, but great care must be taken not to damage blood vessels or lymphatics by this manoeuvre. The denuded submucosa is then fixed over the exposed bivalved glands with interrupted polydioxine or Vicryl sutures (Fig. 10.17). The incisions are closed with suction drainage in the groin wound.

Oral fluid restriction and intravenous fluid administration, with or without nasogastric suction drainage, is maintained for 24–48 hours. The skin sutures are removed 7–10 days later. Patients leave hospital when their small bowel activity has returned to normal, their temperature is normal and they have resumed a normal diet. They should continue to wear elastic stockings and be warned that the beneficial effects of surgery will not become apparent for 3–6 months while the lympho-lymphatic connections are forming, but that a gradual improvement in their limb size can be expected 12–18 months thereafter.

Complications

Wound infection

This can occur as a consequence of noscomial infection, for example with multiply-resistant *Staphlococcus aureus*, or bacterial contamination from the small bowel contents, although these are relatively sterile. We do not routinely give prophylactic antibiotics as our incidence of wound infection has been low.

Small bowel obstruction

This can result from technical problems with the anastomosis or from volvulus around the bridge. If intravenous and nasogastric suction fails to alleviate the problem and a plain radiograph of the abdomen shows the classical signs of obstruction, a re-exploration may be required. The findings at laparotomy will determine the surgery that is required, but it is important not to disturb the bridge.

Small bowel dehiscence

This is a rare but serious complication that we have seen in one patient who had radiotherapy damage to the small bowel following the treatment of Hodgkin's disease affecting his iliac lymph glands, radiotherapy that, in curing his Hodgkin's disease, caused his lymphatic obstruction.

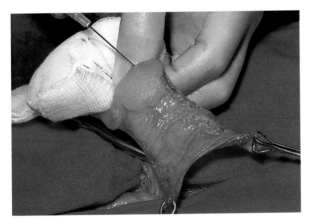

Figure 10.15 *The bowel has been opened along its antimesenteric border. Saline has been injected beneath the mucosa to help its removal by gentle blunt dissection.*

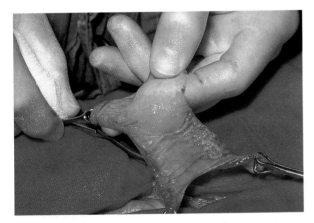

Figure 10.16 *The mucosa of the bowel in the surgeon's fingers has peeled off easily. Sharp dissection is needed where the mucosa is adherent to an underlying Peyer's patch.*

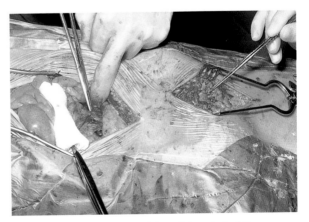

Figure 10.17 *The segment of bowel denuded of its mucosa being sewn down over the opened inguinal lymph glands. The forceps on the left of this photograph is resting beneath the pedicle of lymphatics in the bridge. The forceps on the right is pointing to the serosal surface of the bowel that has been sewn over the opened inguinal lymph glands.*

Signs of peritonitis or free gas under the diaphragm indicated the need for re-exploration.

Deep vein thrombosis, pulmonary embolism and atelectasis

These are complications that may follow any major abdominal surgery. They have not been a problem following this operation at St Thomas'.

Lymphocele and mucocele in the groin

We have not seen these complications, but they are a theoretical risk.

Results

The results of this operation are described in Chapter 11.

MICROSURGICAL PROCEDURES

Chronic lymphoedema develops when the collateral lymphatic circulation becomes insufficient and other compensatory mechanisms, such as the tissue macrophage activity and lymph drainage through spontaneous lymphovenous anastomoses,[37] have been exhausted. Extensive experimental work on the microsurgical reconstruction of the lymphatic circulation to bypass lymphatic obstruction and return lymphatic flow to normal[28–44] has been followed by the clinical application of a number of different microsurgical techniques, for example lymphovenous anastomoses,[28,33,45–55] lymphatic or vein grafts,[56–64] and the free transfer of tissue containing lymph vessels and lymph nodes.[65] Microsurgical lymphovenous reconstructions have also been performed in patients with lymphangiectasia and valvular incompetence.[63,64] In such patients, lymph vessel reconstruction is performed to re-establish the lymph flow of the limb following ligation and excision of the dilated, incompetent abdominal and retroperitoneal lymphatics, which are the pathways for reflux of chyle.

Diagnostic and preoperative evaluation

The investigations described in Chapter 6 are used selectively, depending on the age of the patient, the presentation of the disease and whether or not surgical treatment is planned.[66–68] Computed tomography is important to exclude underlying malignancy, and magnetic resonance imaging is used in patients with suspected congenital vascular malformations. Duplex scanning of the deep veins is used to exclude venous occlusion or venous valvular incompetence. At the Mayo Clinic, lymphoscintigraphy is used as the main diagnostic tool[69–73] and the semiquantitative transport index of Kleinhaus et al. to document the severity of the oedema.[56,71] In our hands, the sensitivity of the semiquantitative interpretation is excellent

(92 per cent), with a specificity of close to 100 per cent for the diagnosis of lymphoedema.[70,71] We reserve X-ray contrast lymphangiography for patients with chylous reflux, abdominal or thoracic chylous fistulae, for evaluation of the thoracic duct and for the preoperative assessment of chronic lymphoedema before lymphatic microsurgery. This method helps to define the anatomy and the exact site of the patent major lymphatic channels. The technique and complications of X-ray lymphangiography are described in Chapter 6.

The main indication for surgical intervention in lymphoedema is impaired function of the limb caused by its size and weight in patients who are not responding sufficiently to intensive medical management. Unfortunately, although the developments in microvascular techniques have allowed surgical attempts at direct lymphatic reconstruction, lymphovenous anastomosis[28,33,45–55] and lymphatic grafting[56–64] (Fig. 10.18), patients with primary lymphoedema usually have diffuse disease and are not considered candidates for direct lymphatic reconstruction.

Lymphovenous anastomosis

Direct lymph vessel-to-vein anastomoses were described in the early 1960s by Jacobson,[38] and lymph node-to-vein anastomoses were reported in 1968 by Nielubowicz and Olszewski.[28] The rationale for the operation is based on the observation that, in patients with chronic lymphoedema, spontaneous lymphovenous anastomosis could occasionally be demonstrated by lymphangiography.[37] Potential candidates for lymphovenous anastomoses include patients with lymphoedema of recent onset secondary to treated lymph gland disease and proximal lymph gland excision without previous episodes of cellulitis or lymphangitis.

All patients should undergo a trial of conservative, non-operative treatment before considering surgery. Venous hypertension is a contraindication to this type of reconstruction. An ideal candidate is a patient with a proximal pelvic lymphatic obstruction with dilated infrainguinal lymph vessels. Anastomoses in the leg are usually performed between the superficial medial lymphatic bundle and tributaries of the saphenous or femoral vein (Figs 10.18a, b and 10.19).

Lymphovenous anastomosis requires a good microsurgical technique and the high-power ($\times 4$–20) magnification of an operating microscope. We have demonstrated with cine-lymphangiography[40] that, in animals, 50 per cent of anastomoses between normal femoral lymph vessels and tributaries of the femoral vein remain patent for between 3 and 8 months.

The effectiveness of similar operations in humans is difficult to prove. In a report on 14 patients who underwent lymphovenous anastomoses at the Mayo Clinic for chronic lymphoedema, only five limbs (36 per cent) maintained the initial improvement at an average of 46 months after surgery.[54] This improvement occurred in four of the

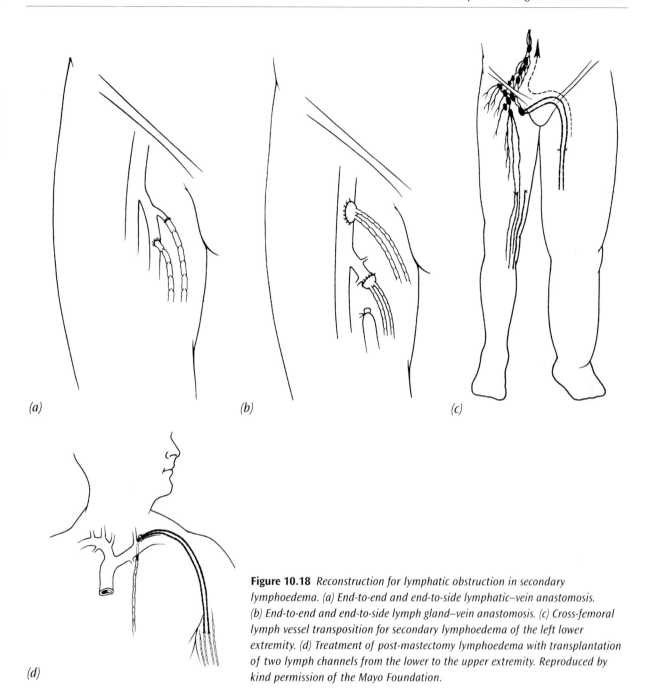

(a)

(b)

(c)

(d)

Figure 10.18 *Reconstruction for lymphatic obstruction in secondary lymphoedema. (a) End-to-end and end-to-side lymphatic–vein anastomosis. (b) End-to-end and end-to-side lymph gland–vein anastomosis. (c) Cross-femoral lymph vessel transposition for secondary lymphoedema of the left lower extremity. (d) Treatment of post-mastectomy lymphoedema with transplantation of two lymph channels from the lower to the upper extremity. Reproduced by kind permission of the Mayo Foundation.*

seven patients with secondary lymphoedema and in only one of the seven patients with primary lymphoedema.

Experience from Asia, Europe and Australia indicates that this operation can produce clinical improvement (Table 10.1).[15,45–53,55] In O'Brien *et al.*'s series from Australia, 73 per cent of patients showed a subjective improvement, and 42 per cent experienced long-term improvement.[55] Campisi and associates [52,53] have reported on 665 patients with obstructive lymphoedema treated with microsurgical lymphovenous anastomoses, documenting a subjective improvement in 87 per cent of their patients.[53] Of the patients, 446 were available for long-term follow-up, and the authors observed a persistent volume reduction in 69 per cent and a discontinuation of

conservative measures in 85 per cent. The authors concluded that microsurgical reconstruction early in the course of lymphoedema is more effective, because the intrinsic contractility of the lymphatics is still present and the chance of returning the lymph circulation to normal is better before significant chronic inflammatory changes have developed in the subcutaneous tissues. There is unfortunately only indirect evidence of the late patency of these anastomoses in humans. Lymphoscintigraphy on Campisi's patients showed an improved lymph transport and a faster disappearance of the tracer at the anastomosis site, but confirmation of long-term patency of lymphovenous anastomoses using X-ray lymphangiography is not available.

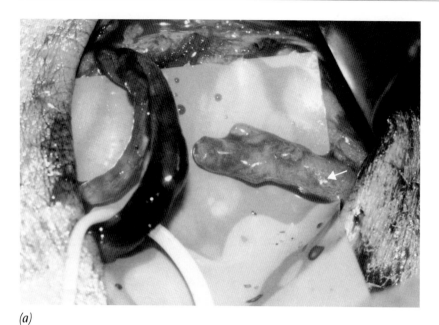

(a)

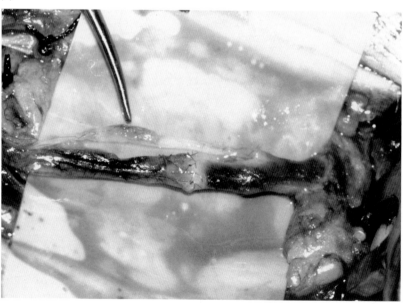

(b)

Figure 10.19 *Microsurgical lymphovenous anastomosis performed at the right groin. (a) Two dissected lymph vessels and a tributary of the saphenous vein (arrow) with a side branch prepared for anastomosis. (b) Patent end-to-end lymphovenous anastomoses. Reproduced by kind permission of the Mayo Foundation.*

We recently reported the results of the medical and surgical treatment of lymphoedema in 35 patients with primary chylous disorders.[64] We performed lymphovenous anastomoses on four patients with lymphangiectasia and reflux of chyle (Fig. 10.20). In two of these patients, we used a saphenous vein interposition graft with competent valves to prevent the reflux of the venous blood into the incompetent lymphatic system. The early results were encouraging.

A lymphovenous anastomosis between the thoracic duct and the azygos vein can be attempted to reconstruct the duct and improve lymphatic transport when the upper thoracic duct is occluded (Fig. 10.21). Through a right posterolateral thoracotomy, an anastomosis is constructed between the lower thoracic duct and the azygos vein, in an end-to-end fashion, with 8/0 or 10/0 non-absorbable

interrupted sutures and magnification using a loupe or the operating microscope. Only a few patients undergoing this operation have been reported.[63,25,75] We have performed it successfully in two patients,[63] and Browse has reported two successes in three patients.[75] Kinmonth suggested that the anastomosis alone is not effective for decompressing the thoracic duct and that ligation of the abnormal mediastinal lymphatics and oversewing of the sites of the lymphatic leak are also necessary.[25]

Lympho-lymphatic anastomosis and lymphatic grafting

The concept of lymphatic grafting is attractive in that it avoids the problems inherent in lymphovenous

Table 10.1 *Clinical results of microsurgical lymphatic reconstructions*

First author (year)	Extremity			Type of operation	Follow-up (months)	Excellent or good clinical results (%)
	Number of patients	Upper	Lower			
Krylov (1982)	50	+		LVA	?	30
Nieuborg (1982)	47	+		LVA	6–12	68
Gong-Kang (1985)	91		+	LVA	24[a]	79
Zhu (1987)	48		+	LVA	6–52	33
	185		+	LVA	6–52	73
Gloviczki (1988)	6	+		LVA	36.6[a]	50
	8		+	LVA		25
O'Brien (1990)	46	+		LVA		54
	30		+	LVA		83
	6[b]	+		LVA	51[a]	33
	8[b]		+	LVA		50
Baumeister (1990)	36	+		LG	>12	33
	12		+	LG	>24	8
Campisi (2001)	231	+		LVA	>7 years[a] in 446 patients	83
	446		+	LVA		
Campisi (2001)	133			LVL	'Long term' in 95 patients, maximum 15 years	81

[a] Mean.
[b] Lymphovenous anastomosis plus excisional procedure.
LVA, Lymphovenous anastomoses; LG, lymphatic grafting; LVL, lymphatic-venous-lymphatic graft with autologous vein.
Adapted from reference 74.

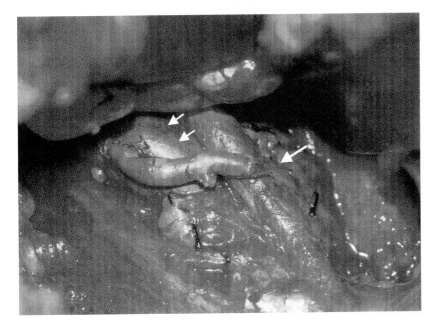

Figure 10.20 *Saphenous vein interposition graft from a dilated lymph vessel (single arrow) to the right common iliac vein (double arrows). This patient had lymphangiectasia, chylous reflux and chylocutaneous fistulae. Reproduced by kind permission of the Mayo Foundation.*

anastomoses caused by blood flowing into the lymphatics and coagulating. Patency of the anastomoses in a lymph-filled system should in theory be better than patency in a blood-filled system. This technique, pioneered by Baumeister, has been offered to patients with unilateral secondary lymphoedema of the lower extremities and to patients with post-mastectomy lymphoedema of the arm (*see* Figs 10.18c, d, 10.22 and 10.23).[56–60] It is important to document the presence of normal lymphatics in the donor leg with lymphoscintigraphy before considering surgery.

In post-mastectomy lymphoedema, two or three lymph vessels from the major lymphatic bundle on the medial

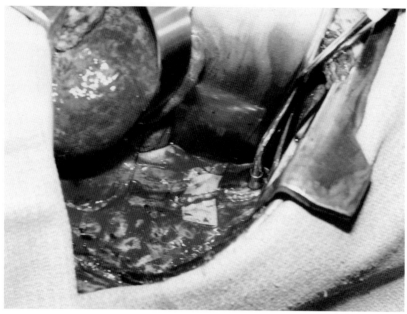

(a)

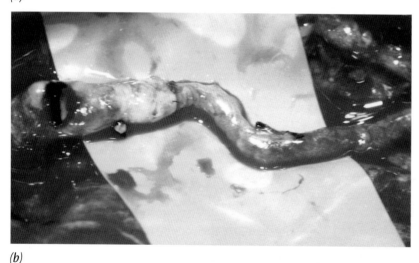

(b)

Figure 10.21a,b *Thoracic duct–azygos vein anastomosis performed through a right posterolateral thoracotomy in an end-to-end fashion with interrupted 8/0 Prolene sutures.*

aspect of the patient's thigh are transplantated into the arm (*see* Fig. 10.18d). The distal anastomoses are fashioned in the upper arm between the distal end of the graft and the epifascial and subfascial lymph vessels in an end-to-end fashion. The proximal anastomoses are best performed in the neck to the larger descending cervical lymphatics.

The procedure for lower limb reconstruction is a transposition of two or three normal lymphatic trunks from the normal thigh to the groin of the diseased limb with lympho-lymphatic anastomoses in the groin (cross-femoral grafting) (*see* Figs 10.18c, 10.22 and 10.23). In a report of 55 patients undergoing such procedures, Baumeister and Siuda recorded that 80 per cent of the patients were improved (a volume reduction) after a mean follow-up of 3 years.[58] An objective documentation of flow through the lymphatic graft can be obtained with lymphoscintigraphy (Fig. 10.24, p. 200).

Since his initial report, Baumeister and colleagues have treated 127 limbs in 122 patients with microsurgical lymphatic grafting, 79 showing arm oedema and 48 lower extremity oedema.[59,60] Most patients with arm oedema experienced a decrease in volume measurement. The authors used both lymphoscintigraphy and indirect lymphography with non-ionic water-soluble contrast injection to demonstrate patent grafts, but the overall graft patency was not recorded. In our limited experience with this operation, we have observed the long-term patency of suprapubic lymphatic grafts (Fig. 10.24), but graft patency was followed by only short-term clinical improvement.

Vein grafting

Campisi *et al.* reported on the use of vein grafting, using microsurgical techniques, to bypass lymphatic obstructions

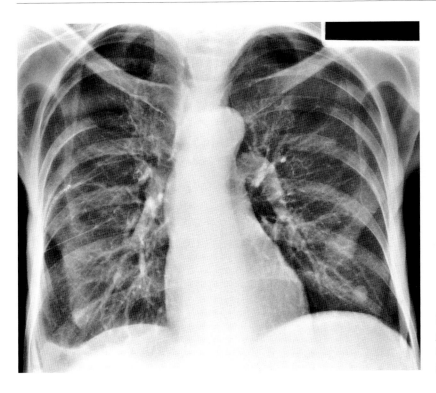

Figure 10.21c *Chest radiograph 2 years later confirming the absence of chylothorax. Reproduced by kind permission of the Mayo Foundation.*

in patients with congenital lymphatic occlusions and acquired segmental lymphatic blocks following excision or radiation of the lymph nodes (Fig. 10.25, p. 200).[61,62] In 133 patients, autologous vein grafts were implanted to bypass lymphatic obstruction at the groin. Volume reduction was higher in those patients who underwent the operation in the early stages of their lymphoedema. Of the entire group, a greater than 75 per cent improvement was noted in 47 per cent of the patients, and a 50–74 per cent improvement in another 34 per cent. The incidence of lymphangitis decreased after surgery. Long-term follow-up was available for 95 patients, but the results of late graft patency, studied with lymphoscintigraphy, were not reported. Clinical evaluation and mean volumetric assessment of the oedema suggested a long-term improvement in 81 per cent of the patients (*see* Table 10.1, p. 195).

Free lymphatic flap autotransplantation

Autotransplantation of normal lymphatic tissue in a free flap to a site deficient of lymph glands and vessels has been used to enhance the lymph transport of limbs affected by lymphoedema. Trevidic and Cormier have autotransplanted free axillary lymph node flaps to the axilla of patients with post-mastectomy lymphoedema.[65] The flap, taken as vascularized pedicle from the contralateral axilla, included the inferior axillary glands, a portion of the latissimus dorsi muscle and a segment of skin. The subscapular artery and vein, which supplied the flap, were anastomosed to the subclavian artery and vein on the recipient side. Only 1 out of 19 grafts failed, and an improvement was documented in 75 per cent of patients.

Lymphoscintigraphy showed improved lymphatic transport in 75 per cent of individuals. X-ray lymphography demonstrated the development of new lympho-lymphatic anastomoses in some patients. Further experience and a longer follow-up of this operation are needed to assess its efficacy.

Comment

Microsurgical reconstructions of the lymphatic system are possible but they are technically challenging because of the small size of the lymph channels. The reported long-term clinical results of microsurgical reconstructions, performed by a very few surgical groups in the world, are described as good or excellent in about two thirds of the patients, but no controlled clinical trials have been published. Although lymphoscintigraphy usually confirms improved lymph transport in patients with clinical improvement, it provides only indirect evidence of the patency of the lymphovenous anastomoses. Postoperative X-ray lymphangiography is the only way to confirm anastomotic patency, but it is invasive and not acceptable to patients as a follow-up study. Patency of the lymphatics in lymphatic grafts can be confirmed by lymphoscintigraphy, but long-term patency rates correlated to clinical improvement have not yet been reported.

Microsurgical lymphatic reconstructions require the expertise of dedicated microvascular surgeons, knowledgeable in the pathology and treatment of lymphoedema. All publications suggest that these operations carry a better chance of success if they are performed in the early stages of obstructive lymphoedema, when the intrinsic contractility

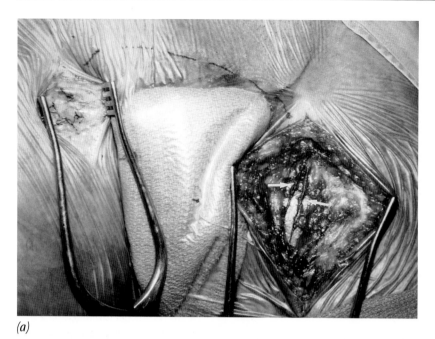

(a)

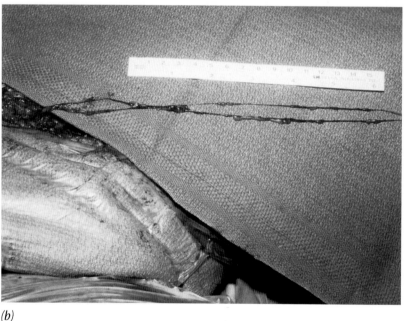

(b)

Figure 10.22 *(a) Exposure of lymph vessels for suprapubic transposition. Note two major lymph vessels of the left thigh that will be used for grafting (arrows). (b) Two lymphatic grafts divided at the distal thigh are prepared for lymphatic grafting. Reproduced by kind permission of the Mayo Foundation.*

of the lymph channels is still intact. Unfortunately, at this stage of the disease, conservative treatment, albeit not a cure, is frequently just as effective a means of control.

Many more controlled experimental and clinical studies are required to prove that lymphatic reconstructions provide long-term benefit. To advance the science of this field and to offer much-needed effective treatment to our patients, future studies should be directed towards answering the following questions:

- Is clinical improvement following surgery superior to results obtained with non-surgical techniques?
- Does restoring the patency of two or three lymph channels at the root of a limb result in the restoration

of an effective lymph transport system for the whole limb?
- Do patent lymphovenous anastomoses or lymphatic grafts reverse the chronic inflammatory changes in the subcutaneous tissue or in the skin?
- Are failed surgical interventions harmful; i.e. when patent lymph vessels used for anastomoses occlude, does the obstruction become worse?

Until these important questions have been answered, microsurgical treatment should be attempted only in carefully selected patients for whom non-operative management has failed. All patients must be made aware of the published results, successes, failures and complications.

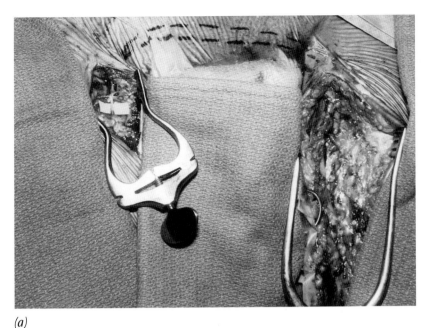

(a)

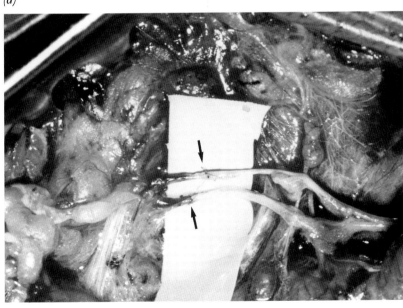

(b)

Figure 10.23 *(a) Completed suprapubic lymph grafting with two lympho-lymphatic anastomoses at right groin. The broken line indicates the position of the suprapubic lymphatic grafts. (b) Magnified photograph of two end-to-end lympho-lymphatic anastomoses (arrows) performed with 11/0 interrupted monofilament sutures. Reproduced by kind permission of the Mayo Foundation.*

ANTI-REFLUX OPERATIONS

The movement of lymph from the initial lymphatics to the junction of the thoracic duct with the great veins in the neck is produced by a number of intrinsic and extrinsic forces (*see* Chapter 3).

The direction of lymph flow depends entirely on the presence of many unidirectional valves. The forces of propulsion – intrinsic and extrinsic – force the lymph in the direction of least resistance, usually centrally, although if the valves are incompetent, lymph may flow peripherally. Gravity will also cause the lymph to flow retrogradely to the most dependent part of the system if the valves are incompetent, for example from the trunk downwards into the lower limbs, and in the upper arm

down to the hand, whenever the individual stands or is semirecumbent.

Valves are present in all but the smallest initial lymphatic capillaries. In the larger lymphatics, they are found 0.5–1.0 cm apart (*see* Chapter 2). Their frequency is presumably a reflection of the relatively weak propulsive forces generated by each lymphangion. True aplasia of valves has not been reported, perhaps because it has not been sought. If it does occur, it is likely to be as rare as it is in the veins.[76] If valves are always present, lymph reflux must always be the result of congenital or acquired vessel dilatation, which, by allowing the valve rings to dilate, makes the valve cusps incompetent.

Retrograde and forward flow in the subcutaneous or retroperitoneal collecting lymphatics is difficult to detect and currently not measurable. The diagnosis of reflux

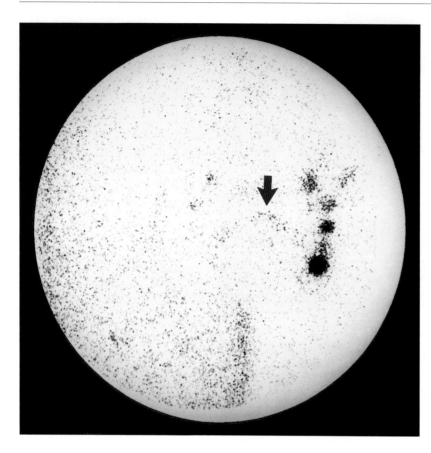

Figure 10.24 *Lymphoscintigram 3 months after suprapubic lymphatic grafting for secondary lymphoedema of the right lower extremity. Labelled colloid was injected into the right foot only. The arrow indicates the suprapubic graft. Note the intense filling of the left inguinal nodes. A preoperative lymphoscintigram in this patient showed no activity at the groin. Reproduced by kind permission of the Mayo Foundation.*

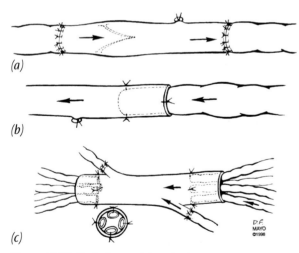

Figure 10.25 *Techniques of lymphatic reconstructions according to Campisi et al.[61,62] (a) Interposition vein graft. (b) Lymphovenous anastomosis. (c) Invagination of multiple lymphatics into the interposition vein graft (lymphatic-venous-lymphatic anastomoses). Reproduced by kind permission of the Mayo Foundation.*

depends on seeing (clinically or on a radiograph) lymph flowing in the wrong direction, for example chyle appearing in vesicles on the skin of the thigh or X-ray contrast medium flowing backwards along the renal lymphatics towards the kidney, or on the assumption that large dilated lymphatics must, because of their abnormal diameter, contain incompetent valves and therefore be the site of reflux. The diagnosis of lymph reflux is therefore usually based upon clinical evidence of reflux supported by a lymphographic demonstration of dilated tortuous vessels and, occasionally, if caught on screen or film, an observation of injected contrast medium flowing in the wrong direction.

Valvular incompetence usually affects all the lymphatics of an anatomical area, such as all the retroperitoneal vessels or all the vessels of a limb. The underlying cause of the incompetence, whether congenital lymphatic ectasia or dilatation below an obstruction, similarly usually affects all the vessels in the affected area, although congenital abnormalities are likely to be more extensive.

The object of treatment is to abolish the reflux or, if this is not possible, to abolish the high intralymphatic pressure that reflux generates. The ways in which this can be achieved are depicted in Fig. 10.26. The ideal way to stop reflux would be to restore valvular competence. This would mean restoring to normal the valve ring dilatation of very many valves and/or correcting any valve cusp abnormality such as laxity or valve cusp eversion. The surgical correction of numerous valves in 1–2 mm diameter lymphatics is beyond our technical abilities at present and may (if the lessons learnt from the veins are any indication[77]) be of questionable and short-term clinical benefit.

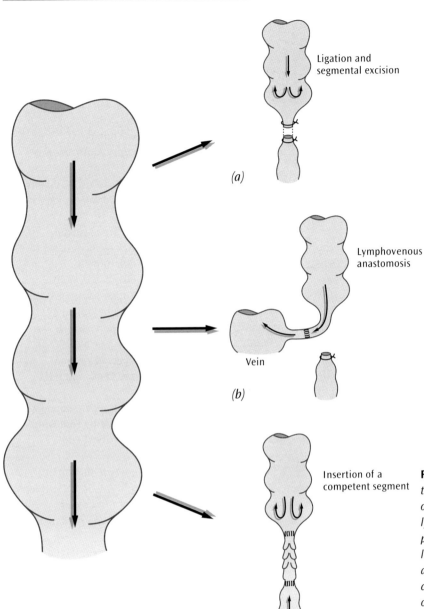

Ligation and segmental excision

(a)

Lymphovenous anastomosis

Vein

(b)

Insertion of a competent segment

(c)

Figure 10.26 *The principles underlying the various operations designed to stop or reduce reflux through incompetent lymphatics. Reflux can theoretically be prevented in three ways – proximal ligation (a), distal lymphovenous anastomoses (b) and the insertion of competent valves (c) – but the last option is not yet a practical proposition.*

An alternative to repairing the valves would be the replacement of a segment of each abnormal lymphatic with a transplanted segment of a normal lymphatic with competent valves. Lympho-lymphatic anastomoses are difficult to perform and often occlude within 1–12 weeks.[43] Furthermore, lymphatics usually run parallel to each other and empty into a common lymph gland without uniting, so any transplant procedure designed to prevent reflux would have to be applied to all or most of the lymphatics that are incompetent. This is an impractical proposition and has not been attempted.

Ligation at the uppermost limit of the abnormality is by far the simplest way of stopping reflux. *All* the abnormal lymphatics must be ligated because the lymphatics draining any area are multiple and, when dilated and incompetent, interconnecting. This approach usually requires an extensive, meticulous dissection across the whole of the retroperitoneal, pelvic or inguinal region. These techniques are described in detail in Chapters 12 and 16.

A thorough dissection and ligation of all the lymphatics draining a single anatomical area such as the pelvis, genitalia or limb carries with it the risk of exacerbating the lymphoedema in the affected region. Patients should be warned of this risk, although it is, surprisingly, infrequent. The swelling does not usually get worse because collateral pathways quickly develop through other normal lymphatics or any incompetent lymphatics that were not ligated. When the surgeon fails to ligate all of the incompetent lymphatics, reflux reappears within 6–12 months. When all the incompetent lymphatics have been ligated and the lymph returns through collateral pathways, these vessels slowly dilate and, as they do, slowly become incompetent. Reflux then returns, although the process usually takes 4–5 years. Ligation therefore has a very worthwhile clinical effect but never provides a permanent cure. Patients must be told that recurrence is likely, but at the same time they should be told that further surgical ligation, when required, is possible. We have patients with genital and limb reflux who have been kept under control with as many as five operations over a 30 year period.

The only alternative to the abolition of reflux is the prevention of the deleterious effects on the distal lymphatics caused by the high intralymphatic pressure generated by reflux and gravity combined. This can be achieved by arranging for the lowermost parts of the refluxing vessels to 'bleed out' into the neighbouring veins. This requires the construction of lymphovenous anastomoses somewhere along, but preferably at the lower end of, the incompetent vessels. Successful anastomoses between the lymphatics and veins remain patent only if the anastomotic stoma is large and the flow of lymph into the vein constant and voluminous. If there is an intermittent or low rate of lymph flow, blood will reflux from the vein into the lymphatic, clot and occlude the anastomosis. This technique thus works best when there is chylous reflux as chyle formation is sustained and copious. The flow of lymph alone without chyle from the lower half of the trunk and lower limb is less copious and intermittent so lymphovenous anastomoses performed in these circumstances are likely to fail. This approach has been used successfully in the treatment of filarial chylous reflux into the genitalia and limbs (see Chapters 12 and 16).

Attempts to vent the high pressure in incompetent lymphatics by making a fistula between the dilated lymphatics and the peritoneal cavity have not succeeded because the fistulae rapidly occlude.

NOTE

The section on liposuction was written with the advice of Dr H. Brorson MD, Consultant Plastic Surgeon, Malmo University Hospital, Malmo, Sweden. Dr P. Gloviczki, MD, Professor of Surgery and Chair, Division of Vascular Surgery, Mayo Medical School and Mayo Clinic, Rochester, Minnesota, USA, wrote the section on microsurgical procedures.

REFERENCES

1. Browse NL. A colour atlas of reducing operations for lymphoedema of the lower limb. London: Wolfe, 1986.
2. Sistrunk WE. Modification of the operation for elephantiasis. Journal of the American Medical Association 1918; 71: 800–3.
3. Homans J. Treatment of elephantiasis of the leg. New England Journal of Medicine 1936; 215: 1099.
4. Thompson N. Surgical treatment of chronic lymphoedema of the lower limb. British Medical Journal 1962; 2: 1566–9.
5. Charles H. In: Latham A, English TC eds. A system of treatment, Vol. 3. London: Churchill, 1912.
6. Teimourian B. Suction lipectomy and body sculpturing. St Louis: CV Mosby, 1987.
7. Nava VM, Lawrence WT. Liposuction on a lymphoedematous arm. Annals of Plastic Surgery 1988; 21: 366–8.
8. Illouz YG. Lymphoedema. In: Illouz YG, de Villiers YT eds. Body sculpturing by lipoplasty. Edinburgh: Churchill Livingstone, 1989: 384–8.
9. Louton RB, Terranova WA. The use of suction curettage as adjunct to the management of lymphoedema. Annals of Plastic Surgery 1989; 22: 345–57.
10. O'Brien BM, Khazanchi RK, Kumar PA, Dvir E, Pederson WC. Liposuction in the treatment of lymphoedema; a preliminary report. British Plastic Surgery 1989; 42: 530–3.
11. Sando WC, Nahai F. Suction lipectomy in the management of lymphoedema. Clinics in Plastic Surgery 1989; 16: 369–73.
12. Brorson H. Liposuction and Controlled Compression in the Treatment of Arm Lymphodema Following Breast Cancer. MD thesis, University of Lund, Sweden, 1989.
13. Brorson H, Svensson H. Complete reduction of lymphoedema of the arm by liposuction after breast cancer. Scandinavian Journal of Plastic and Reconstructive Surgery and Hand Surgery 1997; 31: 137–43.
14. Brorson H, Svensson H. Liposuction combined with controlled compression therapy reduces arm lymphoedema more effectively than controlled compression therapy alone. Plastic and Reconstructive Surgery 1998; 102: 1058–67.
15. Brorson H, Aberg M, Svensson H. Complete reduction of arm lymphoedema by liposuction following breast cancer – 5 year results. Lymphology 1999; 32 (suppl): 250–3.
16. Brorson H, Svensson H. Skin blood flow of the lymphoedematous arm before and after liposuction. Lymphology 1997; 30: 165–72.
17. Larsen OA, Lassen NA, Quaade F. Blood flow through human adipose tissue determined with radioactive xenon. Acta Physiologica Scandinavica 1966; 66: 337–45.
18. Ryan TJ. Lymphatics and adipose tissue. Clinical Dermatology 1995; 13: 493–8.
19. Ryan TJ, Curri SB. Blood vessels and lymphatics. Clinical Dermatology 1989; 7: 25–36.
20. Brorson H, Aberg M, Svensson H. High content of adipose tissue in chronic arm lymphoedema – an important factor limiting treatment outcome. Lymphology 1999; 32 (suppl): 52–4.

21. Brorson H, Svensson H, Norrgren K, Thorsson O. Liposuction reduces arm lymphoedema without significantly altering the already impaired lymph transport. *Lymphology* 1998; **31:** 156–72.

22. Brorson H. Liposuction gives complete reduction of chronic large arm lymphoedema after breast cancer. *Acta Oncologica* 2000; **39:** 407–20.

23. Kondoleon F. Die Dauerresultate der Chirurgischen Behandlung der Elephantiastichen Lymphoedeme. *Münchener Medizine Wochenschrift* 1915; **62:** 154–7.

24. Handley WS. Lymphangioplasty. *Lancet* 1908; **1:** 783–4.

25. Kinmonth JB. *The lymphatics.* London: Arnold, 1982.

26. Gillies HD, Fraser FR. The treatment of lymphoedema by plastic operation. *British Medical Journal* 1935; **1:** 96–8.

27. Nielubowicz J, Olszewski W. *Journal of Cardiovascular Surgery,* Special issue for the XVth Congress of ESCVS, 1966: 384–5.

28. Nielubowicz J, Olszewski W. Surgical lymphaticovenous shunts in patients with secondary lymphoedema. *British Journal of Surgery* 1968; **55:** 440–3.

29. Politowski M, Bartkowski S, Dynowski J. Treatment of lymphoedema of the limbs by lymphatico-venous fistula. *Surgery* 1969; **66:** 639–43.

30. Goldsmith HS. Longterm results of omental transposition for chronic lymphoedema. *Annals of Surgery* 1974; **180:** 847–9.

31. Lanzara A. Surgical treatment of lymphoedema by omental transplantation. *Journal of Cardiovascular Surgery,* Special issue for the XVIIth Congress of the ECVS, 1968: 122.

32. Degni M. New technique of lymphatico-venous anastomosis (buried type) for the treatment of lymphoedema. *Vasa* 1974; **3:** 479–81.

33. O'Brien BMcC, Shafiroff BB. Microlymphaticovenous and resectional surgery in obstructive lymphoedema. *World Journal of Surgery* 1979; **3:** 3–15.

34. Pugnaire M. Lifangioplastia mesenterica en al tratamiento de las elefantiasis de les membros inferiores. *Angiologia* 1968; **20:** 146–52.

35. Hurst PA, Kinmonth JB, Rutt DL. A gut and mesentery pedicle for bridging lymphatic obstruction. *Journal of Cardiovascular Surgery* 1978; **19:** 589–96.

36. Kinmonth JB, Hurst PA, Edwards JM, Rutt DL. Relief of lymph obstruction by use of a bridge of mesentery and ileum. *British Journal of Surgery* 1978; **65:** 829–33.

37. Edwards JM, Kinmonth JB. Lymphovenous shunts in man. *British Medical Journal* 1969; **4:** 579–81.

38. Jacobson JH. Discussion. In: Danese C, Bower R, Howard J eds. Experimental anastomoses of lymphatics. *Archives of Surgery* 1962; **84:** 9.

39. Laine JB, Howard JM. Experimental lymphatico-venous anastomosis. *Surgical Forum* 1963; **14:** 111–12.

40. Gloviczki P, Hollier LH, Nora FE, Kaye MP. The natural history of microsurgical lymphovenous anastomoses: an experimental study. *Journal of Vascular Surgery* 1986; **4:** 148–56.

41. Yamada Y. The studies on lymphatic venous anastomosis in lymphedema. *Nagoya Journal of Medical Science* 1969; **32:** 1.

42. Gilbert A, O'Brien BM, Vorrath JW, Sykes PJ. Lymphaticovenous anastomosis by microvascular technique. *British Journal of Plastic Surgery* 1976; **29:** 355–60.

43. Shaper NJ, Rutt DR, Browse NL. Use of Teflon stents for lymphovenous anastomosis. *British Journal of Surgery* 1992; **79:** 633–6.

44. Kinjo O, Kusara A. Lymphatic vessel-to-isolated-vein anastomosis for secondary lymphedema in a canine model. *Surgery Today* 1995; **25:** 633–9.

45. Puckett CL, Jacobs GR, Hurvitz JS, Silver D. Evaluation of lymphovenous anastomoses in obstructive lymphedema. *Plastic and Reconstructive Surgery* 1980; **66:** 116–20.

46. Huang GK, Ru-Qi H, Zong-Zhao L, Yao-Liang S, Tie De L, Gong-Ping P. Microlymphaticovenous anastomosis for treating lymphedema of the extremities and external genitalia. *Journal of Microsurgery* 1981; **3:** 32–9.

47. Jamal S. Lymphovenous anastomosis in filarial lymphedema. *Lymphology* 1981; **14:** 64–8.

48. Krylov V, Milanov N, Abalmasov K. Microlymphatic surgery of secondary lymphoedema of the upper limb. *Annales de Chirurgie et Gynécologie* 1982; **71:** 77–9.

49. Nieuborg L. *The role of lymphaticovenous anastomoses in the treatment of postmastectomy oedema.* Alblasserdam, Netherlands: Offsetdrukkerij Kanters, 1982.

50. Ho LC, Lai MF, Kennedy PJ. Micro-lymphatic bypass in the treatment of obstructive lymphoedema of the arm: case report of a new technique. *British Journal of Plastic Surgery* 1983; **36:** 350–7.

51. Gong-Kang H, Ru-Ai H, Zong-Zhao L, Yao-Liang S, Tie De L, Gong-Ping P. Microlymphaticovenous anastomosis in the treatment of lower limb obstructive lymphedema: analysis of 91 cases. *Plastic and Reconstructive Surgery* 1985; **76:** 671–85.

52. Campisi C, Tosatti E, Casaccia M, *et al.* Lymphatic microsurgery [in Italian]. *Minerva Chirurgica* 1986; **41:** 469–81.

53. Campisi C, Boccardo F, Zilli A, Maccio A, Napoli F. Long-term results after lymphatic-venous anastomoses for the treatment of obstructive lymphedema. *Microsurgery* 2001; **21:** 135–9.

54. Gloviczki P, Fisher J, Hollier LH, Pairolero PC, Schirger A, Wahner HW. Microsurgical lymphovenous anastomosis for treatment of lymphedema: a critical review. *Journal of Vascular Surgery* 1988; **7:** 647–52.

55. O'Brien BMcC, Mellow CG, Khazanchi RK, Dvir E, Kumar V, Pederson WC. Long-term results after microlymphatico-venous anastomoses for the treatment of obstructive lymphedema. *Plastic and Reconstructive Surgery* 1990; **85**: 562–72.

56. Kleinhaus E, Baumeister RGH, Hahn D, *et al.* Evaluation of transport kinetics in lymphoscintigraphy: follow-up study in patients with transplanted lymphatic vessels. *European Journal of Nuclear Medicine* 1985; **10**: 349–62.

57. Baumeister RG, Siuda S, Bohmert H, Moser E. A microsurgical method for reconstruction of interrupted lymphatic pathways: autologous lymph-vessel transplantation for treatment of lymphedemas. *Scandinvian Journal of Plastic and Reconstructive Surgery* 1986; **20**: 141–6.

58. Baumeister RG, Siuda S. Treatment of lymphedemas by microsurgical lymphatic grafting: what is proved? *Plastic and Reconstructive Surgery* 1990; **85**: 64–74.

59. Baumeister RGH, Frick A, Hofmann T. 10 years experience with autogenous microsurgical lymphvessel-transplantation. *European Journal of Lymphology* 1991; **6**: 62.

60. Baumeister RGH, Fink U, Tatsch K, Frick A. Microsurgical lymphatic grafting: first demonstration of patent grafts by indirect lymphography and long term follow-up studies. *Progress in Lymphology* 1994; **27**: 787.

61. Campisi C, Boccardo F, Alitta P, Tacchella M. Derivative lymphatic microsurgery: indications, techniques, and results. *Microsurgery* 1995; **16**: 463–8.

62. Campisi C, Boccardo F, Zilli A, Maccio A, Napoli F. The use of vein grafts in the treatment of peripheral lymphedemas: long-term results. *Microsurgery* 2001; **21**: 143–7.

63. Gloviczki P, Noel AA. Lymphatic reconstructions. In: Rutherford RB ed. *Rutherford's vascular surgery*, 5th edn. Philadelphia: WB Saunders, 2000: 2159–74.

64. Noel AA, Gloviczki P, Bender CE, Whitley D, Stanson AW, Deschamps C. Treatment of primary chylous disorders. *Journal of Vascular Surgery* 2001; **34**: 785–91.

65. Trevidic P, Cormier JM. Free axillary lymph node transfer. In: Cluzan RV ed. *Progress in lymphology*, Vol. 13. Amsterdam: Elsevier Science, 1992: 415–20.

66. Browse NL. The diagnosis and management of primary lymphedema. *Journal of Vascular Surgery* 1986; **3**: 181–4.

67. Gloviczki P, Wahner H. Clinical diagnosis and evaluation of lymphedema. In: Rutherford RB ed. *Vascular surgery*, 5th edn. Philadelphia: WB Saunders, 2000: 2123–42.

68. Rockson SG. Lymphedema. *American Journal of Medicine* 2001; **110**: 288–95.

69. Stewart G, Gaunt JI, Croft DN, Browse NL. Isotope lymphography: a new method of investigating the role of the lymphatics in chronic limb oedema. *British Journal of Surgery* 1985; **72**: 906–9.

70. Gloviczki P, Calcagno D, Schirger A, *et al.* Noninvasive evaluation of the swollen extremity: experiences with 190 lymphoscintigraphic examinations. *Journal of Vascular Surgery* 1989; **9**: 683–9.

71. Cambria RA, Gloviczki P, Naessens JM, Wahner HW. Noninvasive evaluation of the lymphatic system with lymphoscintigraphy: a prospective, semiquantitative analysis in 386 extremities. *Journal of Vascular Surgery* 1993; **18**: 773–82.

72. Williams WH, Witte CL, Witte MH, McNeill GC. Radionuclide lymphangioscintigraphy in the evaluation of peripheral lymphedema. *Clinical Nuclear Medicine* 2000; **25**: 451–64.

73. Witte CL, Witte MH. Diagnostic and interventional imaging of lymphatic disorders. *International Angiology* 1999; **18**: 25–30.

74. Gloviczki P. The management of lymphatic disorders. In: Rutherford RB ed. *Vascular surgery*, 5th edn. Philadelphia: WB Saunders, 1995: 1883–949.

75. Browse NL. The surgery of lymphedema. In: Veith FJ ed. *Current critical problems in vascular surgery*. St Louis: Quality Medical Publishing, 1989: 408–9.

76. Lindvall N, Lodin A. Congenital absence of venous valves. *Acta Chirurgica Scandinavica* 1962; **124**: 310–19.

77. Browse N, Burnand KG, Irvine AT, Wilson NM. Chronic deep vein incompetence. *Diseases of the veins*. London: Arnold, 1988.

PART 2

Management of clinical problems

Management of lymphoedema of the lower limb

Primary lymphoedema affects the lower limb much more often than the upper limb. Genetic factors almost certainly play a major role in its aetiology (*see* Chapter 5). The signs of the disorder may be present at birth or appear at any age throughout life, although the teenage years and early twenties are the most common times for presentation. Late-onset lymphoedema, particularly after the age of 40, should always be considered to be secondary to another disease, such as metastatic carcinoma, until proved otherwise (*see* Chapter 7). Many patients, particularly those with lipodystrophy or venous disease, are referred with a mistaken provisional diagnosis of 'lymphoedema' so it is important to confirm the diagnosis with objective investigations whenever possible (*see* Chapter 6).

LYMPHOEDEMA PRESENTING AT OR SOON AFTER BIRTH

Lymphoedema of the lower limb that is present at birth in a child who has a clear family history of lymphoedema may be categorized as Milroy's disease, but there are cases in which the family history cannot be confirmed and other forms of congenital lymphoedema that are not familial. The genetic abnormality in Milroy's disease has now been established as missense mutations in *VEGFR-3* – the gene responsible for lymphangiogenesis (*see* Chapter 5), and it may soon be possible to test for the gene abnormality of this and other congenital syndromes.

Presentation

The condition is usually noticed soon after birth when one limb appears enlarged in comparison to its fellow.

Detection of the swelling may be delayed if both lower limbs are swollen. Congenital familial and non-familial lymphoedema may be associated with other congenital abnormalities such as Turner's, Proteus, Noonan's and Pierre Robin syndromes, cardiac abnormalities and hydroceles (*see* Chapter 5). Some infants also have swelling of one or both upper limbs. Apart from the limb swelling, these children do not exhibit other problems unless another associated genetic disorder is present.

Physical signs

Inspection of the limbs should confirm soft tissue swelling, usually maximal over the dorsum of the foot, with an associated Stemmer's sign (*see* Chapter 6). The subcutaneous tissues usually have a doughy consistency and resist deformation, but firm prolonged compression on the dorsum of the foot *always* produces a pit. Failure to produce a pit should make the clinician reconsider the diagnosis of lymphoedema.

An increased leg length or the presence of a capillary naevus should suggest a diagnosis of Klippel–Trenaunay syndrome (*see* Chapter 18). General tissue overgrowth suggests a diagnosis of local gigantism (sometimes associated with hemihypertrophy) Proteus or Parkes Weber syndrome. The latter diagnosis is supported by the presence of machinery murmurs over the leg or a positive Branham's sign (a slowing of the pulse rate produced by arterial occlusion at the root of the limb by hand or with a tourniquet). The limb should be measured to establish its real and apparent length and its diameter in relation to fixed bony points. Clinical photographs of the limbs make a useful permanent record for future comparison. To exclude the presence of other associated genetic disorders, the general examination should focus on the face, the eyelids, the chest and the heart.

Investigation

Confirmation of the diagnosis in neonates is difficult. Tiny children rarely co-operate with isotope lymphography, and a general anaesthetic for X-ray lymphography is rarely indicated on the basis of risk versus benefit. If the child will co-operate, computed tomography or magnetic resonance imaging can be used to confirm that the swelling is subcutaneous and mainly water. Chromosomal abnormalities should be looked for if other congenital anomalies exist.

Management

The parents should be told that the provisional diagnosis is lymphoedema but that final confirmation of the diagnosis should await later childhood or the teenage years, when the child will be better able to tolerate and understand the purpose of any investigations and participate in management decisions. The parents' attention often focuses on any associated genetic disorders (whose management may take precedence) and on the risks of the same problems developing in further offspring. They must be told about the condition's pattern of inheritance and its clinical nature, and, if they wish, be referred to a clinical geneticist. Congenital lymphoedema is often less severe than other types of lymphoedema. Parents can be reassured that the condition rarely reduces the quality of life and, to the best of our knowledge, does not reduce life expectancy.

Compression hosiery and manual massage can be discussed and tried but are often impractical in young children. Drug therapy is rarely beneficial. Surgical reduction is rarely indicated; it is extremely unusual to have to perform a reducing operation on a child less than 12 years old. A 'wait and watch' policy with 'masterly inactivity' is usually all that is indicated. Some parents press for definitive investigations when the child is young, but this should be resisted if the child is growing normally and is fully active. Yearly follow-up consultations give the parents an opportunity to discuss new therapies and developments, and enable the clinician to measure the limb and take new clinical photographs. In late childhood or early adolescence, the child or teenager may consent to lymphoscintigraphy, which can also be performed on other members of the family if a genetic trait is thought to be likely. The subsequent management then depends on the size of the limb, the degree of disability and the result of the lymphoscintigram.

The prognosis of congenital lymphoedema is usually very good, although it is currently incurable. Most patients have a completely satisfactory existence with little therapy except for compression therapy and massage (*see* Chapter 9). Some, however, suffer a progressive deterioration and, by the time they reach their third or fourth decade, require vigorous treatment and sometimes surgical reduction. Genetic manipulation may be feasible in the years ahead.

LYMPHOEDEMA PRESENTING AROUND THE TIME OF PUBERTY

Approximately one third of patients who present with peri- and post-pubertal lymphoedema, i.e. in their teenage years or early twenties, have a family history, but this group differs from the congenital lymphoedema group in that the lymphoedema affects about three females to every one male. Although a gene has been identified for one rare form of pubertal-onset lymphoedema, the lymphoedema–distichiasis syndrome, the most common form of pubertal lymphoedema (Meige's disease) has no associated features. The pathological abnormality is a distal lymphatic obliteration with a normal or reduced number of lymphatics in the upper thigh, groin and torso.

Presentation

Affected individuals, mostly women, first complain of the swelling of one foot or ankle that appears quite suddenly and often seems to have followed an insect bite or an episode of trauma such as a sprained ankle. The swelling may be intermittent at first but quite rapidly becomes permanent. It usually resolves partially or completely at night only to reappear over the course of the next day. It is not usually associated with pain, except transiently at the onset, but it may cause a 'stiffness' and 'heaviness' of the affected limb. The swelling eventually affects both legs in about one third of patients. The diagnosis is rarely made at the patient's first medical consultation, especially if the swelling is unilateral; at this stage it is usually misdiagnosed as a deep vein thrombosis or torn muscle.

The first presentation is occasionally with a severe attack of cellulitis (erysipelas), in which the patient suddenly develops a fever, malaise and rigors, and the limb becomes red, hot and swollen (*see* Chapter 6); it is therefore important to remember the possibility of underlying lymphoedema when a patient presents with a cellulitis of unknown cause. In such patients, an associated area of athlete's foot is often the portal of entry for the infecting organism, commonly a *Streptococcus*.

Severe pain and swelling in the absence of cellulitis is rarely caused by lymphoedema. A deep vein thrombosis, a ruptured Baker's cyst, a torn plantaris muscle, a ruptured gastrocnemius muscle, a septic or rheumatoid arthritis, an intramuscular or intra-articular haemorrhage, a rapidly growing soft tissue or bony sarcoma, and a pathological or stress fracture are the important differential diagnoses that must be excluded by careful examination and appropriate investigations. A history of a surgical block dissection or previous irradiation of the local lymph glands points to the possibility of a secondary rather than a primary lympheodema.

Physical signs

The presenting physical sign is usually unilateral pitting oedema of one or both feet, ankles and calves. (It should be noted here that lymphoedema always pits if the pressure is sufficient and sustained!) The toes are usually square in appearance because they have been compressed within shoes, and Stemmer's sign may be present. A systemic cause of oedema must be carefully excluded if the swelling is bilateral at the first presentation. A careful clinical examination may detect the presence of chronic liver disease, malnutrition or extensive protein loss, cardiac failure or renal failure. The presence of other causes of oedema should be suspected if pitting is easy to elicit. Firm pressure is usually required if the oedema has a lymphatic cause, presumably related to the relatively greater concentration of protein within the interstitial fluid. The genitalia and upper limbs must be examined for the presence of oedema, although oedema of these areas is rare in these patients.

The presence of varicose veins, lipodermatosclerosis, ulceration and venous flares suggests that venous disease rather than primary lymphoedema is the cause of the swelling, but the two conditions can co-exist and overlap. Investigation of the veins is then indicated. The eyelids should be examined for distichiasis as the lymphoedema–distichiasis syndrome often presents with peri-pubertal lymphoedema. Other types of lymphoedema should be suspected if ascites, genital oedema and cutaneous lymph vesicles (lymphangiectasia) are present (*see* Chapter 7).

Investigation

Simple blood tests (serum proteins, liver function tests, urea and electrolytes, and creatinine level), chest radiography, electrocardiography and echocardiography should be used to exclude hepatic, cardiac and nutritional diseases if these are considered to be possible alternative diagnoses. Many patients are diagnosed solely on clinical grounds as having mild, stable lymphoedema and remain under the care of their general practitioner. No further steps are required for these patients other than the prescription of regular elastic support, unless they request that the diagnosis be confirmed by an objective investigation.

We request an isotope lymphogram on all patients referred to us for a second opinion. This allows us to support or refute the referring physician's diagnosis with confidence and assess the lymphatics of the other limb in cases of unilateral oedema. The diagnosis is confirmed if the lymphoscintigraph shows an uptake of less than 0.3 per cent of the initial pedal dose in the groin 'region of interest' at 30 minutes and little further increase in uptake at 1 hour.[1] An above normal uptake of isotope in the inguinal glands suggests the presence of significant venous disease, which can be confirmed by duplex scanning, ascending venography or a test of calf pump function.[2]

The combination of clinical suspicion, confirmatory isotope lymphography and the exclusion of any venous or medical disease is usually sufficient to establish the diagnosis in the majority of cases. X-ray lymphography (*see* Chapter 6) is only indicated if the diagnosis remains equivocal after isotope lymphography or if the results of the test are at variance with the clinical findings, but the patient must understand that, in such circumstances, the investigation is only being performed to confirm or refute the diagnosis and is unlikely to have any bearing on future therapy. Other diagnostic tests such as skin biopsy and chromosomal analyses currently have little part to play. Magnetic resonance imaging and computed tomography scanning are only relevant if other pathologies are suspected.

Management

The majority of patients with confirmed peri-pubertal lymphoedema caused by distal lymphatic obstruction can be managed conservatively. The nature of the condition should be explained to the patient gently and tactfully, stressing its remediable albeit incurable prognosis.

Many patients require nothing more than advice, elastic compression and massage (*see* Chapter 9). In spite of stressing the importance of these measures and the need to apply them diligently for the rest of their life, some quickly give them up or use them haphazardly because they interfere with their normal daily routine or because they find elastic hosiery cosmetically unacceptable. Drugs are largely ineffective, but it is important to check for the presence of athlete's foot and treat this, if it is present, with local antifungal agents. Antibiotics may be required for attacks of cellulitis.

Bypass surgery is usually impossible as the lymphatic obliteration is of the distal collecting lymphatics. Reducing operations are rarely required in the teens and twenties, especially if the patient applies the conservative treatment diligently, but some limbs get steadily larger in spite of elastic compression and massage to such an extent that a Homans' or Charles's operation is the only possible treatment (*see* Chapter 10). The results of these operations are set out in Chapter 11.

PATIENTS PRESENTING WITH WHOLE-LEG LYMPHOEDEMA IN ADULT LIFE

This condition is usually unilateral and often starts in the thigh. The cause of the lymphoedema in many of these patients is an obstruction in the inguinal or iliac lymph glands without any distal lymphatic obliteration. Combined proximal and distal lymphatic obstruction/obliteration may also cause a steadily progressive swelling of the whole limb.

Presentation

Proximal obstruction alone is equally common in males and females, and does not appear to have a genetic basis.

It normally presents in adulthood. It rarely presents at birth but can develop in early childhood and in the teens and twenties, when it can usually be differentiated from mild distal lymphatic obstruction by its rapid onset and the fact that the swelling involves the whole limb, often beginning in the thigh. The relative or complete sparing of the foot in these patients indicates that the lymphatic collecting vessels in the lower leg are functioning normally. This form of more proximal oedema must be differentiated from that caused by venous obstruction, acquired arteriovenous fistulae, metastatic lymph gland involvement and pelvic tumours (see Chapter 7).

Combined proximal and distal lymphatic obliteration is more common in females, which suggests that it is a severe form of obliteration, similar to that seen in Meige's disease, beginning in the peripheral lymphatics but slowly progressing up the limb, gradually involving the proximal vessels.

Investigation

A lymphoscintigraph showing a slightly delayed clearance of isotope from the foot, with normal filling of the inguinal lymph glands but no filling of the iliac lymph glands, suggests the presence of a proximal obstruction. The normal or high 30 and 60 minute radioactivity of the inguinal glands, which may increase still further over the second hour, is sometimes erroneously reported as indicating normal lymphatic flow; however, the failure of the isotope to progress to the iliac and aortic glands, and a high concentration of radioactivity in the groin, should suggest the correct diagnosis, especially when the scintigraphs are reviewed in the light of the clinical findings. Any doubt about the diagnosis should be resolved by performing an X-ray lymphograph. This investigation will also help the clinician to assess the possibility of performing an enteromesenteric bypass operation, an operation that should be performed early in the course of the disease before the distal vessels become obliterated.[3]

Management

Proximal obstruction/obliteration should first be treated conservatively with massage and compression (see Chapter 9), but if it increases and the swelling becomes severe, it should be treated by a bypass operation before distal obliteration develops. The enteromesenteric bypass operation (see Chapter 10) is our procedure of choice for proximal obstruction/obliteration. It may be used for primary and secondary proximal obstruction provided the underlying cause of any secondary obstruction is under control. The results of this operation are described on p. 215.

Combined proximal and distal obstruction should also be treated vigorously with massage and compression as the only other treatment is a reducing operation.

Reducing operations should only be used when the limb has stabilized and the size, weight and appearance are seriously interfering with normal daily work and social activity. The patient and surgeon must choose between a below-knee Homans' procedure, which can be performed on both sides (medial and lateral) of the limb, and a Charles's operation combined with some form of thigh reduction (see Chapter 10). Homans' operation gives a better cosmetic result, especially if the skin is healthy, but Charles's operation is better for massive lower leg swelling with unhealthy skin. The choice must be made with informed input from the patient, who should have the opportunity to study pre- and postoperative photographs of similar patients and, if possible, meet others who have undergone the procedures.

Comment

Bypass surgery and reducing operations are very much a last option for patients with severe lymphoedema who have failed conservative management. The number of patients with lower limb lymphoedema whom we have advised to have surgical treatment is only 5 per cent of the already selected population who are referred to our clinic.

RESULTS OF REDUCING OPERATIONS FOR LYMPHOEDEMA OF THE LOWER LIMB

It is difficult to apply objective methods of assessment to the results of reducing operations as this form of surgery is essentially a 'cosmetic' procedure, each patient's subjective assessment being as important as the surgeon's physical assessment. When the limb is massive, the skin unhealthy and mobility restricted, we have been impressed by the ability of a Charles's procedure, combined with thigh reduction, to enable patients to return to work and cast off a sedentary or even a wheelchair existence. For less severe disease, Homans' operation is more appropriate and can be repeated. Few, if any, patients are made worse, and we are unaware of any fatalities following the St Thomas' Hospital, London, series of operations.

In 1975, Kinmonth et al.[4] published the results of 74 operations – 56 Thompson's and 12 Homans' procedures – and six experimental operations in which the denuded flap was not buried but sewn beneath the opposing flap. The follow-up period varied from 1 to 15 years. The results were classified as poor, moderate and good:

- A poor result occurred when the limb remained the same size or became larger, judged by measurements of circumference and a study of pre- and postoperative photographs (even though most of these patients thought they were better).
- A moderate result was when the circumference was less and the patient and surgeon were pleased with the result.

- *A good result* was viewed as being when there was a major improvement that was considered satisfactory by both patient and surgeon.

The result in 13 patients (17.5 per cent) was thought to be poor. The result in 45 patients (55 per cent) was moderate, whereas in 16 patients (27.5 per cent) it was good. Overall, 80 per cent of the patients considered that the result was satisfactory and were glad that the reduction had been carried out. Primary healing occurred in 38 patients (51 per cent) and delayed healing in 36 (49 per cent). The delayed healing group included 18 patients with major skin necrosis, i.e. necrosis requiring excision, re-suture or skin grafting. Infection occurred in only two patients.

Two years later, Sakulsky et al.[5] published the results of the surgical treatment of lower limb lymphoedema carried out at the Mayo Clinic, Rochester, USA. They reported that they had operated on 64 patients between 1936 and 1964 and presented the results of a 1–22 year follow-up of 56 patients. The data in this paper are difficult to interpret as the numbers of patients, legs and operations are mixed together, but the majority – approximately 53 individuals (80 per cent) – underwent a Homans' operation and 9 (17 per cent) a Charles's operation. The results were classified as excellent, good, fair and poor. Of the 56 patients followed up, 13 (23 per cent) had an excellent result, 22 (39 per cent) a good result, 8 (14 per cent) a fair result and 13 (23 per cent) a poor result. These results are almost identical to those recorded by Kinmonth.

In 1990, we reviewed the results of all the more recent St Thomas' reducing operations. Between 1956 and 1990, we saw more than 5000 patients with lymphoedema of the lower limb, and during this period Professors Kinmonth and Browse performed reducing operations on 218 patients, approximately 4 per cent of all the patients referred over this time. The results were collected from the records of the annual follow-up visit and a postal questionnaire. No information beyond the operation could be obtained for 42 patients, most of whom had left the UK, leaving a study group of 176:121 females and 55 males. The type of lymphoedema and age of onset are presented in Table 11.1.

Preoperative investigations revealed that 136 patients (77 per cent) had distal lymphatic obliteration, 19 (11 per cent) proximal and distal obliteration and 21 (12 per cent) incompetent megalymphatics. The main indications for operation were severe swelling causing heaviness, aching, functional impairment, disfigurement and social and cosmetic embarrassment. No operations were performed solely for cosmetic reasons. Homans' and Thompson's operations were used rather than the Charles's operation whenever possible, but we abandoned the Thompson buried dermis flap operation in 1980 because of its late complications and failure to promote superficial-to-deep lymphatic connections. The median weight of tissue removed by the Homans' operation was 596 g. The Thompson procedure removed a median weight of 710 g and the Charles's operation 3466 g.

Early (within 3 months) postoperative complications

The general postoperative complications were limited to one patient who developed a deep vein thrombosis in the calf.

Primary wound healing occurred in 77 per cent of the 228 operations (some patients having more than one procedure). Skin flap necrosis occurred after 28 operations (12 per cent) (Table 11.2). Excision and skin resuturing was possible in 20 limbs, but 8 needed a skin graft to close the defect. Eight operations were complicated by wound abscesses that required drainage under general anaesthesia. Minor wound infection occurred in another 16 limbs. The overall rate of healing was 81 per cent.

There was no significant difference in the incidence of early wound complications between the Homans' or Thompson's operations. Skin-edge necrosis requiring excision, resuturing or skin grafting did not occur in any of the Homans' operations performed after 1985, when we increased the thickness of the flaps and slightly shortened their length. This contrasts with the 12 cases of skin necrosis that occurred before 1985. Approximately 90 per cent of the skin grafts applied after the Charles's

Table 11.1 *Type of lymphoedema and age of the patients at the time of onset of their lymphoedema in a consecutive series of 176 patients who underwent reducing operations at St Thomas' Hospital, London, between 1956 and 1990*

Type of lymphoedema	Number of patients and time of onset
Primary lymphoedema	156
Within 3 years of birth	25
3–35 years	111 (mean age 20, SD $\pm$ 8)
36–70 years	20 (mean age 45, SD $\pm$ 9)
Secondary lymphoedema	20
After treatment of a benign disease	9 (mean age 31, SD $\pm$ 13)
After treatment of a malignant disease	11 (mean age 33, SD $\pm$ 11)

SD, standard deviation.

Table 11.2 *Postoperative wound complications following 130 Homans' and 98 Thompson's operations*

Complications	Homans' operation (n = 130)	Thompson's operation (n = 98)
Necrosis requiring skin excision and re-suturing	12	8
Necrosis requiring skin excision and skin grafting	3	5
Major infection (requiring surgical drainage or cleaning)	5	3
Minor infection (requiring only dressing)	7	9
Total complications delaying healing	27 (21%)	25 (26%)

excision took 'per primum', but all patients needed wound cleaning and many required one or two small additional split-skin grafts to obtain 100 per cent healing. The donor sites, usually on the good leg but occasionally on the back or abdomen, caused no significant problems.

Late complications

There were no significant late complications following the Homans' operations. The wounds remained well healed and did not show keloid change (Fig. 11.1).

The principal problem with the Thompson buried dermis flap operation was the development of pilonidal sinuses in the buried flap. These produced tender lumps deep to the longitudinal scar, which eventually ruptured on to the skin surface and discharged hair and sebaceous material. They often became infected and could only be cured by excision. It was this annoying complication and the fact that the buried flap appeared to serve no purpose that made us decide in 1980 to abandon this procedure and use only the simpler Homans' operation.

The majority of the skin grafts applied after the complete excision of skin and subcutaneous tissues (the Charles's operation) became stable and smooth. Figure 11.2a shows a limb 10 years after a Charles' operation, with good-looking skin grafts but also an annoying, but avoidable, feature, a 'pantaloon' effect caused by a marked change in diameter between the untreated tissues around and above the knee and the excised and grafted area below. This can be avoided (Fig. 11.2b and c) by carefully cutting thin anterior and posterior flaps just below the knee (*see* Chapter 10).

Some skin grafts, especially if meshed, unfortunately become keloid (Fig. 11.3). The keloid scars become prominent, almost papillomatous, and the cracks and crevices between the keloid protuberances become infected. This is less likely to occur if the skin grafts are always kept firmly compressed. When it does happen, the only treatment is excision of the keloid protuberances. If this is done with a Syme's knife, the many normal areas of skin between the lumps can be preserved and will quickly re-epithelialize the raw areas. Large raw areas have to be re-grafted.

Lumps beneath the skin grafts may appear if fat is left on the deep fascia. These can usually be excised without damaging the graft.

Late results

We assessed our late results as:

- *Good*: Patient fully satisfied and glad to have had the operation, plus a documented reduction in limb size.
- *Moderate*: Patient not wholly satisfied but of the opinion that the operation was worthwhile, plus a documented decrease in limb size.
- *Poor*: Patient dissatisfied and/or no reduction or an increase in the limb size.

The median follow-up period was 5 years (range 0.5–32 years). Over half the patients were followed up for more than 5 years and another third for 1–5 years. The mean reduction in the limb circumference at calf level, 15 cm below the patella, after the Homans' and Thompson's operation was similar, being 9.2 and 7.7 cm respectively. Those who underwent a Charles's operation had a mean reduction of calf circumference of 16.5 cm (Table 11.3). Only 15 patients in the whole series had an increase in the circumference of their limbs, this ranging from 1 to 11 cm (mean 4.5 cm). The median follow-up interval in these 15 patients was 3.6 years.

The patients' overall opinion of their result is shown in Table 11.4. There were no significant differences between the results when they were subdivided according to the different types of operation, nor were the results significantly affected by the different underlying pathological causes of the lymphoedema (Table 11.5). It must be remembered, however, that these results relate in some patients to a series of procedures rather than necessarily a single operation, and occasionally to different types of operation. Only three out of the 78 patients who diligently used their compression stocking after their operation thought that they had had a poor result. The surgeons' assessment of the results was almost identical to that of the patients, the surgeons considering that 77 per cent of the results were good.

These results show that, although reducing operations are only indicated for a very small proportion (approximately 5 per cent) of patients with lymphoedema, they are worthwhile. Provided patients fully understand the risks as well as the possible benefits of the procedure, they are usually satisfied with the result and prepared to have the operation repeated 5–10 years later if the limb deteriorates.

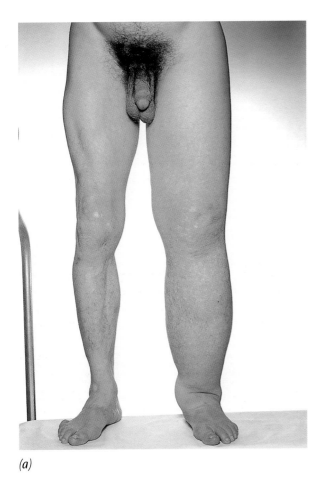

(a)

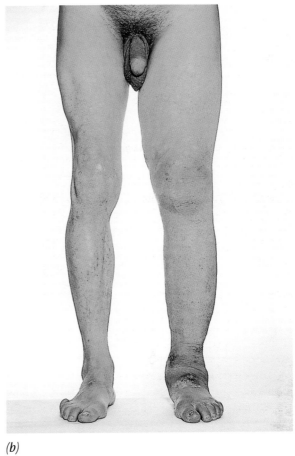

(b)

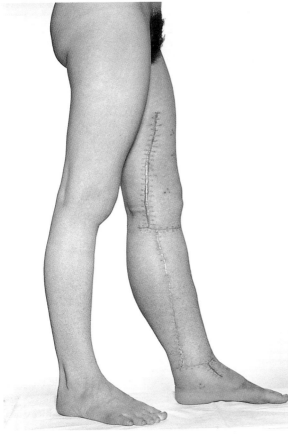

(c)

Figure 11.1a,b *Before (a) and after (b) a medial below-knee and thigh Homans' operation. (c) A well-healed scar 3 years after a Homan's operation.*

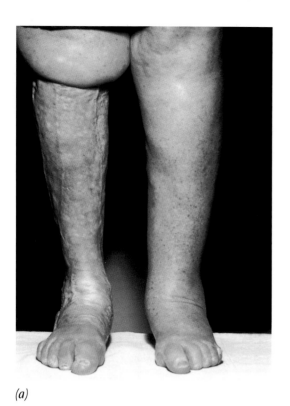

(a)

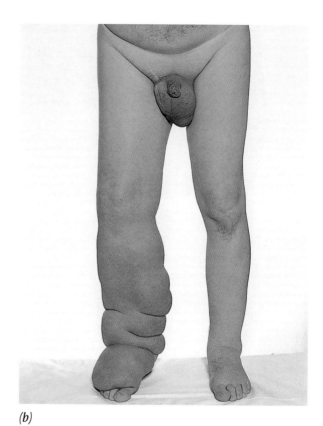

(b)

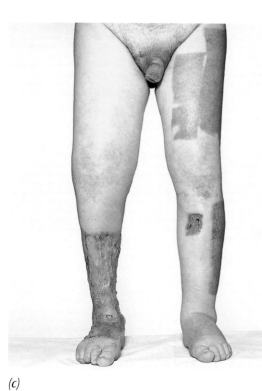

(c)

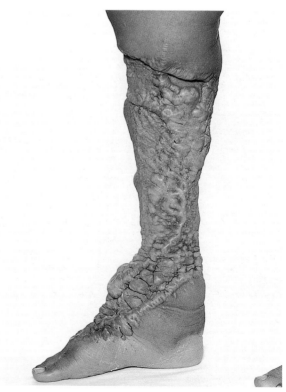

Figure 11.2 *(a) Ten years after a Charles's operation. The skin grafts are smooth and healthy. This patient did not have a proper reduction of the tissues just below the knee so she has been left with a 'pantaloon' effect. (b) Before and (c) 1 month after a Charles's operation, showing how the below-knee 'pantaloon' effect can be avoided by thinning the anterior and posterior below-knee flaps and suturing their edges down to the deep fascia. (This patient also had a scrotal reduction.)*

Figure 11.3 *Excessive keloid scaring over the forefoot following a Charles's operation. These keloid protuberances can be excised and the raw areas left to re-epithelialize or be regrafted.*

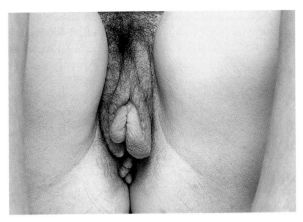

Figure 12.2 *Female genital lymphoedema (lithotomy position). This patient had been resting in bed for 2 days before this photograph was taken, but the swelling of the labia, especially the labia minora, is clearly visible. There are also some oedematous peri-anal condylomata.*

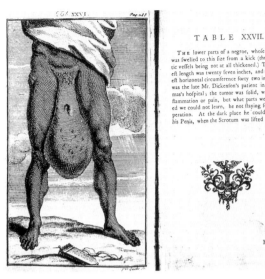

Figure 12.3 *An illustration of an enormously swollen scrotum, taken from the fourth edition of* Cheselden's Anatomy, *published in 1730. The cause was unknown but was almost certainly lymphoedema. In Cheselden's time, the role of the lymphatics in the absorption of interstitial fluid was not known (see Chapter 1).*

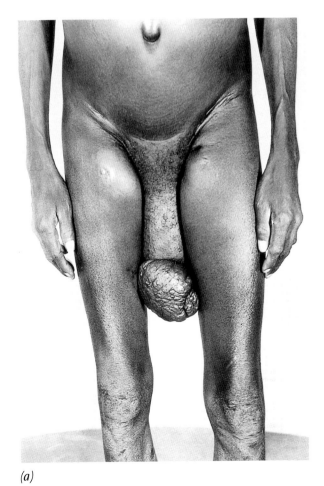

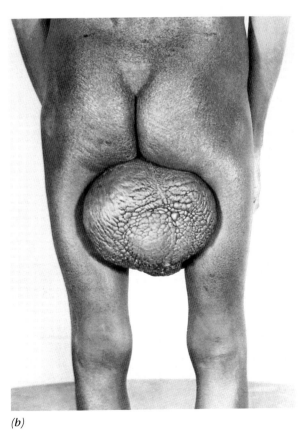

(a)   *(b)*

Figure 12.4 *These photographs of gross genital lymphoedema, probably caused by the tuberculous inguinal lymph glands visible in the upper thighs, was taken by Professor J.B. Kinmonth in Ibadan in 1959. The swelling was so gross that it hung most comfortably behind the thighs (b). The penis is not visible (a) but was not swollen. Micturition was possible only after pulling the scrotum upwards and forwards, and extracting the penis from the subpubic skin.*

it exacerbates any pre-existing phimosis, especially in young children, causes difficulty with micturition and may precipitate secondary balanoposthitis.

The oedema often extends up into the subcutaneous tissues of the lower abdomen, especially when there is lymphoedema of one or both limbs.

Hyperkeratosis and condylomata

Long-standing lymphoedema causes thickening and hyperkeratosis of the overlying skin.[17] Hyperkeratosis of the scrotum accentuates the ridges of the rugae and leads to the development of papillomata. These changes take many years to occur.

'Vesicles': dilated intradermal lymphatics

Obstruction to the outflow of lymph from the scrotum, or the reflux of lymph into it through incompetent megalymphatics, causes progressive dilatation of the many small tributaries of the collecting vessels and ultimately dilatation of the minute lymphatics of the dermis.

As these dilate in an irregular and patchy manner close to the epidermis they look like intradermal vesicles. They are not true vesicles (closed, fluid-filled spaces) but connect with and are part of the intradermal lymphatic plexus. Sometimes only one or two are visible, but sometimes they cover the whole surface of the scrotum. When they are filled with lymph, they have a transparent, pale yellow appearance, but when filled with chyle they are opaque and white (Fig. 12.5).

Because the overlying epidermis is thin, vesicles often break open and leak lymph or chyle. If they are caused by an obstruction at the neck of the scrotum, they leak for a few hours or days and then dry up, but if they are caused by reflux from the ilio-inguinal lymphatics they leak continuously and voluminously. Constant leaks cause softening, excoriation and secondary infection of the skin.

Cellulitis

Attacks of cellulitis are common in oedematous scrotal skin.[4] The scrotal skin harbours many organisms, which

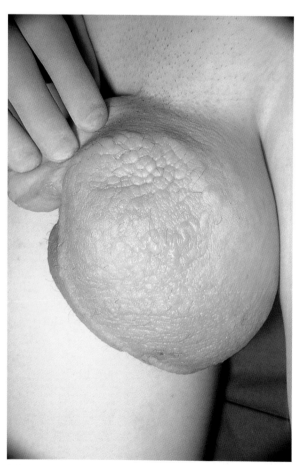

(a)

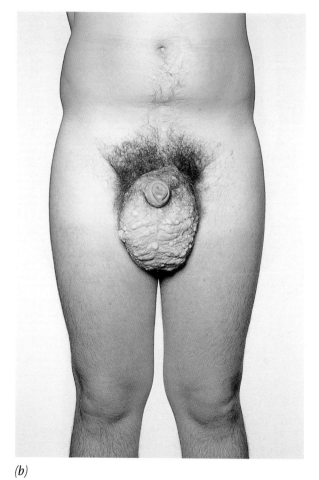

(b)

Figure 12.5 *Two examples of dilated intradermal scrotal lymphatics. (a) An almost transparent, tortuous, dilated intradermal lymphatic on an oedematous scrotum caused by obstruction to the outflow of lymph from the scrotum (see Fig. 12.10b). (b) Dilated intradermal lymphatics full of chyle that has refluxed down incompetent aortic and iliac megalymphatics (see Fig. 12.10c).*

quickly invade the oedematous tissues through small abrasions in the warm cracks and crevices of the scrotal skin. The organisms proliferate in the protein-rich oedema fluid, and infection spreads rapidly throughout the scrotum, causing redness, pain and more swelling (Fig. 12.6). True streptococcal erysipelas is not uncommon.

After an attack of cellulitis, the swelling rarely returns to its previous size. Some patients give a very clear history of their genital oedema beginning after an attack of cellulitis. Lymphangiographs of these patients often show a localized occlusion of the collecting lymphatics in the neck of the scrotum, suggesting that the blockage and subsequent oedema was caused by the attack of lymphangitis.

Sexual dysfunction

A grossly swollen scrotum partially enveloping the penis, and/or a swollen penis or swollen labia, invariably interferes with sexual intercourse. In our own patients,[15] 12 out of the 31 men (40 per cent) complained of impotence caused by the swelling, problems with erection or pain during intercourse. All of our female patients complained of discomfort during intercourse, three (30 per cent) being unable to have intercourse because of severe pain.

Wet sore skin, sometimes associated with an unpleasant smell around leaking vesicles, is also a serious disincentive to sexual enjoyment.

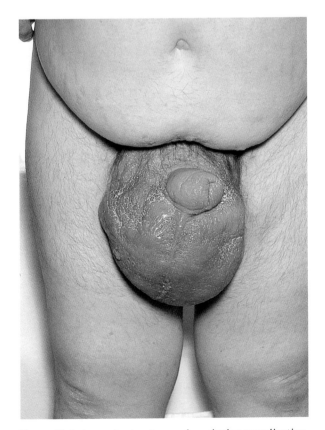

Figure 12.6 *An acute streptococcal erysipelas complicating a mild genital lymphoedema beginning to subside after 3 days of penicillin.*

Inguinal lymphadenopathy

The inguinal lymph glands are often slightly enlarged and tender if there have been attacks of cellulitis. These glands are almost always enlarged if they are a site of filariasis or tuberculosis.

Other lymphatic problems

Seventy per cent of our patients with primary genital lymphoedema, both male and female, had other lymphatic problems at the time they presented with swelling of their genitalia. All had oedema of one or both limbs, which the majority had noticed before the age of 20 (Fig. 12.7). The limb swelling usually preceded the genital swelling by about 10 years, but sometimes both began at the same time. We have not seen a patient with a primary genital lymphoedema that preceded the appearance of lower limb oedema. The clinical features and aetiology of the limb oedema in patients with genital lymphoedema have the same pattern as those of patients with limb oedema alone.

In our own series of patients,[15] approximately 12 per cent also had chylous ascites, and 10 per cent had protein-losing enteropathy. Some of the patients with chylous ascites had leaking vesicles on their genitalia and/or legs. We have also seen patients with concommitent chylothorax, lymphoedema of the face and lymphoedema of the arm. Because of the possibility of the existence of other lymphatic abnormalities, all the bodily system of patients presenting with genital lymphoedema must be thoroughly examined and investigated.

INVESTIGATIONS

It is important to use all the current radiological, ultrasound, biochemical and haematological investigations to exclude other lymphatic abnormalities and discover whether they are causing any systemic disturbances, such as the hypoproteinaemia caused by protein-losing enteropathy. Filariasis must be excluded if the patient has lived in or visited an area where this condition is endemic; for this, the simplified antigen test or nighttime smears (*see* Chapter 15) can be used. Confirmed filariasis must be treated before considering the surgical treatment of any genital oedema.

Lymphograms

Effective treatment depends upon a precise demonstration of the underlying lymphatic abnormality.[18]

Isotope lymphographs

Isotope lymphographs following the bipedal injection of a radioactive colloid (*see* Chapter 6) do not provide

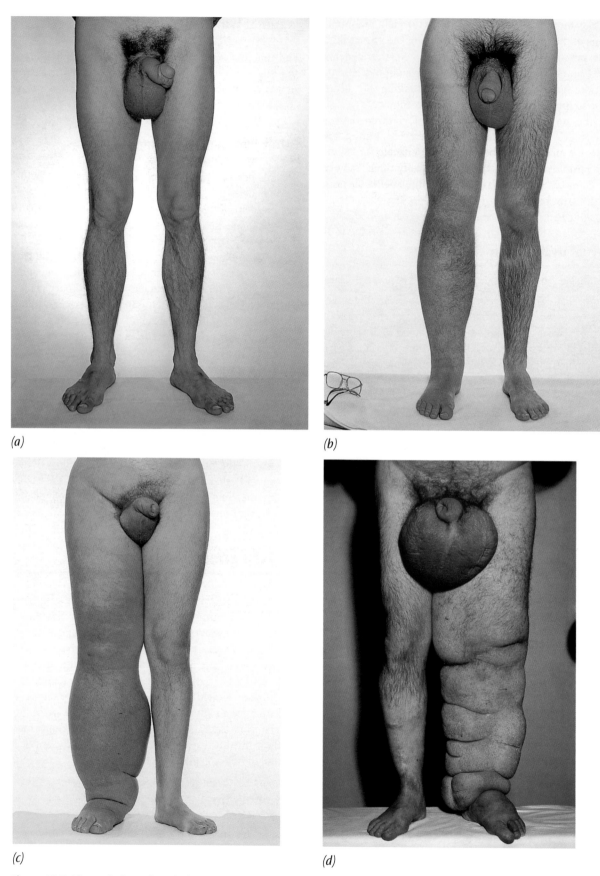

Figure 12.7 *The variations of genital oedema associated with limb oedema. (a) Primary genital lymphoedema with normal lower limbs. (b) Mild limb oedema with moderate scrotal oedema. (c) Moderate/severe limb oedema with minimal scrotal oedema. (d) Severe limb and scrotal oedema.*

sufficient information because they do not give clear pictures of the number, size and valvular function of the inguinal, pelvic and lumbar lymphatics, although they can be used to demonstrate the lymphatic function of the lower limb.

Bilateral pedal X-ray contrast lymphogram

Such a lymphogram (*see* Chapter 6) is usually an essential investigation. After injecting 5–7 mL Ultrafluid Lipiodol into a lymphatic on the dorsum of each foot, X-rays should be taken to illustrate the lymphatics and lymph nodes of the upper thigh, inguinal and external iliac regions (Fig. 12.8a). To expedite the movement of Lipiodol to the groin, the patient is normally tilted head-down, but once the Lipiodol has reached the ilio-inguinal region the tilt should be reversed to encourage the demonstration of any reflux into the scrotum or labia (Fig. 12.8b). The testes should be protected with a lead screen while films are taken of the ilio-inguinal region. To minimize the radiation dose, the total number of films taken should be kept to a minimum consistent with obtaining the desired information.

Films of the lower abdomen and scrotum or labia should be taken 1, 2 and 24 hours after completing the injection.

Scrotal lymphangiogram

A scrotal lymphangiogram should be performed, whenever possible, by injecting Lipiodol into a vesicle on the skin surface (Fig. 12.9). It is sometimes difficult to keep the tip of the needle in the centre of a vesicle, and the oil may leak out around the puncture site. Leakage and movement may be prevented or reduced by spraying the vesicle puncture site with an adhesive wound coating such as Mastasol or Nobecutane. Multiple punctures should be avoided because the oil will leak out of the puncture sites and not move onwards through the lymphatics. The dilated lymphatics of a swollen scrotum will be filled by an injection of 2–3 mL. If there is no exit route, the puncture site will then leak. If the vesicle is part of a system of dilated megalymphatics, 5–6 mL may be injected because the Lipiodol will pass onwards with ease into the ilio-inguinal vessels. A large, capacious lymphatic plexus in the pelvic region can be visualized after injecting 5–6 mL Lipiodol by changing the contrast medium to a non-ionic, water-soluble contrast medium such as Hypaque, but this will diffuse out of the lymphatics in a few hours.

Figure 12.10 illustrates the three common lymphatic abnormalities revealed by lymphographs that cause genital lymphoedema: inguinal/iliac lymph vessel and lymph gland fibrosis or diseases such as filariasis and secondary malignant disease (*a*), occlusion of the outflow lymphatics of the scrotum, cause unknown (*b*) and dilated incompetent megalymphatics allowing the reflux of lymph and/or chyle into the scrotum (*c*).

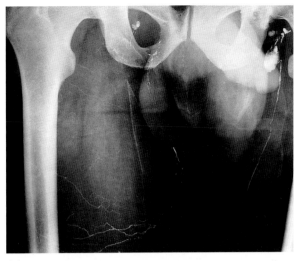

(a)

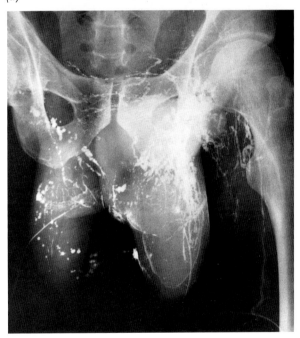

(b)

Figure 12.8 *Ascending bipedal lymphographs of the upper thigh and groin of two patients with associated oedema of the leg, showing the two commonly found abnormalities. (a) Proximal lymphatic obliteration of the lymphatics of the upper thigh and fibrosis of the inguinal (and iliac) lymph nodes both obstructing the outflow of lymph from the scrotum, which can be seen to be significantly swollen. (b) Dilated incompetent megalymphatics in the upper thigh, inguinal and iliac regions with Lipiodol refluxing into dilated lymphatics on the left side of the scrotum. A vesicle on the right side of the scrotum is also being injected and beginning to fill dilated vessel draining towards the right groin.*

Inguinal gland biopsy

Any desire to perform an excisional biopsy of an enlarged inguinal lymph gland must be resisted unless it is essential

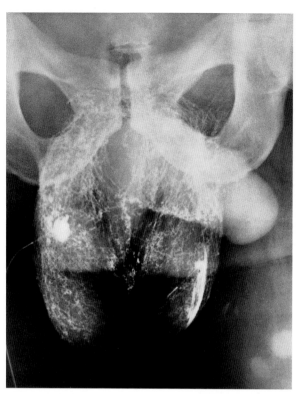

Figure 12.9 *A scrotal lymphograph, obtained by injecting Lipiodol directly into an intradermal lymphatic, showing no outflow vessels from the scrotum to the inguinal lymph glands. This patient had no leg swelling and normal leg lymphatics (see Fig. 12.7a, p. 222). His scrotal swelling began after an attack of scrotal cellulitis, which presumably caused a permanent obstruction of the lymphatics in the neck of the scrotum.*

to establish that disease in the glands, such as filariasis, tuberculosis, lymphogranuloma or secondary malignant disease, is the cause of the oedema. Excising a whole lymph gland in a patient with primary lymphoedema of the scrotum or limb carries a significant risk of exacerbating the swelling. A wedge or Tru-cut biopsy is acceptable.

Skin and lymph cultures

Even when there is no clinical evidence of active infection, bacteriological swabs should be taken from the skin and any fluid draining from vesicles as resident organisms may be a source of postoperative wound infection. Blood cultures should be obtained if there is any evidence of active cellulitis.

TREATMENT

Conservative treatment

Conservative treatment is suitable for many patients if there are no leaking vesicles. Women can wear elasticated corsets/roll-ons, which provide considerable upward support to the labia, sometimes helped by the inclusion of an old-fashioned type of sanitary pad.

The scrotum and penis should be held up and pressed against the pubis and mons veneris as high as possible with well-fitting pants of the Y-front variety or the smooth elasticated pantyhose (Spandex) that stretch from the lower abdomen to the upper thighs and are now worn by many athletes. Compression of the scrotum with an elasticated scrotal support can help mild cases, but it must be of the triangular athlete's jockstrap design rather than a bag with an elasticated edge, which might constrict the neck of the scrotum. Patients who also have swollen legs can get custom-made tights that compress both the lower abdomen, perineum and limb.

Diligent hygiene is essential. Washing with an antibacterial soap, drying carefully and powdering all help to reduce the risk of cellulitis. Any tinea cruris that develops between the scrotum and the thigh must be vigorously treated with antifungicides. Patients who have suffered repeated attacks of cellulitis may need to take long-term prophylactic antibiotics (*see* Chapter 9).

Surgical treatment

There are three categories of surgical treatment: operations to stop reflux, bulk-reducing operations and miscellaneous bypass operations.

Anti-reflux operations

Anti-reflux operations are described in Chapters 10 and 16. The reflux usually comes from the medial ilio-inguinal lymphatics. These can be exposed and ligated where they lie in the retroperitoneum via an oblique suprainguinal, lower abdominal incision. After displaying the vessels with a subcutaneous injection into the groin of Patent Blue Violet, every vessel must be carefully dissected and doubly ligated with a fine non-absorbable material, at least 2–3 cm apart, so that the intervening section can be excised. Care must be taken not to leave punctured vessels unligated as these will leak and produce lymphoceles.

Ligating incompetent vessels at the neck of the scrotum does not give good long-term results as collaterals soon develop in the surrounding tissues.

Scrotal reduction

Genital-reducing operations have been used for the past 150 years,[19,20] and the surgical journals contain descriptions of many different techniques.[2,4,21–37] The method described below and illustrated in Fig. 12.11 is the simplest and, in our hands, the most effective.

After ensuring that the scrotal and preputial skin is as clean and bacterium free as possible, patients are given preoperative cover with a suitable antibiotic. The patient

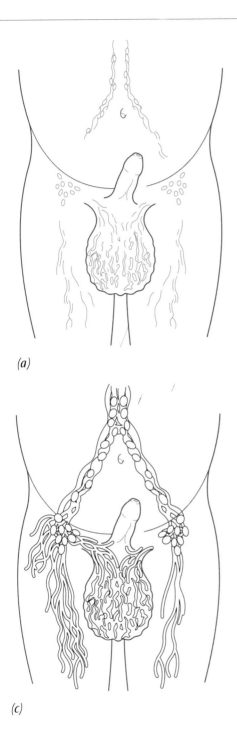

(a)

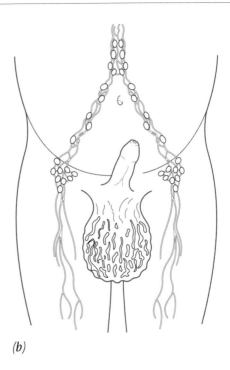

(b)

(c)

Figure 12.10 *The three lymphographic abnormalities commonly found in patients with genital lymphoedema. (a) Upper thigh, inguinal and iliac lymph vessel obliteration and lymph gland fibrosis or disease such as filariasis or secondary malignant disease – 60 per cent. These patients usually have lymphoedema of one or both limbs. (b) Obliteration of the outflow lymphatics of the scrotum with normal limb, inguinal and iliac lymphatics and lymph glands: 20–25 per cent. These patients have normal legs. (c) Dilated, incompetent aortic, iliac, inguinal and sometimes limb lymphatics (the distal extent of the abnormality being variable), allowing reflux of lymph and chyle into the scrotum: 15–20 per cent.*

is anaesthetized and placed supine on an operating table with a foot board that allows the legs to be spread wide apart. The lower abdomen, penis, scrotum, perineum and thighs are painted with a coloured antiseptic solution. Ordinary iodine is unsuitable because it burns the skin if it lies in a puddle between the rugae of the scrotum or in the creases of the perineum. We use chlorhexidene or povidone iodine. The drapes are placed to give full access to the posterior aspect of the scrotum but fixed so that the anus is excluded from the operative field. The drapes over the legs should be arranged so that the legs can be moved or lifted out of the way when working on the posterior aspect of the scrotum.

Two incisions are made, just through the skin, each beginning above and lateral to the pubic tubercles and superficial inguinal rings and then extending downwards and posteriorly, either side of the scrotum, in the corrugated scrotal skin close to the junction between that skin and the smooth skin at the base of the scrotum that lies between it and the perineum (Fig. 12.11a). The object is to remove all or as much as possible of the corrugated scrotal skin. These incisions are curved convexly forwards to ensure that there will be, when dissected out, two semilunar skin flaps long enough to cover the testes and be sutured to each other. These two incisions meet posteriorly in the midline 3–5 cm anterior to the anal

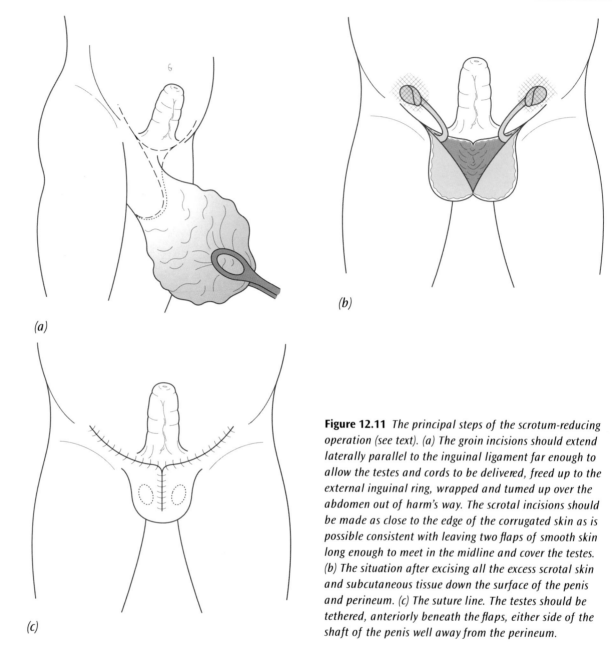

(a)

(b)

(c)

Figure 12.11 *The principal steps of the scrotum-reducing operation (see text). (a) The groin incisions should extend laterally parallel to the inguinal ligament far enough to allow the testes and cords to be delivered, freed up to the external inguinal ring, wrapped and turned up over the abdomen out of harm's way. The scrotal incisions should be made as close to the edge of the corrugated skin as is possible consistent with leaving two flaps of smooth skin long enough to meet in the midline and cover the testes. (b) The situation after excising all the excess scrotal skin and subcutaneous tissue down the surface of the penis and perineum. (c) The suture line. The testes should be tethered, anteriorly beneath the flaps, either side of the shaft of the penis well away from the perineum.*

verge. At this stage, it is wise to cut the flaps too long, as short, inadequate flaps can present a most difficult surgical problem. The upper ends of the incisions are then deepened to expose the cords of the testes, both testes then being defined. After opening the tunica vaginalis (which often contains hydrocele fluid), the testes are delivered out of the scrotum, wrapped in warm moist swabs and laid up on the lower abdomen out of harm's way (Fig. 12.11b).

After identifying and protecting the testes, the penis is pulled firmly forwards and upwards and the two incisions joined by a third horizontal incision which runs across and convexly downwards 1–2 cm below the skin covering the base of the shaft of the penis. If there is abdominal oedema, a 'melon slice' of lower skin and

subcutaneous tissue may be removed at this stage. The two lateral flaps of skin and a thin layer of subcutaneous tissue are then fashioned by reflecting the skin down to the perineum and then medially to the side of the perineal part of the corpora cavernosa. Large vessels should be ligated; complete haemostasis is essential. The excess skin and subcutaneous tissue can then be removed by continuing the dissection from either side and above, across the surface of the perineal part of the penis.

At this stage of the operation, the two testes lie isolated on the lower abdominal wall, and there are two, thin, semilunar skin flaps on either side of the perineum. The perineal part of the penis and the perineum either side of it are totally exposed, having been completely denuded of subcutaneous tissue (Fig. 12.11b).

The testes are then unwrapped and inspected. If a hydrocele is present, all the tunica vaginalis is removed or, in children, opened, everted and fixed around the epididymis (the Jaboulay procedure). Even when there is no hydrocele, the tunica is opened and partially excised so that a postoperative hydrocele cannot form. The testes are then placed on either side of the base of the penis and held in this position with one or two small sutures. They must not be fixed too far back where they might be compressed or damaged when sitting.

The skin flaps are then sutured together over the testes to produce a Y-shaped suture line (Fig. 12.11c). It is important that the flaps are not slack but hold the testes firmly on either side of the shaft of the penis without compressing them. The skin flaps may have to be trimmed at this stage. Two suction drains are placed one either side of the testes and brought out just above the upper ends of the suture line lateral to the mons veneris.

Postoperatively, firm pressure is applied to the scrotum and perineum by the use of a large pad of wool and a T-bandage or a triangular scrotal support. A urethral catheter is inserted if the penis has been reduced so that difficulty with micturition in the presence of a bulky compression dressing can be avoided. We have not found it necessary to insert a urethral catheter after simple scrotal or labial reductions.

Penis reduction

The method used to reduce the penis should be varied according to the degree of swelling. In many instances, nothing more is required than a circumcision. On occasions, however, a strip of the penile skin and a much more extensive portion of the oedematous subcutaneous tissue can be removed through a vertical eliptical incision down the shaft of the penis. Whenever possible, this incision should not run along the whole length of the penis lest the scar impede or distort erection. If a long incision is unavoidable, it should be made in the form of a lazy-S.

In some cases, gross swelling or unhealthy skin may make a reduction impossible without removing all of the skin and subcutaneous tissue. In these circumstances, all the skin and subcutaneous tissue covering the shaft of the penis should be removed and the exposed fascia covering the corpora cavernosa and spongiosa covered with split-skin grafts[38] (Fig. 12.13).

Patients sometimes find it easier if the scrotum is reduced first and the penis reduced a few weeks or months later.

Labial reduction

Labial reduction is achieved by simply excising the oedematous labia including some of the underlying perineal fat. In the majority of patients, most of the swelling is in the labia majora, and the labia minora can be left intact. This gives a better and sexually more acceptable result. If both the major and minor labia have to be reduced, the cosmetic effect is better if the excisions and suture lines of each labium are kept separate. A wide elliptical excision of both labia with a single suture line is more likely to leave a sensitive scar in a position that is rubbed during intercourse.

Suction drainage is not necessary after a labial excision, except in those patients who have megalymphatics with reflux, because, unlike the case with the scrotum, the subcutaneous tissues can be sutured together to obliterate any potential space beneath the sutured skin. Compression is maintained postoperatively with a large wool pad and T-bandage.

Other operations

None of the many operations designed to improve lymph drainage (see Chapter 10), such as the insertion of polythene tubes,[39,40] skin bridges and pedicles,[41,42] pedicles of omentum,[43,44] lymph node-to-vein anastomoses[45] and complex reconstructions,[46,47] have been successful in our hands.

Huang and colleagues[48,49] have reported a good reduction in oedema and the abolition of chylorrhoea and skin vesicles in a series of six patients with vulval lymphoedema caused by incompetent megalymphatics that they treated by microsurgical lymphatic-to-vein anastomoses within the labia. Their follow-up was short, mostly less than 1 year. Five patients were improved. No evidence was presented to confirm postoperative patency of the anastomoses.

The problem with anastomosing incompetent lymphatics to veins is the reflux of blood into, and its subsequent thrombosis in, the lymphatics. Long-term patency therefore depends upon the existence of a higher pressure in the lymphatic and a steady volume of lymph flow into the vein. These difficult procedures require further critical evaluation.

RESULTS OF REDUCING OPERATIONS

We have been unable to find any publications that describe the long-term results of a large series of genital-reducing operations for primary lymphoedema other than those from our own unit.[15] Between 1958 and 1990, we saw more than 70 patients with genital lymphoedema. A number, most with filarial oedema, came from foreign countries and were lost to follow-up, leaving us with 41 patients (31 male and 10 female) available for study in depth. Nine of these patients (5 male and 4 female) were treated conservatively, and 32 patients surgically. Of the 26 men treated surgically, 15 (58 per cent) had a peno-scrotal reduction, 10 (38 per cent) a scrotal reduction – 2 following the ligation of incompetent megalymphatics – and 1 (4 per cent) a penile reduction. Six of the 10 women underwent a labial reduction.

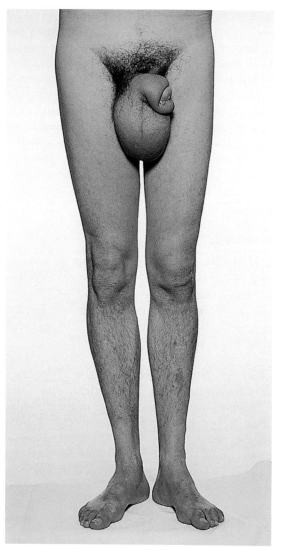

(a)

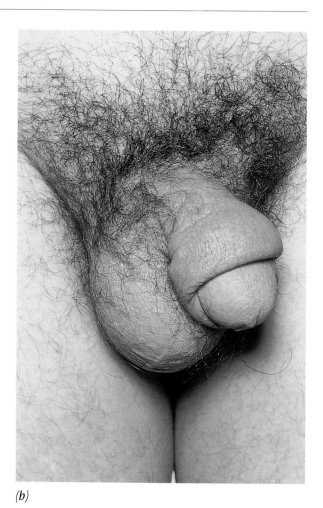

(b)

Figure 12.12 *The pre- and postoperative appearances of a scrotal reduction. (a) Moderate scrotal swelling before treatment by the excisional operation as illustrated in Fig. 12.11. (b) The appearance of the scrotum 5 years later. Two years later the patient asked for the penis to be reduced.*

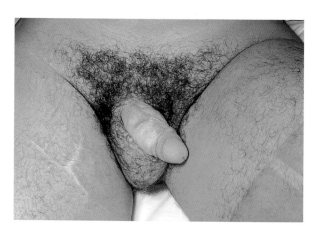

Figure 12.13 *Six months after a peno-scrotal reduction (the scrotum being reduced using the standard operation). The penis was reduced by excising all the skin and oedematous tissue, and covering the denuded area with split-skin grafts. This patient shows the scars of a reducing operation on the right leg.*

The results at a mean of 10 years after operation, assessed in a special follow-up clinic, showed that reducing operations always produced a significant improvement (Figs 12.12 and 12.13) but that a slow gradual recurrence was common. At a mean of 10 years after their initial operation, 15 (57 per cent) of the men considered that they were cured of their swelling and concomittent symptoms, but 4 (15 per cent) had had to have two operations, the second taking place approximately 7 years after the first. Similarly, although 11 (43 per cent) thought that they were significantly improved, 8 (30 per cent) had had to have a second operation 5–7 years after the first.

These results show that one half of patients with penoscrotal lymphoedema and its symptoms can expect to be cured or adequately improved for at least 10 years by a single simple reducing operation, but the other half will develop recurrent swelling after 5–7 years and require a second operation, which will usually be effective for at least another 7 years.

We have not yet had to perform a third scrotal reduction on any patient, although we have had to perform more than two operations on the penis, for example a circumcision followed by a shaft subcutaneous excision, followed by a total skin and subcutaneous tissue excision and skin graft.

The long-term results of labial reduction is better. In two thirds of women, a single operation will provide a 'cure' lasting at least 10 years. The other third will have to have a second operation approximately 5–7 years after the first. More women than men have a long-lasting cure, probably because recurrent labial lymphoedema is easier to prevent with well-fitting pants. None of our patients, male or female, considered that their operation(s) had made them worse.

We found no relationship between the results and the underlying lymphatic abnormality, duration of symptoms before operation or any other lymphatic problem. Swelling and leaking vesicles tended to recur in the same area from which they had been excised. Removing tissues from the scrotum did not exacerbate penis swelling, or vice versa.

HYDROCELE

Many patients with scrotal lymphoedema are found at operation to have small, soft hydroceles, and the fact that approximately a quarter of males, of all ages, with lymphoedema of the lower limb have a soft hydrocele suggests that hydroceles might be caused by an abnormality of the lymphatics draining the testis and its coverings.

When Patent Blue Violet is injected just below the coverings of the testis or into the epididymis, it appears rapidly in the lymphatics in the spermatic cord and around the vas deferens, respectively.[50] When similar injections are given to patients with *primary* hydroceles, the dye injected into the testis appears in the spermatic cord lymphatics in two thirds of cases, but dye injected into the epididymis does not appear in the lymphatics around the vas deferens.[1] This observation suggests that hydroceles may in part be caused by a failure of the lymphatics of the epididymis and coverings of the testis that drain to the inguinal lymph glands. Lymphographs following the injection of Lipiodol into the spermatic cord lymphatics of patients with hydroceles show one or two vessels passing upwards to join the para-aortic lymph glands or sometimes bypassing these glands and running directly into the pre-aortic plexus and cisterna chyli.[51]

Lymphograms cannot be performed on the lymphatics of the vas deferens in patients with hydroceles as these vessels are not visualized by the injection of the Patent Blue Violet, but lymphographs of normal vas deferens lymphatics show that they usually drain into the ilio-inguinal glands.[51]

Although a lymphatic deficiency probably plays a role in the aetiology of primary hydrocele, it is unlikely to be the sole cause. The rapid accumulation of fluid within the tunica vaginalis after aspiration, and the high pressures and high protein concentrations that quickly develop,[52] suggest a concurrent abnormality of fluid filtration and reabsorption by the capillaries of the tunica vaginalis. Furthermore, the possibility of an active secretory mechanism cannot be excluded.

The treatment of primary hydrocele, whatever the causative mechanism, is ablation of the potential space around the testis by excising the parietal layer of the tunica vaginalis using one of the accepted surgical techniques.

REFERENCES

1. Kinmonth JB. *The lymphatics*, 2nd edn. Baltimore: Arnold, 1982.
2. Dandapat MC, Mohapatro SK, Patro SK. Elephantiasis of the penis and scrotum. A review of 350 cases. *American Journal of Surgery* 1985; **149:** 686–90.
3. Partono F. The spectrum of disease in lymphatic filariasis. *Ciba Foundation Symposium* 1987; **127:** 15–31.
4. Geyer H, Geyer A, Schubert J. Erysipelas and elephantiasis of the scrotum, surgery and drug therapy. *Urology International* 1997; **58:** 243–6.
5. Ngu V, Konstan PG. Chronic lymphoedema in Western Nigeria. *British Journal of Surgery* 1964; **51:** 101–4.
6. Wright RA, Judson FN. Penile veneral edema. *Journal of the American Medical Association* 1979; **241:** 157–8.
7. Konety BR, Cooper T, Flood HD, Futrell JW. Scrotal elephantiasis associated with hidradenitis suppurativa. *Plastic and Reconstructive Surgery* 1996; **97:** 1243–5.
8. Ebri B, Portoles A, Munoz JR, Cimorra G, Madrid G, Hilario J. Hereditary genital lymphedema of the Milroy–None type. *Rev Clin Espana* 1983; **171:** 333–6.
9. Dijkstra JW, Bergfeld WF, Kay R. Congenital lymphedema of genitalia and extremities. *Cleveland Clinical Quarterly* 1984; **51:** 553–7.
10. Ross JH, Kay R, Yetman RJ, Angermeier K. Primary lymphedema of the genitalia in children and adolescents. *Journal of Urology* 1998; **160:** 1485–9.
11. Bolt RJ, Peelen W, Nikkels PG, de Jong TP. Congenital lymphoedema of the genitalia. *European Journal of Pediatrics* 1998; **157:** 943–6.
12. Hashem FK, Ahmed S. Idiopathic scrotal lymphoedema in Down's syndrome. *Australian and New Zealand Journal of Surgery* 1999; **69:** 75–7.
13. Kinmonth JB, Wolfe JH. Fibrosis in the lymph nodes in primary lymphoedema. *Annals of the Royal College of Surgeons* 1980; **62:** 344–54.
14. Browse NL, Stewart G. Lymphoedema: pathophysiology and classification. *Journal of Cardiovascular Surgery* 1985; **26:** 91–106.
15. Browse NL, Russo F, Wilson NM, Burnand KG. The aetiology, management and long-term results of treatment of lymphoedema of the external genitalia (in preparation).

16. Gorshkov SZ. Vulval elephantiasis. *Akush Ginekol (Mosk)* 1974; **2:** 71–3.

17. Skoog SJ. Verrucous elephantiasis of the scrotum: an unusual variant of genital lymphedema. *Journal of Urology* 1986; **135:** 799–800.

18. May AR, Kinmonth JB. Proceedings: Lymphographic studies of primary genital lymphoedema. *British Journal of Surgery* 1976; **63:** 655.

19. Larrey, 1803. Cited in Dandapat MC, Mohapatro SK, Patro SK. Elephantiasis of the penis and scrotum. A review of 350 cases. *American Journal of Surgery* 1985; **149:** 686–90.

20. Delpech JM. *Chirurgie clinique de Montpelier.* Paris, 1820.

21. Morales PA, O'Connor JJ, Gordon SG. Surgical treatment of severe lymphedema of penis. *Journal of Urology* 1954; **72:** 880–5.

22. Prpic I. Severe elephantiasis of penis and scrotum. *British Journal of Plastic Surgery* 1966; **19:** 173–8.

23. Khanna NN. Surgical treatment of elephantiasis of male genitalia. *Plastic and Reconstructive Surgery* 1970; **46:** 481–7.

24. Vaught SK, Litvak AS, McRoberts JW. The surgical management of scrotal and penile lymphedema. *Journal of Urology* 1975; **113:** 204–6.

25. McKay HA, Meehan WL, Jackson AC, LeBlanc GA. Surgical treatment of male genital lymphedema. *Urology* 1977; **9:** 284–7.

26. Holman CM Jr, Arnold PG, Jurkiewicz MJ, Walton KN. Reconstruction of male external genitalia with elephantiasis. *Urology* 1977; **10:** 576–8.

27. Feins NR. A new surgical technique for lymphedema of the penis and scrotum. *Journal of Pediatric Surgery* 1980; **15:** 787–9.

28. Tapper D, Eraklis AJ, Colodny AH, Schwartz M. Congenital lymphedema of the penis: a method of reconstruction. *Journal of Pediatric Surgery* 1980; **15:** 481–5.

29. Das S, Tuerk D, Amar AD, Sommer J. Surgery of male genital lymphedema. *Journal of Urology* 1983; **129:** 1240–2.

30. Hirshowitz B, Peretz BA. Bilateral superomedial thigh flaps for primary reconstruction of scrotum and vulva. *Annals of Plastic Surgery* 1982; **8:** 390–6.

31. Yormuk E, Sevin K, Emiroglu M, Turker M. A new surgical approach in genital lymphedema. *Plastic and Reconstructive Surgery* 1990; **86:** 1194–7.

32. Apesos J, Anigian G. Reconstruction of penile and scrotal lymphedema. *Annals of Plastic Surgery* 1991; **27:** 570–3.

33. Ollapallil JJ, Watters DA. Surgical management of elephantiasis of male genitalia. *British Journal of Urology* 1995; **76:** 213–15.

34. Steinberg J, Kim ED, McVary KT. A surgical approach to penoscrotal lymphedema. *Journal of Urology* 1996; **156:** 1770.

35. Benchekroun A, Abakka T, Lakrissa A, Faik M, Taghy A. Elephantiasis of the external genital organs in the male. Apropos of 18 cases. *Journal of Urology (Paris)* 1986; **92:** 297–300.

36. Morey AF, Meng MV, McAninch JW. Skin graft reconstruction of chronic genital lymphedema. *Urology* 1997; **50:** 423–6.

37. Servelle M. Surgical treatment of lymphoedema. A report of 652 cases. *Surgery* 1987; **101:** 485–95.

38. Ketterings C. Lymphedema of penis and scrotum. *British Journal of Plastic Surgery* 1968; **21:** 381–386.

39. Truc, 1954. Cited in Dandapat MC, Mohapatro SK, Patro SK. Elephantiasis of the penis and scrotum. A review of 350 cases. *American Journal of Surgery* 1985; **149:** 686–90.

40. Stenberg, 1955. Cited in Dandapat MC, Mohapatro SK, Patro SK. Elephantiasis of the penis and scrotum. A review of 350 cases. *American Journal of Surgery* 1985; **149:** 686–90.

41. McDonald DF, Huggins C. The surgical treatment of elephantiasis. *Journal of Urology* 1950; **63:** 187–90.

42. Gillies H, Fraser FR. The treatment of lymphoedema by plastic operation: a preliminary report. *British Medical Journal* 1935; **1:** 96–101.

43. Goldsmith HS, De Dos Santos R. Omental transplantation in primary lymphoedema. *Surgery, Gynecology and Obstetrics* 1967; **125:** 607–11.

44. Goldsmith HS. Long term evaluation of omental transposition for chronic lymphoedema. *Annals of Surgery* 1974; **180:** 847–9.

45. Nielubowicz J, Olszewsky W, Sokolowski J. Surgical lymphovenous shunts. *Journal of Cardiovascular Surgery* 1968; **9:** 262–7.

46. Martinez RE, Couchell SH, Raffel B, Swaetz WM. Primary lymphoedema of the scrotum: surgical treatment and reconstruction. *Annals of Plastic Surgery* 1988; **21:** 354–7.

47. Chitale VR. Role of tensor fascia lata musculocutaneous flap in lymphedema of the lower extremity and external genitalia. *Annals of Plastic Surgery* 1989; **23:** 297–305.

48. Huang GK, Hu RQ, Liu ZZ, Pan GP. Microlymphaticovenous anastomosis for treating scrotal elephantiasis. *Microsurgery* 1985; **6:** 36–9.

49. Huang GK, Hu RQ, Yao-Liang S, Gong-Ping P. Microlymphaticovenous anastomosis for lymphoedema of external genitalia in females. *Surgery, Gynecology and Obstetrics* 1986; **162:** 429–32.

50. Kinmonth JB. Lymphangiography in clinical surgery. *Annals of the Royal College of Surgeons* 1954; **15:** 300–8.

51. McBrian MP, Edwards JM, Kinmonth JB. Lymphography of the testis and adnexa in the normal and in idiopathic hydrocele. *Archives of Surgery* 1972; **104:** 820–5.

52. Witte CL, Witte MH, Drach GW, Butler C. On the protein of hydrocele fluid. *Surgery* 1973; **73:** 347–52.

Management of lymphoedema of the upper limb

Primary and secondary lymphoedema of the upper limb is much less common than lymphoedema of the lower limb. This is almost certainly related to the greater influence of gravity on the lower limb. Secondary lymphoedema of the arm is much more common than primary lymphoedema because it is a not infrequent complication of carcinoma of the breast and its treatment.

Upper limb lymphoedema is not difficult to diagnose if it develops following axillary lymphadenectomy for cancer or occurs in the presence of lymphoedema elsewhere, such as in a child with congenital lymphoedema of the lower limb, but when upper limb swelling occurs for no obvious reason, lymphoscintigraphy is the investigation of choice to confirm that the oedema is of lymphatic origin. Lymphoscintigraphy does not necessarily reveal the origin of the oedema: other investigations may be required to identify the underlying cause.

DIFFERENTIAL DIAGNOSIS

In the absence of an obvious cause, consideration must be given to the nature of the swelling, i.e. whether it is composed of fluid or excess tissue constituents (Table 13.1). Chronic oedema associated with venous outflow obstruction, one of the most common causes of upper limb swelling, tends to have a bluish hue, mottled discoloration, venous telangiectasia and dilated veins. Chronic venous outflow obstruction eventually manifests with collateral veins around the shoulder and across the anterior surface of the chest. Venous abnormalities often co-exist with lymphoedema in advanced malignancy, particularly metastatic axillary lymph gland disease.

BREAST CANCER-RELATED LYMPHOEDEMA

Lymphoedema of the arm is a common complication of the treatment of breast cancer. Breast cancer-related lymphoedema, also known as post-mastectomy oedema, causes disfigurement and reduced mobility as well as aching, heaviness and tightness in the arm (Fig. 13.1).[1] In addition to chronic oedema, the lymphatic insufficiency predisposes to episodes of infection, particularly acute streptococcal cellulitis, other acute inflammatory episodes and lymphangitis – all of which can be recurrent – and very rarely to malignant change, i.e. lymphangiosarcoma (Stewart–Treves syndrome) (Fig. 13.2).

Breast cancer-related lymphoedema was first described as a side-effect of surgical mastectomy operations by Halstead in 1921 (hence the term post-mastectomy oedema).[2] The introduction of more conservative surgery for carcinoma of the breast has reduced the prevalence and severity of postoperative arm swelling yet it remains a common iatrogenic problem and the most frequent cause of upper limb lymphoedema. Breast cancer may, albeit rarely, present with arm swelling. To do so requires advanced axillary lymph gland and/or chest wall metastatic disease often associated with venous outflow obstruction. Recurrent breast cancer should always be borne in mind in any patient considered to be in remission following initial curative treatment who develops arm swelling.

Epidemiology

A questionnaire survey of an entire population of breast cancer patients in one health district revealed a 28 per cent

Table 13.1 *Causes of chronic upper limb swelling*

LYMPHATIC
Congenital
Lymphoedema: usually associated with abnormalities of
the central lymphatics (Milroy's disease does not cause
upper limb swelling)
Diffuse lymphangiomatosis
Amniotic bands

Acquired
Cancer treatment (axillary surgery ± radiotherapy)
Malignant disease (apical lung cancer, axillary metastatic
disease – Kaposi's sarcoma)
Infection (cellulitis, lymphangitis, lymphadenitis)
Accidental trauma (degloving injury)
Inflammatory disorders (rheumatoid arthritis, psoriasis,
chronic hand dermatitis)
Yellow nail syndrome
Factitious lymphoedema (Secretan's syndrome)

VASCULAR
Congenital
Klippel–Trenaunay syndrome
Venous (cavernous) haemangioma
Parkes Weber syndrome (multiple arteriovenous fistulae)
Other congenital vascular malformations
Maffucci's syndrome

Acquired
Axillary/subclavian vein thrombosis
External compression of vein by malignant disease
Venous and lymphatic damage following intravenous
drug abuse

OTHER
Congenital
Hemihypertrophy/gigantism
Fat hypertrophy/lipomatosis
Plexiform neurofibroma
Proteus syndrome

Acquired
Reflex sympathetic dystrophy (chronic regional pain
syndrome)
Pretibial myxoedema
Tumours/hamartomata
Musculoskeletal disorders (arthritis, joint effusions)

lifetime prevalence of arm swelling in 1077 unilateral cases.[3] A similar figure was obtained from a hospital series of 200 consecutive patients, arm oedema, measured objectively, being found in 26 per cent.[4] Axillary clearance and radiotherapy produced the highest prevalence of 38 per cent.

Lymphoedema is twice as common in women treated by radiotherapy than not (38 per cent versus 20 per cent), and more common after mastectomy than after wide local excision (29 per cent versus 19 per cent).[3] There is a significant increase in prevalence in patients who receive postoperative radiotherapy as the time interval after the radiotherapy increases.

Pathophysiology

Although the fundamental cause of breast cancer-related lymphoedema is interference to lymph drainage via the lymph collectors and lymph glands by surgery and radiotherapy, particularly in the axilla, the exact pathophysiology is not well understood.[5] For example:

- Why do some women but not others develop breast cancer-related lymphoedema?
- Why is there a variable latent period before the onset of established swelling?
- Why is there variation in the distribution of oedema, in some patients, for example, the hand being predominantly affected whereas in others it is spared?

The pathogenesis at first seems self-evident, namely that damage to the axillary lymphatic system causes lymph obstruction in a 'stopcock' manner. Lymphangiography during the latent phase (post-surgery but before swelling) shows dilatation of the main collecting lymphatics in the arm with extravasation of contrast medium and 'hold-up' at the axilla.[6] It is therefore assumed that lymph flow from the arm is reduced. Whereas arm oedema may develop rapidly, it eventually, once it has become established, adopts a relatively 'steady state' when the reduction in lymph flow (and protein clearance) is matched by a reduction in net capillary filtration (J_V) and a rise in interstitial protein (C_i) through adaption of the Starling forces. Interstitial pressure (P_i) rises, as expected, from $-2\,\mathrm{cm}$ to $+2\,\mathrm{cmH_2O}$.[7] Surprisingly, the measured C_i has been found to be reduced, rather than increased, in breast cancer-related lymphoedema when compared with the contralateral unaffected arm. Moreover, the ratio of interstitial protein concentration to plasma (total) protein concentration correlates negatively and significantly with severity, i.e. volume of arm swelling.[8] Breast cancer-related lymphoedema does not therefore appear to be a 'high-protein' oedema.

One explanation for a fall in C_i would be an increase in J_V. All oedema is caused by impaired lymph drainage and/or increased microvascular filtration. To assess the latter in breast cancer-related lymphoedema, J_V was studied in the oedematous forearm and found to be lower (as would be expected in lymphoedema) rather than higher. However, when differences in arm volume on the two sides were taken into account, the total fluid load on the lymphatic system of each arm (normal and abnormal) was not significantly different.[9] This indicates that the filtration load in breast cancer-related lymphoedema remains relatively constant, arguing against a significant haemodynamic contribution to its pathophysiology. The low C_i in the subcutis remains unexplained. As filtration rate is matched by lymph flow in a steady state, the above studies suggest that lymph flow in post-mastectomy oedema is reduced.

It is unfortunate that the measurement of lymph flow in absolute units is not yet possible. It is often assumed

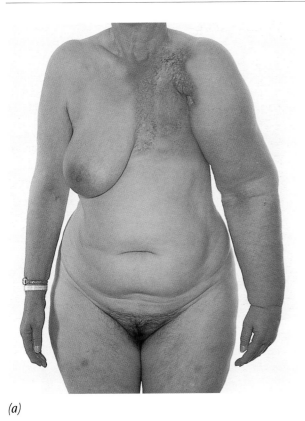

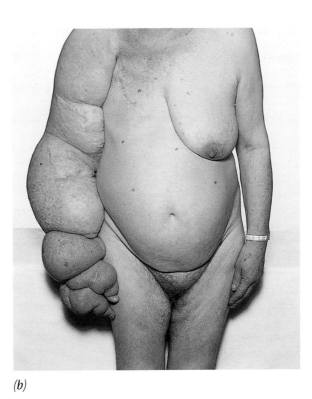

(a)   *(b)*

Figure 13.1 *(a) Moderate degree of oedema affecting the upper arm more than the hand. The skin is healthy, and there are no deep creases at the joints. This degree of oedema responds well to vigorous, lifelong manual lymphatic drainage and elastic compression. Also illustrated is the extensive scarring and skin damage that occurs in the region of the axilla after a radical mastectomy followed by radiotherapy. (b) A severely oedematous arm, following a radical mastectomy and radiotherapy, involving the forearm and hand more than the upper arm. This swelling did not respond to conservative treatment but could be treated with a reducing operation.*

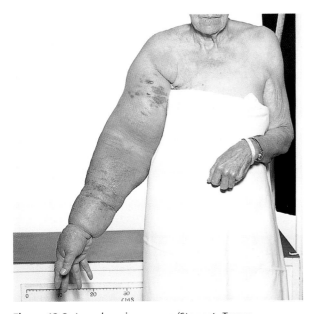

Figure 13.2 *Lymphangiosarcoma (Stewart–Treves syndrome) arising in a long-standing lymphoedematous arm. Neoplastic nodules can be seen in the lower forearm and just below the axilla. Two months later similar nodules appeared on the chest wall, and the patient died a few weeks later with disseminated metastases.*

that the dilated lymphatics seen on lymphangiographs indicate a reduced lymph flow, but flow is the product of lymphatic vessel cross-sectional area and velocity so the assumption of a reduced rate of flow may be erroneous.

Quantitative lymphoscintigraphy can be used as an indirect measure of lymph flow. Information from the regional lymph gland uptake of a radiolabelled tracer cannot be used in breast cancer-related lymphoedema because the lymph glands have been removed or irradiated. The removal rate constant (k) from a peripheral subcutaneous depot, for example in the hand or forearm, is a measure of *local* lymph flow i.e. mL/min/unit volume of tissue, providing the volume of distribution (V_D) is known.

In order to test the hypothesis that local differences in lymph drainage contribute to the regionality of the swelling, for example a spared hand, local lymph flow (k) was measured in the oedematous proximal forearm and in the unaffected hand (on the swollen side) (Fig. 13.3). V_D was assessed from the image width of depot size. Contralateral upper limbs served as controls. The value of k was 25 per cent lower in the oedematous forearm tissue than in the control forearm, and V_D was greater. In the non-oedematous hand of the breast cancer-related

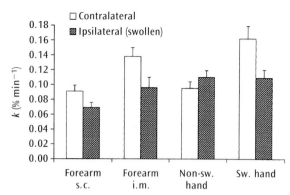

Figure 13.3 *Column chart showing removal rate constants (k, mean + SEM) for ^{99m}Tc-HIG injected into the ipsilateral and contralateral arms of women with breast cancer-related lymphoedema. Forearm injections were performed subcutaneously (s.c.) and intramuscularly (i.m.). Hand injections (s.c.) were performed in women with sparing of the hand itself but with forearm involvement (Non-sw. hand) and in women with hand (and forearm) swelling (Sw. hand). Note that, in the non-swollen hand group, k for the ipsilateral hand was not decreased relative to the contralateral hand.*

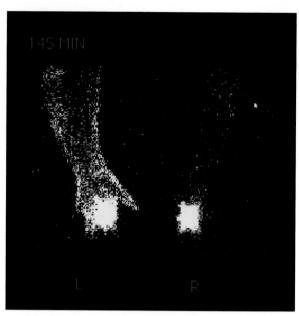

Figure 13.4 *Lymphoscintigram showing the hands and forearms, and the depot of ^{99m}Tc-HIG (in the second web space of the hand), 145 minutes after injection in a woman with breast cancer-related lymphoedema affecting the left arm (left side of image). The forearm was swollen, but the hand itself was spared of swelling. The image shows diffuse activity, peripherally concentrated, in the affected forearm and extending into the hand. This indicates the rerouting of lymph along dermal routes, i.e. dermal collateralization of flow, more commonly called dermal backflow.*

lymphoedema arm, k was 18 per cent higher than in the control hand and 59 per cent higher than forearm k on the breast cancer-related lymphoedema side. The V_D of the two sets of hands was the same.

One possible interpretation is that the hand is spared in some patients because local lymph flow is increased and diverted along collateral dermal routes (Fig. 13.4). These results support the hypothesis that regional differences in surviving lymphatic function determine the distribution of swelling.[10] Published studies of subfascial lymph flow from the muscle compartment where swelling does not occur have demonstrated k to be significantly reduced. The value of k shows a striking inverse correlation with swelling of the whole limb, i.e. the lower the subfascial lymph flow, the greater the epifascial oedema (Fig. 13.5).

The pathophysiology of breast cancer-related lymphoedema is therefore more complex than merely being a 'stopcock' effect from axillary lymphatic obstruction. The basic rule that all oedemas arise from an imbalance between capillary filtration and tissue (lymph) drainage demands consideration of the microcirculation as well as the lymphatic system. There is some evidence that total arm blood flow[11] and size of the vascular bed[12] increase in breast cancer-related lymphoedema, but it is likely that these are a consequence rather than a cause of the swelling. There is no evidence to suggest that regulation of the microvascular blood flow and, by implication, capillary pressure fails.[13]

Our current working hypothesis is that the active contractile lymphatic collectors of the arm have to work against increased resistance following damage to the

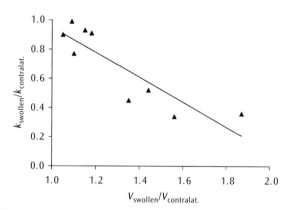

Figure 13.5 *Scattergram showing the correlation between the removal rate constant in the subfascial intramuscular compartment of the forearm and the total arm volume in breast cancer-related lymphoedema. The removal rate constant in the ipsilateral swollen forearm ($k_{swollen}$) relative to the contralateral forearm ($k_{contralat.}$) is plotted against the volume of the swollen arm ($V_{swollen}$) relative to the contralateral arm ($V_{contralat.}$) for nine women. The linear regression line is shown. The correlation was highly significant (r = -0.88, P = 0.002).*

axillary lymph glands by surgery and radiotherapy. The distribution of the swelling within a limb appears to depend upon the fatigue and eventual pump failure of the constitutionally weakest vessels, which may be those draining the mid-arm region. In regions where local collectors have not undergone failure, no oedema appears.

One of the problems in/of studying breast cancer-related lymphoedema is that patients are investigated at one moment in time during an evolving process. Pathological changes must be developing before the oedema becomes manifest, but non-swollen arms on the side of breast cancer treatment have not been studied in detail. One study of the skin lymphatic networks using fluorescence microlymphography has shown no abnormalities whatsoever in non-swollen forearms but enhanced dermal lymphatic networks (in terms of lymph vessel density and size) in the skin of swollen forearms, an observation in keeping with the dermal collateralization seen on lymphoscintigraphic images[14] and lymphangiographs (see Fig. 13.7b).

Risk factors

Postoperative complications such as wound infection, haematoma and skin flap necrosis are twice as likely to have occurred in patients who develop breast cancer-related lymphoedema.[15] Other risk factors include the extent of the surgery and radiotherapy, the dominant arm and the presence of metastases in the lymph glands. Obesity also increases the risk, as may venepuncture. Patients should be told not to have intravenous injections or infusions into the arm on the side of the treated cancer, even though the statistical risk of such interventions on inducing oedema is not known.

Diagnosis

A transient oedema of the arm develops in approximately 7 per cent of patients with breast cancer within 2 months of their surgery or radiation. Oedema that develops more than 3 months after treatment tends to be permanent. The swelling may develop rapidly, for example overnight. When it does, it is important to exclude infection and venous thrombosis as possible causes. Infection in the form of cellulitis may be difficult to diagnose because the classical features, for example rash, may be minimal, be atypical or postdate any systemic complaints such as fever or flu-like symptoms.

Whereas most patients develop swelling of the whole limb, a proportion develop oedema limited to the hand, forearm or upper arm. Mild, limited swelling may well be missed by both patient and doctor unless objective volume or arm circumference measurements are made. Differences between the dominant and non-dominant arms may serve to confuse, and some lymphoedematous

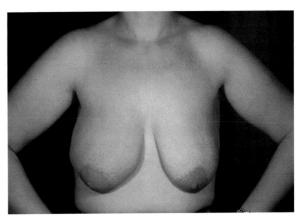

Figure 13.6 *Breast lymphoedema. The right breast is swollen and engorged despite the partial mastectomy.*

limbs may actually be smaller than the unaffected side because of tissue reactions or fibrosis.

Lymphoedema of the breast

The axillary lymph glands receive lymph not only from the upper limb, but also from the adjoining quadrant of the trunk, including the breast. The upper torso is therefore also at risk of developing lymphoedema after the treatment of breast cancer, and although it does not suffer to the same extent as the arm, presumably because of the greater availability of collateral lymph drainage pathways, lymphoedema can frequently be detected in the posterior axillary fold.

Since the introduction of breast-conserving treatments, the incidence of lymphoedema within the breast itself has increased (Fig. 13.6).[16] This may occur immediately after the axillary lymphadenectomy but often resolves spontaneously. Persistent oedema is more likely to follow irradiation of the breast itself. The affected breast becomes swollen, heavy and larger than the contralateral normal breast despite the reducing effect of the initial lumpectomy or partial mastectomy. Women with large breasts seem more at risk, possibly because of the added risk of 'dependency oedema' in a large, congested, pendulous breast. Persistent redness and pain suggest cellulitis, which can be difficult to settle with antibiotics. It is important to exclude the possibility that these symptoms are being caused by recurrent carcinoma before accepting a diagnosis of simple secondary lymphoedema. A breast biopsy may be required to achieve this.

Associated complications in the upper limb following breast cancer treatment

Other consequences of breast cancer treatment include limited shoulder movements, venous outflow obstruction and neurological deficits, all of which can cause or exacerbate arm oedema. Poor shoulder abduction inevitably leads to longer periods with the limb held dependent. Any sustained increase of venous and capillary pressure caused by these complications will increase capillary filtration and consequently the interstitial fluid load on an already compromised lymph drainage system. A flaccid arm resulting from brachial plexus neuropathy has a similar effect. Neurological traction deficits can also be caused by the weight of a swollen arm pulling on the cervical nerve roots. Lymphoedema also increases the likelihood of developing a carpal tunnel syndrome.

Abnormal venous anatomy following mastectomy was first described in 1938 using phlebography.[17] Other studies have subsequently confirmed that venous obstruction contributed to, or even caused, the swelling of breast cancer-related lymphoedema. In a more recent study using colour duplex Doppler imaging, only 30 per cent of the swollen arms of 81 patients with breast cancer-related lymphoedema and no sign of recurrent cancer had a normal venous outflow,[18] whereas 57 per cent had evidence of venous obstruction and a further 14 per cent had signs of venous 'congestion'. The contralateral arm

of the same patients and both arms of 28 control breast cancer patients who had similar treatment but no swelling were normal, and direct measurements of venous pressure in similar patients have also been found to be normal.[7] Because of the risk of venous thrombosis in cancer patients and the risk of external compression of the axillo-subclavian vein from fibrosis or tumour being significantly greater than normal, a colour-coded duplex Doppler ultrasound examination is indicated at an early stage.

Investigation

It is rarely necessary to confirm that the swelling is caused by lymphatic insufficiency when there is a history of lymph gland metastases, surgical lymphadenectomy or axillary irradiation, but, if thought necessary, the diagnosis can be confirmed with lymphoscintigraphy. X-ray lymphangiography is indicated only when complex

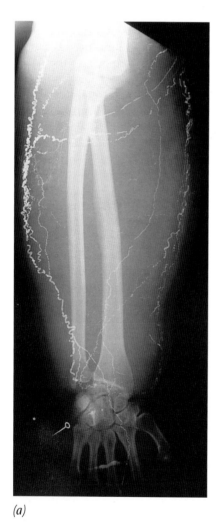

(a)

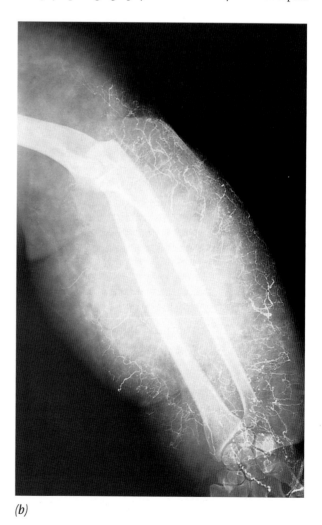

(b)

Figure 13.7 *(a) Lymphangiograph obtained 6 months after an axillary block dissection for malignant melanoma, showing dilated lymphatic collecting trunks. (b) Lymphangiograph of a swollen lymphoedematous arm, 5 years after a radical mastectomy and axillary radiotherapy. All the subcutaneous collecting lymphatics have occluded ('die-back'[19]), leaving a multitude of irregular, dilated lymph vessels just below the dermis.*

procedures such as lympho-lymphatic anastomoses or pedicles are being considered (*see* Chapter 11). The lymphographs of limbs that have reached the size of those shown in Fig. 13.1, p. 233 show either a few tortuous, dilated, subcutaneous collecting lymphatics (Fig. 13.7a) or a total absence or obliteration of the subcutaneous vessels ('die-back'[19]) with an extensive network of dilated subdermal vessels (Fig. 13.7b).

An ultrasound or phlebographic study of the axillary and subclavian veins is important if any form of surgical treatment is being considered. Surgery in the presence of an occluded axillary or subclavian vein is inadvisable.

Treatment

There is currently no cure for breast cancer-related lymphoedema. Until staging procedures avoid axillary lymph gland sampling or, for that matter, any form of axillary intervention, the risk of arm lymphoedema will remain. Even the removal of a single 'sentinel' gland does not preclude its development.

Physical therapy

Treatment aims to reduce or delay progression of swelling, restore limb shape and prevent associated infection. First-line treatment is, as for most forms of lymphoedema, physical therapy (compression, exercises, massage and elevation at night) to stimulate lymph flow (*see* Chapter 9). Prolonged elevation by suspending the arm in a roller towel fixed to a drip stand for a number of days does reduce the swelling,[6] probably by producing a sustained reduction in venous pressure. There is no objective evidence that elevation improves the rate of lymph drainage, but the flow of the oedema fluid to lower parts of the elevated limb that is effected by gravity moves the fluid into areas with a better lymph drainage, for example the trunk. Comfortable positioning of the arm at heart level or above when at rest, during the day and night, does have some effect on the overall size of the limb.

Despite the known effect of active and passive movements on enhancing lymph flow, there are no published randomized controlled clinical trials that have evaluated the benefit of exercise in relieving arm oedema. Sustained isometric muscle contraction such as gripping can increase oedema. The higher oxygen demand that occurs during this exercise increases blood flow and consequently fluid filtration, and the isometric muscle contractions do not generate the intermittent changes in tissue pressure needed for the propulsion of the lymph along the collecting lymphatics. Patients thus frequently comment that tasks such as carrying suitcases or shopping increase the swelling.

Drug therapy

Drug therapy is largely unhelpful. A randomized controlled cross-over trial of a preparation of oxerutins (hydroxyethylrutosides), taken as a daily dose of 3 g for 24 weeks, reduced arm volume by a statistically significant but clinically unimportant amount (4 per cent).[20]

Oral coumarin (5,6-benzo-[α]-pyrone) 400 mg daily for 6 months has been claimed to be effective in reducing arm oedema following breast cancer treatment,[21] but a more recent trial has cast doubt on its efficacy and also reported a significant risk of hepatotoxicity.[22]

Liposuction

Liposuction (*see* Chapter 10) has been shown by Brorson to achieve a complete reduction of arm swelling provided it is used in conjunction with high-quality compression hosiery, otherwise the oedema returns immediately (Fig. 13.8).[23,24] Part of the reason for the success of liposuction for arm, as opposed to leg, lymphoedema is to be found in the fact that chronic lymphoedema in the arm appears to stimulate fat cell growth and fat accumulation so there is more fat to suck out than in a normal arm. As this is a comparatively minor surgical procedure, we would advise its use for any patient in whom compression alone does not produce an acceptable result, provided the patient has used compression therapy diligently. It should not be used on patients who are not prepared or able to use good compression therapy after the liposuction because it has no long-term value when used alone.

Reducing operations

Reducing operations (*see* Chapter 10) should be reserved for very severe lymphoedema. We have treated eight

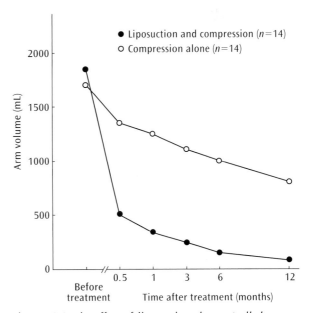

Figure 13.8 *The effect of liposuction plus controlled compression therapy in 14 patients (●), and controlled compression therapy alone in 14 patients (○), with post-mastectomy lymphoedema of the arm. Adapted from Brorson and Svensson[23] and Brorson.[24]*

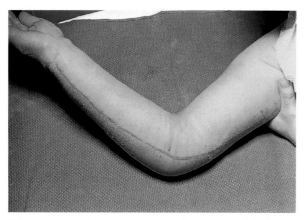

(a)

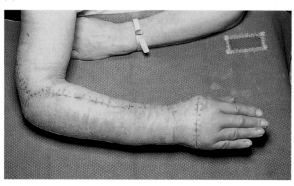

(b)

Figure 13.9 *Healed incisions from an arm-reducing operation. (a) Medial incision 9 months after operation. (b) Lateral incision, 3 weeks after the operation shown in (a). The swelling on the back of the hand was reduced through a transverse incision. It is essential to continue to use elastic compression after a reducing operation.*

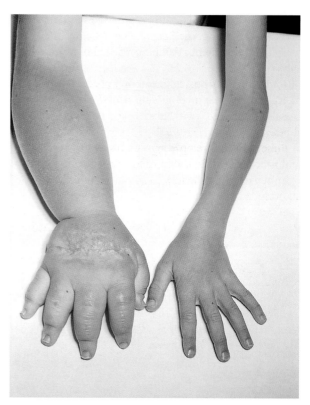

Figure 13.10 *An example of a patient with mild swelling of the forearm but severe swelling of the fingers and the back of the hand. An attempt to reduce the swelling on the back of the hand was partially successful, but her fingers were still very swollen and stiff.*

patients with the Homans' form of reducing operation over the past 30 years, all of whom were patients who had had a radical mastectomy and radiotherapy 10–20 years earlier.

The upper arm and forearm are technically easy to reduce. It is wise to perform the reduction in two stages, beginning with the medial aspect of the limb, to ensure that the skin flaps are viable. Three or 4 months later, the lateral aspect may be reduced (Fig. 13.9). Care must be taken to preserve the subcutaneous nerves. Patches of numbness on the forearm appear to be more troublesome to patients than the numb areas on the leg that may follow leg reductions. Fortunately, the sensory nerves of the skin of the hand are not at risk as they do not appear in the subcutaneous tissues above the wrist. As with surgical reduction of the lower limb, careful lifelong external compression, exercise and massage must be continued.

It is far more difficult to reduce the size of the hand. An enlarged bulging mass of oedematous tissue on the back of the thigh can be excised through a transverse convex-distal incision, but it is almost impossible to obtain a satisfactory reduction of the fingers (Fig. 13.10). Patients must continue to use an elasticated glove and

make sure that no constriction is caused by the arm sleeve at the lower end of the forearm reduction.

Lymphatic transplantation

Despite the apparent improvement in lymph drainage, as assessed by lymphoscintigraphy, there is little evidence that lymph vessel transplants (*see* Chapter 10) used to re-route lymph drainage[25] provide any long-term benefit.

MALIGNANT MELANOMA-RELATED LYMPHOEDEMA

The management of lymphoedema that follows the treatment of malignant melanoma is poorly documented. Although melanoma that has metastasized to the inguinal or axillary lymph glands can present with lymphoedema, the most common form of lymphoedema associated with malignant melanoma is that which arises from the surgical excision of involved glands. The risk of lymphoedema appears to be greater after block resection of the inguinal rather than the axillary glands,[26,27] but, interestingly, the risk of lower limb lymphoedema appears to be no higher following ilio-inguinal lymph gland clearance than following superficial inguinal gland clearance.[27]

In recent years, sentinel gland biopsy has become a regular part of the investigation of patients with malignant melanoma, but this seemingly minor procedure is not without risk. Between 1997 and 2000, 40 patients (17 per cent) from a series of 230 patients treated for malignant melanoma (29 lower limb, 11 upper limb) at St George's Hospital, London, were referred to the lymphoedema clinic for the management of their lymphoedema. Eleven of these 40 had developed lymphoedema as a result of a sentinel gland biopsy alone (B.W. Powell, pers. comm.), one after an axillary sentinel gland biopsy and 10 after an inguinal sentinel gland biopsy.

Although little evidence exists to indicate the best treatment for lymphoedema arising from the treatment of malignant melanoma, our recommended guidelines for its prevention after surgery are:

- elevation of the limb at rest;
- exercising little and often;
- good skin hygiene to minimize infection;
- once any drains or stitches have been removed, the fitting of compression hosiery as soon as any sign of oedema appears.

Many surgeons prescribe immediate postoperative compression hosiery in the absence of any sign of oedema as a prophylactic measure.

LYMPHOEDEMA ASSOCIATED WITH CHRONIC INFLAMMATORY DISORDERS

Rheumatoid and psoriatic arthritis

There are many published case reports demonstrating an apparent association between lymphoedema and rheumatoid arthritis or psoriatic arthritis.[28,29] In all cases, the oedema has been peripheral and was either followed by or occurred coincidentally with the onset of inflammatory polyarthritis of the rheumatoid type. Proof of a causal relationship is, however, lacking. The severity of the oedema does not correlate with the duration or the severity of arthritis. Furthermore, the oedema does not usually resolve following spontaneous or pharmacological resolution of the arthritis, although improvement can occur following steroid treatment.

Lymph drainage has been shown, using lymphoscintigraphy, to be significantly reduced in a group of 10 patients with inflammatory arthritis (8 rheumatoid and 2 psoriatic) and upper limb oedema but normal in 18 rheumatoid arthritis patients with no oedema.[28] Although the swelling was confirmed to be lymphoedema, no relationship could be demonstrated between it and the arthritis or the change in lymph drainage, indicating that inflammatory arthritis alone does not impair lymphatic drainage.

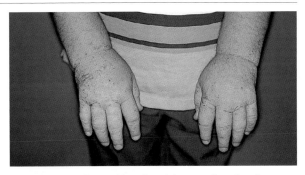

Figure 13.11 *Bilateral hand and forearm lymphoedema secondary to chronic hand dermatitis.*

When anti-inflammatory measures fail to influence the oedema, other conventional treatments also appear to be relatively ineffective. Joint pain and tenderness may make the wearing of compression hosiery unacceptable and prohibit exercise. The firm, brawny nature of the oedema, particularly in the hands, seems particularly resistant to treatment.

Chronic hand dermatitis

Upper limb swelling may occur after chronic hand dermatitis with or without documented evidence of lymphangitis (Fig. 13.11).[30] Hand dermatitis such as atopic eczema is very common, but the association with lymphoedema is rare, suggesting that an additional abnormality is necessary to produce the swelling.

Once established, exacerbations of the oedema tend to follow outbreaks of the eczematous dermatitis and lymphangitis/cellulitis. Increasingly frequent attacks of secondary infection lead to a downhill spiral of worsening oedema and more cellulitis. Consequently, if control of the swelling is to be obtained, it is essential that infection be prevented and the dermatitis cleared. This may require aggressive treatment with prophylactic antibiotics and long-term immunosuppressant drugs. Patients in whom an occupational contact allergy exists as the cause of the dermatitis, for example a florist allergic to certain plants, may need to change employment.

Pretibial myxoedema

Pretibial myxoedema rarely affects the upper as well as the lower limb. The swelling has, in the past, been attributed to the deposition of mucopolysaccharide within the skin, but studies using lymphoscintigraphy have demonstrated that there is an associated reduction of lymph drainage. Fluorescence microlymphography fails to demonstrate functioning skin lymphatics, and it has been postulated that the deposited mucin interferes with initial lymphatic uptake from the affected tissues.[31] This may explain why pretibial myxoedema can bear a striking resemblance to lymphoedema. Pretibial myxoedema can unfortunately be exacerbated by successful treatment of the thyrotoxicosis.

Yellow nail syndrome

The oedema of the yellow nail syndrome (yellow nails, bronchiectasis and chronic sinusitis) was alleged to be lymphatic in origin on the basis of some morphological abnormalities observed on lymphography (*see* Chapter 5). However, only in cases with severe oedema do the clinical features resemble those of lymphoedema. Furthermore, the oedema can come and go (as can the nail abnormality), whereas lymphoedema is characteristically permanent.

One study using lymphoscintigraphy has demonstrated reduced lymph drainage in patients with yellow nail syndrome compared with normal controls, but not to the very reduced levels seen with established lymphoedema.[32] The mechanism that gives rise to the oedema associated with yellow nail syndrome therefore remains unclear.

PRIMARY LYMPHOEDEMA

Lymphoedema occurring in the upper limb(s) in childhood for no obvious cause is not unreasonably attributed to a congenital or genetic cause. As described in Chapter 7, lymphatic abnormalities present at birth can be caused by aplasia, hypoplasia, ectasia or hyperplasia of the limb collecting vessels or malformations of the central (thoracic) lymphatics with extension of the process into the limbs. At the time of publication, mutations for three independent genetic syndromes associated with lymphatic maldevelopment have been described:

- The *VEGFR-3* gene is involved in Milroy's disease, in which there is hypoplasia of the peripheral lymphatics and the clinical phenotype appears *not* to involve the upper limb.
- Similarly, the lymphoedema–distichiasis syndrome, involving the *FOXC2* gene, which appears to cause hyperplasia of the leg collecting lymphatics,[33] does not affect the upper limb.
- Mutations in the *NEMO* (NF-κB essential modulator) gene have been found responsible for lymphoedema of both legs and one arm associated with immunodeficiency and intestinal lymphangiectasia[34] in a male infant with incontinentia pigmenti (an X-linked dominant disorder and therefore normally lethal in males), the mechanism probably being a failure in the balance between endothelial proliferation and apoptosis during lymphatic development.

Although most forms of childhood lymphoedema are caused by genetic factors, not all are inherited. A family history will indicate an inherited aetiology, but some mutations arise for the first time and therefore have no past family history. Inherited lymphoedemas caused by germline mutations usually display bilateral involvement, whereas sporadic cases caused by somatic mutations

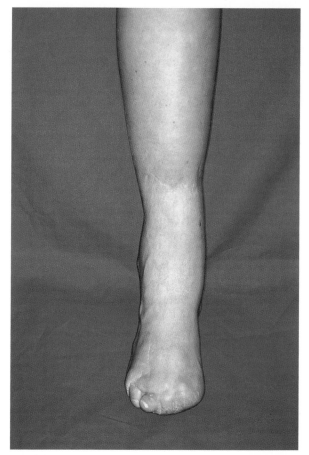

(a)

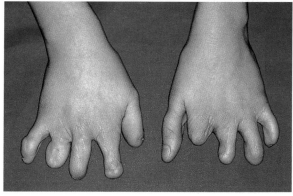

(b)

Figure 13.12 *Amniotic band syndrome. (a) Congenital fibrotic constriction encircling the lower leg and causing distal lymphoedema. Note the auto-amputation of the toes resulting from other amniotic bands. (b) The hands of the same patient were similarly affected.*

are usually strikingly asymmetrical and often affect only one limb.

Most forms of childhood lymphoedema of the upper limb are sporadic – having no family history – and are associated with lower limb lymphoedema and other lymphatic abnormalities, sometimes involving the face. Abnormalities such as congenital heart disease may co-exist. One example is Turner's syndrome, which is caused by the absence of one X chromosome.

Upper limb swelling in the absence of oedema or abnormalities elsewhere may be lymphoedema, but consideration must be given to other causes of enlargement, such as hemihypertrophy, plexiform neurofibromatosis, proteus syndrome or muscle hamartoma. Lymphoedema of one arm may be caused by an isolated lymphatic abnormality but is more often than not just one part of a mixed vascular malformation. Local gigantism and cutaneous angiomata suggest a diagnosis of Klippel–Trenaunay syndrome.

A slow progressive enlargement of the arm may be caused by an intrinsic proliferative process in deep cavernous or diffuse lymphangiomatosis (see Chapter 19) as opposed to extension caused by a raised hydraulic pressure (lymphangiectasia). These abnormalities typically present in children and, in a significant proportion of cases, are confined to one limb with or without bone involvement.[35] Involvement of the visceral organs, as opposed to soft tissue and bone, is associated with a poor prognosis.[36] Lymphangiomatosis in soft tissues presents as a diffuse, fluctuant swelling that may have surface lymphangiomatous vesicles.

A child may be born with a swollen limb or digit caused by a constricting amniotic band (Fig. 13.12). These are fibrous strands that encircle a digit or limb in utero, obstruct the lymph flow and may even lead to an auto-amputation in utero. It is assumed that the band arises from an adhesion between the amniotic sac and the surface of the fetus. In utero diagnosis is now possible using ultrasound or magnetic resonance imaging.[37,38]

REFERENCES

1. Arm oedema following breast cancer treatment. *Drugs and Therapeutics Bulletin* 2000; **38**: 41–3.

2. Halstead WS. The swelling of the arm after operations for cancer of the breast – elephantiasis chirgica – its cause and prevention. *Bulletin of the Johns Hopkins Hospital* 1921; **32**: 309–13.

3. Mortimer PS, Bates DO, Brassington HD, Stanton AWB, Strachan DP, Levick JR. The prevalence of arm oedema following treatment for breast cancer. *Quarterly Journal of Medicine* 1996; **89**: 377–80.

4. Kissin MW, Querci della Rovere G, Easton D, Westbury C. Risk of lymphoedema following the treatment of breast cancer. *British Journal of Surgery* 1986; **73**: 580–4.

5. Stanton AWB, Levick JR, Mortimer PS. Current puzzles presented by postmastectomy oedema (breast cancer related lymphoedema). *Vascular Medicine* 1996; **1**: 213–25.

6. Hughes JH, Patel AR. Swelling of the arm following radical mastectomy. *British Journal of Surgery* 1966; **53**: 4–15.

7. Bates DO, Levick JR, Mortimer PS. Subcutaneous interstitial fluid pressures and arm volume in lymphoedema. *International Journal of Microcirculation* 1992; **11**: 359–73.

8. Bates DO, Levick JR, Mortimer PS. Changes in macromolecular composition of interstitial fluid from swollen arms after breast cancer treatment, and its implications. *Clinical Science* 1993; **85**: 737–46.

9. Stanton AWB, Holroyd B, Mortimer PS, Levick JR. Comparison of microvascular filtration in human arms with and without postmastectomy oedema. *Experimental Physiology* 1999; **84**: 405–19.

10. Stanton AWB, Svensson WE, Mellor RH, Peters AM, Levick JR, Mortimer PS. Differences in lymph drainage between swollen and non swollen regions in arms with breast cancer-related lymphoedema. *Clinical Science* 2001; **101**: 131–40.

11. Svensson WE, Mortimer PS, Tohno E, Cosgrove DO. Increased arterial inflow demonstrated by Doppler ultrasound in arm swelling following breast cancer treatment. *European Journal of Cancer* 1994; **30**: 661–4.

12. Roberts CC, Stanton AWB, Pullen J, Bull RH, Levick JR, Mortimer PS. Skin microvascular architecture and perfusion studied in human postmastectomy oedema by intravital video-capillaroscopy. *International Journal of Microcirculation* 1994; **14**: 327–34.

13. Stanton AWB, Levick JR, Mortimer PS. Assessment of cutaneous vascular control in the arms of women with postmastectomy oedema. *Experimental Physiology* 1996; **81**: 447–64.

14. Mellor RH, Stanton AWB, Azarbod P, Sherman MD, Levick JR, Mortimer PS. Enhanced cutaneous lymphatic network in the forearms of women with postmastectomy oedema. *Journal of Vascular Research* 2000; **37**: 510–12.

15. Mozes M, Papa MZ, Karasik A, Reshef A, Adar R. The role of infection in post-mastectomy lymphoedema. *Surgical Annals* 1987; **14**: 73–83.

16. Hughes LL, Styblo TM, Thoms WW, et al. Cellulitis of the breast as a complication of breast conserving surgery and irradiation. *American Journal of Clinical Oncology* 1997; **20**: 338–41.

17. Veal JR. The pathological basis for swelling of the arm following radical amputation of the breast. *Surgery, Gynecology and Obstetrics* 1938; **67**: 752–60.

18. Svensson WE, Mortimer PS, Tohno E, Cosgrove DO. Colour Doppler demonstrates venous flow abnormalities in breast cancer patients with chronic arm swelling. *European Journal of Cancer* 1994; **30**: 657–60.

19. Fyfe NCM, Wolfe JHN, Kinmonth JB. Die-back in primary lymphoedema. *Lymphology* 1982; **15**: 66–9.

20. Taylor HM, Rose KE, Twycross RG. A double blind clinical trial of hydroxyethylrutosides in obstructive arm oedema. *Phlebology* 1993; **8 (suppl. 1)**: 22–8.

21. Casley-Smith JR, Morgan RG, Piller NB. Treatment of lymphoedema of the arms and legs with 5,6-benzo-[α]-pyrone. *New England Journal of Medicine* 1993; **329:** 1158–63.

22. Loprinzi CL, Kugler JW, Sloan JA, *et al.* Lack of effect of coumarin in women with lymphoedema after treatment for breast cancer. *New England Journal of Medicine* 1999; **340:** 346–50.

23. Brorson H, Svensson H. Complete reduction of lymphoedema of the arm by liposuction after breast cancer. *Scandinavian Journal of Plastic and Reconstructive Surgery* 1997; **31:** 137–43.

24. Brorson H. Liposuction and Controlled Compression Therapy in the Treatment of Arm Lymphoedema following Breast Cancer. MD thesis, University of Lund, Sweden, 1998.

25. Baumeister RG, Siuda S. Treatment of lymphoedemas by microsurgical lymphatic grafting: what is proved? *Plastic and Reconstructive Surgery* 1990; **85:** 75–6.

26. Karakousis CP, Driscoll D. Groin dissection in malignant melanoma. *British Journal of Surgery* 1994; **81:** 1771–4.

27. Hughs TM, Thomas JM. Combined inguinal and pelvic lymph node dissection for stage III melanoma. *British Journal of Surgery* 1999; **86:** 1493–8.

28. Kiely PDW, Bland JM, Joseph AEA, Mortimer PS, Bourke BE. Upper limb lymphatic function in inflammatory arthritis. *Journal of Rheumatology* 1995; **22:** 214–17.

29. Mulherin DM, Fitzgerald O, Bresnihan B. Lymphoedema of the upper limb in patients with psoriatic arthritis. *Seminars in Arthritis and Rheumatism* 1993; **22:** 350–6.

30. Worm AM, Staberg B, Thomsen K. Persistent oedema in allergic contact dermatitis. *Contact Dermatitis* 1983; **9:** 517–18.

31. Bull RH, Coburn PR, Mortimer PS. Pre-tibial myxoedema: a manifestation of lymphoedema. *Lancet* 1993; **341:** 403–4.

32. Bull RH, Fenton DA, Mortimer PS. Lymphatic function in the yellow nail syndrome. *British Journal of Dermatology* 1996; **134:** 171–80.

33. Dale RF. Primary lymphedema when found with distichiasis is the type defined as bilateral hyperplasia by lymphography. *Journal of Medical Genetics* 1987; **24:** 170–1.

34. Mansour S, Woffendin H, Mitton S, *et al.* Incontinentia pigmenti in a surviving male is accompanied by hypohidrotic ectodermal dysplasia and recurrent infection. *American Journal of Medical Genetics* 2001; **99:** 172–7.

35. Sing H, Gomez C, Calonje E, Browse NL. Lymphangiomatosis of the limbs: clinicopathologic analysis of a series with a good prognosis. *American Journal of Surgical Pathology* 1995; **19:** 125–33.

36. Ramani P, Shah A. Lymphangiomatosis. Histological and immunohistochemical analysis of four cases. *American Journal of Surgical Pathology* 1992; **16:** 764–71.

37. Tadmor OP, Kriesberg GA, Achiron R, Porat S, Yagel S. Limb amputation in amniotic band syndrome: serial ultrasonographic and Doppler observations. *Ultrasound in Obstetrics and Gynaecology* 1997; **10:** 312–15.

38. Laor T, Burrows PE. Congenital anomalies and vascular birthmarks of the lower extremities. *Magnetic Resonance Imaging Clinics of North America* 1998; **6:** 497–519.

14

Management of lymphoedema of the head and neck

Lymphoedema of the face is uncommon because the face has an extensive bilateral lymph drainage and there are no gravitational factors to compound any lymphatic insufficiency. Pure lymphatic abnormalities of the face are very rare, most cases of facial oedema being associated with an increased lymph load from excessive capillary filtration. Although such cases are of mixed aetiology, i.e. both vascular and lymphatic, chronic oedema would not occur unless there were a significant impairment of lymphatic outflow. This chapter will therefore discuss all forms of chronic facial oedema (Table 14.1).

CONGENITAL/GENETIC DISORDERS

It is unusual to observe primary facial lymphoedema in a child or young adult without involvement of either the upper or the lower limbs. Facial involvement is usually asymmetrical and may be intermittent or even appear to resolve (Fig. 14.1). If the peri-orbital tissues are affected, conjunctival oedema can frequently be seen as fluid-filled sacs underneath the conjunctiva. Apart from the disfigurement, facial lymphoedema causes few problems except when the chronic eyelid swelling is severe enough to close the palpebral fissure or cellulitis occurs as a result of the lymphatic insufficiency.

Swelling is not usually associated with port wine stain (naevus flammeus), but should it occur, a cavernous component to the angioma is the probable cause. Nevertheless, facial lymphoedema secondary to lymph-angiectasia has been described.[1]

An unusual congenital cause of facial lymphoedema is an oblique facial cleft. One patient out of the three described by Mishima and colleagues[2] displayed ring constriction and an occipital encephalocele to which an

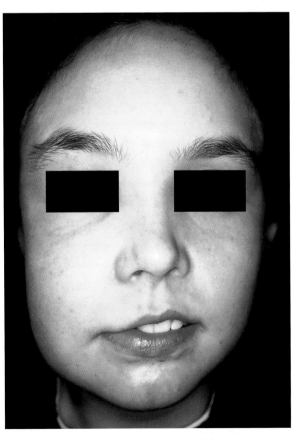

Figure 14.1 *Facial lymphoedema in a child.*

Table 14.1 *Causes of chronic facial oedema*

Name	Cause	Manifestations
Genetic		
?Trisomy 21		Nuchal and thoracic lymphangiomatosis
?Turner syndrome	Chromosome XO	Webbed neck
?Noonan syndrome	Autosomal dominant	Nuchal swelling in utero, webbed neck, ptosis, hypertelorism, low-set ears and possibly hairline
Hennekam syndrome (lymphangiectasia–lymphoedema syndrome)	?Autosomal recessive	Flat face and nasal bridge, hypertelorism, epicanthic folds (resembling Down's syndrome)
	Sporadic (somatic mutation or recessive)	Hemi-oedema of face and swelling of one or more limbs. Congenital heart defects, pharyngeal problems at birth
Incontinentia pigmenti		Immunodeficiency, ectodermal dysplasia, protein-losing enteropathy
?Proteus syndrome		Gigantism
Mixed vascular malformations, naevus flammeus, haemangioma		Port wine stain
Lymphangioma		Surface vesicles (lymph blisters)
Oblique facial cleft (amniotic bands)	Amnion rupture sequence	Ring constriction, pseudodyndactyly, occipital encephalocele (to which amniotic band attached)
Trauma		
Lymphadenectomy, radiotherapy, blunt injury to face, burns		
Systemic conditions		
Nephrotic syndrome	Hypoproteinaemia	
Superior vena caval obstruction	Mediastinal tumours	Chemosis, suffused face
Graves' disease	Autoimmune	Exophthalmos, eyelid swelling
Dermatomyositis		Eyelid swelling with heliotrope discolouration and telangiectasia
Local inflammatory conditions		
Rosacea	?	Fixed facial redness, pimples/pustules, flushing
Morbihan's disease	?Rosacea	Fixed facial redness, no signs of acne
Sarcoidosis	Dermal granulomata	Cutaneous granulomata (may not be visible)
Orofacial granulomatosis	Granulomatous disease ?Sarcoid ?Crohn's disease	Lip swelling ± scrotal tongue. Facial palsy
Infection		
(a) Cellulitis/erysipelas	May require pre-existing lymphatic insufficiency	Fever, flu-like symptoms, relapsing attacks
(b) Dental abscess	Sepsis	Pain, unilateral swelling
(c) Leprosy	*Mycobacterium leprae* granulomata	Nodules
(d) Filariasis/onchocerciasis		
(e) Tularaemia (oculoglandular type)	*Francisella tularensis*	Lid oedema, severe redness and chemosis of conjunctivae, lymphadenopathy
(f) Lympogranuloma venereum	*Chlamydia*	Lid oedema, chemosis, lymphadenopathy
Angioedema		Recurrent acute exacerbations of oedema
Chronic dermatitis		
(a) Contact allergy		Eczematous rash
(b) Atopy		
(c) Head lice		
Malignancy		
Angiosarcoma	Endothelial cell tumour	Bruise discolouration in skin, usually forehead and scalp, ±nodules
Kaposi's sarcoma	Herpes virus 8 (usually in AIDS)	Dark plum red-to-black plaques in skin
Recurrent head and neck cancer (squamous cell carcinoma, non-Hodgkin's lymphoma)	Recurrent tumour in collateral lymphatics following bilateral neck dissection ± radiotherapy	Severe swelling resistant to lymphoedema treatment
Degenerative		
Blepharochalasia		

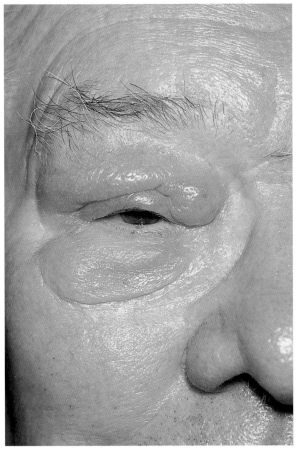

Figure 14.2 *Peri-orbital lymphoedema arising from a blunt injury and depressed fracture.*

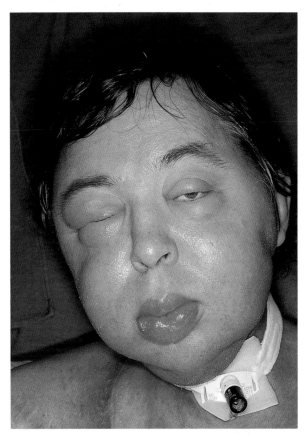

Figure 14.3 *Gross facial lymphoedema following bilateral neck dissections and radiotherapy for squamous cell carcinoma with covert local recurrence, which proved fatal.*

amniotic band was attached at birth. The cause was considered to be an amnion rupture sequence.

TRAUMA

Blunt trauma can rarely be a cause of facial swelling. In such cases, the injury is usually severe and associated with an underlying fracture (Fig. 14.2). The cause of the oedema is damage to the local skin and subcutaneous lymphatics. It is not known whether the development of the oedema depends upon the lymphatic vessels being abnormal prior to the injury.

Lymphoedema of the head and neck can develop following the surgical removal of lymph glands and after fibrosis as a result of irradiation. Bilateral obstruction of the lymph drainage pathways, be it from cancer, surgery or radiotherapy, is usually necessary to generate permanent swelling (Fig. 14.3).

The absence of a satisfactory collateral lymphatic drainage may cause a reduction in aqueous humour outflow and a rise of intra-ocular pressure.[3]

SYSTEMIC CAUSES

It is of the utmost importance to consider the systemic and potentially treatable causes of facial swelling. *Nephrotic syndrome* with hypoproteinaemia and *Graves' disease* are easily excluded by the appropriate blood tests. *Dermatomyositis* need not possess the myositis component, i.e. the creatine kinase level may be normal, so the diagnosis depends on the cutaneous features with or without skin biopsy. Any swelling is likely to be very responsive to steroid therapy, but consideration should always be given to the possibility of underlying *systemic malignant disease*.

LOCAL INFLAMMATORY CONDITIONS

Rosacea

Rosacea is by far the most common cause of facial lymphoedema (Fig. 14.4). Conversely, lymphoedema is a rare complication of (acne) rosacea. Rosacea is a chronic skin disorder of unknown cause that is characterized by

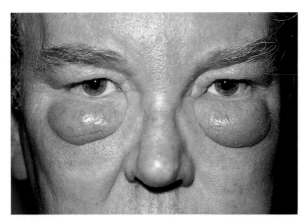

Figure 14.4 *Rosaceous lymphoedema. The swelling is always associated with a red complexion caused by persistent erythema and telangiectasia.*

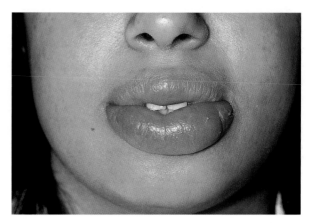

Figure 14.5 *Orofacial granulomatosis giving rise to swelling of the lower lip.*

persistent redness and telangiectasia, and punctuated by episodes of inflammation (pimples and pustules). The redness and telangiectasia preferentially affect the convexities of the face. Swelling in rosacea is of two kinds: intermittent, related to episodes of inflammation; and persistent, attributed to lymphoedema.

Rosaceous lymphoedema develops in one or more areas of the face and does appear to be related to the episodes of inflammation. The forehead, cheeks and/or peri-orbital tissues are the sites usually affected. The swollen area is often indurated – solid facial oedema. Although there may be some fluctuation in intensity, the swelling is remarkably persistent.

Histopathologically, the only consistent features are vascular ectasia, dermal oedema and connective tissue disorganization. Features of acne (folliculitis) are not always present, indicating that the vascular abnormalities (and consequently the clinical redness) are an essential component. Lymphoscintigraphy has demonstrated that the swelling is in part lymphatic, although there is also likely to be excessive capillary filtration from the dilated, damaged skin blood microvessels.

The treatment of rosaceous lymphoedema is extremely difficult. The first objective must be to bring any inflammation under control using antibiotics such as oxytetracycline 500 mg twice daily for a minimum of 6 weeks. If antibiotic treatment fails, consideration should be given to the vitamin A analogue isotretinoin. Dermatological expertise is necessary at this stage.

Measures should also be introduced that discourage the erythema and high blood flow to the face. A cool environment, particularly in the bedroom, and the avoidance of alcohol, hot beverages and spicy foods are recommended. The regular use of a moisturiser containing a sunblock with a sun protection factor of at least 15 is advisable as exposure to ultraviolet light serves only to excerbate the redness (and may be a causal factor in the first place). There is unfortunately little treatment specifically for the lymphoedema. Massage, although theoretically helpful,

can increase the redness if it is directed to the affected sites. Blepharoplasty is indicated if vision is compromised despite adequate medical treatment for the rosacea.

Morbihan's disease was first reported as a distinct entity in 1957 by Degos who described a chronic persistent erythema and oedema of the upper half of the face. The condition is probably a variant of the lymphoedema associated with rosacea.

OROFACIAL GRANULOMATOSIS (MELKERSSON–ROSENTHAL SYNDROME, GRANULOMATOUS CHEILITIS)

The combination of facial oedema and facial palsy was first described in 1928 by Melkersson, the feature of lingua plicata or scrotal tongue being added in 1931 by Rosenthal. The mean age of onset of the condition is 33 years, and it has an equal sex distribution.[4] Orofacial oedema is accepted as the dominant manifestation. Swelling tends to affect the lip and peri-oral tissues, extension into the mouth involving the tongue and buccal mucosa (Fig. 14.5).[5] Granulomatous cheilitis is a limited form of the syndrome affecting only the lip(s).

Histologically, non-caseating epitheloid granulomatous inflammation is characteristic, although granulomata are not always identified. Consistent in their presence are oedema and dilated vessels, which have at times been shown to contain granulomata within their lumen, indicating their lymphatic nature.[6] The term 'orofacial granulomatosis' was coined to emphasize the hallmark feature of granulomata and to indicate the similarity to Crohn's disease.[7] Indeed, a number of reports cite orofacial granulomatosis with intestinal Crohn's disease, although bowel involvement is more often than not absent.

The suggestion that orofacial granulomatosis is a variant of sarcoidosis has not been confirmed. Sarcoid granulomata are typically well formed, unlike the less discrete granulomata of orofacial granulomatosis and Crohn's disease, which are similar. There is little evidence to support an infectious aetiology, and *Toxoplasma*, mycobacteria, herpes simplex and *Borrelia burgdorferi* have been excluded. A report linking the food additives cinnamaldehyde carnosine, monosium glutamate, cocoa, carbone and sunset yellow has not been substantiated.[8]

Orofacial granulomatosis is extremely resistant to treatment; the range of therapies cited in anecdotal reports claiming success only testifies to the difficulty. Treatment with antibiotics such as erythromycin can help, but this may indicate a contribution from secondary infection entering through lip cracks and fissures. High-dose systemic steroids can have a dramatic initial benefit that unfortunately wanes, relapse occurring as the steroid dosage is necessarily reduced. Repeated local injections of triamcinolone can be successful. Clofazimine 100 mg twice daily for 10 days, reducing to twice weekly, appears to help the majority of patients.[9] Surgical reduction (cheiloplasty) has a high rate of relapse unless combined with local steroid injections.

Sarcoid

Although doubt exists regarding the role of sarcoid in causing orofacial granulomatosis, lymphoedema associated with sarcoid, usually involving a limb, is well described. Distinguishing sarcoid as a cause of facial swelling from orofacial granulomatosis is difficult, although one report cites a positive Kweim test.[10]

INFLAMMATION/INFECTION

The relationship between lymphoedema and infection is agreed, but which comes first is less clear. Infection can certainly result from lymphatic insufficiency, presumably because of the disturbance to local immunosurveillance mechanisms. Infection as a cause of lymphoedema is described, but to what extent latent lymphatic abnormalities must exist prior to the initial infection if swelling is to persist is uncertain.

Persistent or recurrent inflammation without overt infection is a possible cause of lymphoedema. Recurrent angioedema can eventually lead to chronic swelling. Similarly, a chronic eczematous dermatitis from a contact allergy or atopic dermatitis can cause long-term oedema. Lymphoedema of the external ear has been described following head louse infestation.[11]

Erysipelas/cellulitis

Recurrent infection at one site, such as the face (Fig. 14.6), implies an underlying lymphatic problem. With each acute inflammatory episode, further lymphatic damage occurs and a vicious cycle is established. In these circumstances,

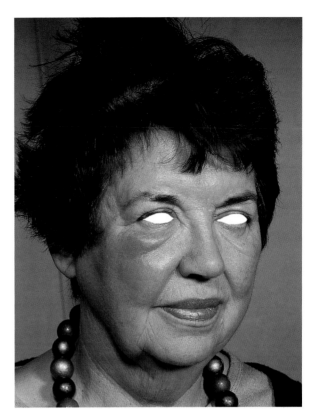

Figure 14.6 *Recurrent facial erysipelas associated with underlying lymphatic insufficiency.*

prophylactic antibiotics, for example phenoxymethylpenicillin 250–500 mg twice daily, are indicated. Such treatment should not only stop the recurrent attacks in the majority of cases, but also frequently permit swelling to subside as the inflammatory drive has now been removed.

Filariasis and onchocerciasis

Chronic eyelid swelling arising from both filariasis and onchocerciasis is described but as a consequence of ocular involvement.

MALIGNANCY

Lymphoedema may arise because of direct *de novo* infiltration of the cutaneous lymphatics by tumour (angiosarcoma or Kaposi's sarcoma), or through a local or lymph gland recurrance of metastatic head and neck cancer. Radical surgery or radiotherapy without tumour recurrence rarely gives rise to lymphoedema of the head and neck, owing to the excellent opportunities for collateral lymph drainage.

Angiosarcoma

Angiosarcoma is a rare lethal tumour arising from vascular endothelium. It characteristically affects the skin of the scalp in an elderly patient, manifesting itself as a bruise-like patch with ill-defined borders that advances rapidly. Oedema is a consistent feature and usually involves the scalp, forehead and eyelids. Radiotherapy is the treatment of choice, but relapse rates are high and the prognosis is poor.

Kaposi's sarcoma

Kaposi's sarcoma is well described with lymphoedema. There is some evidence to suggest that the process origin-ates from either lymphatic endothelium or 'stem cell' vascular endothelium (which has lost its phenotypic differentiation). Extensive Kaposi's sarcoma, as can occur with AIDS (autoimmune deficiency syndrome), may involve the face, leading to widely dilated cutaneous lymphatics and lymphoedema. In one report, treatment with alpha-interferon led to a partial regression of the Kaposi's sarcoma and the lymphoedema.[12]

BLEPHAROCHALASIA

Extremely lax eyelid skin can be associated with chronic oedema. In blepharochalasia, the elastic fibres of the eyelid skin degenerate. Elastic fibres probably play an important role in the functioning of cutaneous lymphatics, not only in the entry of interstitial fluid into the initial lymphatics, but also in maintaining tissue compliance. Compliance influences interstitial fluid pressure, one of the important buffers against oedema. Consequently, loose baggy eyelids swell more easily. The only treatment is blepharoplasty, which, by tightening the eyelid, improves tissue compliance.

REFERENCES

1. Mahler V, Kiesewetter F, Hornstein OP. Einseitige Lidschwellung bei Naevus flammeus faciei. Problematiken der Differential-diagnose unilaterater Lidsschwellungen. *Hautartz* 1994; **45:** 792–8.
2. Mishima K, Sugahara T, Mori Y, Sakuda M. Three cases of oblique facial cleft. *Journal of Crano-maxillo-facial Surgery* 1996; **24:** 372–7.
3. Hollo G. Bilateral intraocular pressure elevation and decrease of facility of aqueous humour outflow as a consequence of regional lymphedema of head and neck. *Acta Ophthalmologica* 1993; **71:** 415–18.
4. Greene RM, Rogers RS III. Melkersson–Rosenthal syndrome: a review of patients. *Journal of the American Academy of Dermatology* 1989; **21:** 1263–70.
5. Zimmer WM, Rogers RS III, Reeve CM, *et al.* Orofacial manifestations of Melkersson–Rosenthal syndrome: a study of 42 patients and review of 220 cases from the literature. *Oral Surgery, Oral Medicine, Oral Pathology* 1992; **74:** 610–19.
6. Nozicka Z. Endovasal granulomatous lymphangitis as a pathogenetic factor in cheilitis granulomatosa. *Journal of Oral Pathology* 1985; **14:** 363–5.
7. Wisenfield D, Ferguson MM, Mitchell DN, *et al.* Orofacial granulomatosis: a clinical and pathological analysis. *Quarterly Journal of Medicine* 1985; **54:** 101–13.
8. Rogers RS III. Granulomatous cheilitis, Melkersson–Rosenthal syndrome, and orofacial granulomatosis. *Archives of Dermatology* 2000; **136:** 1557–8.
9. Neuhofer J, Fritsch P. Cheilitis granulomatosa: therapy with clofazimine. *Hautartz* 1984; **35:** 459–63.
10. Shehade SA, Foulds JS. Granulomatous cheilitis and a positive Kweim test. *British Journal of Dermatology* 1986; **115:** 619–22.
11. Manzoon S, Azadeh B. Elephantiasis of the external ear: a rare manifestation of pediculosis capitis. *Acta Dermatologica et Venereologica* 1983; **63:** 363–5.
12. Bossuyt L, Van Den Oord JJ, Degreef H. Lymphangioma-like variant of AIDS-associated Kaposi's sarcoma with pronounced oedema formation. *Dermatology* 1995; **190:** 324–6.

15

Management of filariasis and its lymphatic complications

TERENCE RYAN

Lymphatic filariasis is the term given to the most common cause of lymphoedema worldwide.[1] It is a disease that has mostly been the concern of experts in tropical medicine and insufficiently attracted the interest of experts on the lymphatic system. The 'lymphologist' is often an anatomist or physiologist interested in the normal function of the lymphatics, or a practitioner earning a living from the management of lymphoedema, which in general means dealing with the problems of Western medicine such as the consequences of cancer and its treatment. But there are important questions that arise from the study of lymphatic filariasis that should be of interest to lymphologists, and the management of the morbidity consequent on filarial infection should reflect recent advances in medical knowledge – especially those concerned with the management of lymphoedema.

FILARIASIS

Parasitology

Filariasis is an invasion of man by *Wuchereria bancrofti*, *Brugia malayi* or *Brugia timori*, two of the species of the nematode (round worm) family called the Filariide. Their life cycle is divided between man – the vector – and five different genera of mosquito (in different areas of the world) – the intermediate host.[2] *Wuchereria bancrofti* does not have an alternative animal vector, whereas *Brugia malayi* and *Brugia timori* are believed to infect some other animals.

In man, the worms live in the lymph glands and lymph vessels. The male worm is 30–40 mm long, the female worm 75–100 mm long. The worms (the macrofilariae) produce many embryos (larvae or microfilariae), which, for reasons unknown, are released into the bloodstream at night, a time that coincides with the biting habits of the mosquito. There are three larval forms, the third-stage larva being the one injected back into man when the mosquito bites through the skin and sucks up human blood. The term 'filariae' refers to both the macrofilariae, the adult worms that do not live in the blood, and the microfilariae, which live and circulate in the blood.

Geographical pathology

There are two common diseases caused by the filariides: one is onchocerciasis, which produces an itching skin and blindness, and the other is lymphatic filariasis. Onchocerciasis occurs mainly in rural villages and is associated with rivers because the life cycle of the filariae while they are in the mosquito requires warmth and the mosquito needs water. Lymphatic filariasis is increasingly seen in urban and peri-urban areas and is less tightly distributed along rivers.

The prevalence of both these diseases is increasing because urbanization has led to the introduction of new sources of water and reduced the distance the mosquitoes have to fly to find a human to bite, pick up the microfilariae and become carriers. It is estimated that some 120 million people are affected by lymphatic filariasis in at least 73 countries throughout the tropics and subtropics (Fig. 15.1),[3] but *1.1 thousand million people* (20 per cent of the world's population) are at risk by living in regions where infection is a possibility (Box 15.1).

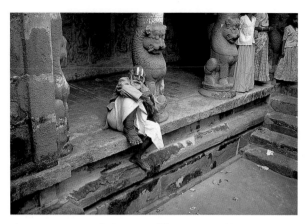

Figure 15.1 *One of the 120 million people afflicted by filariasis. Sitting on the temple steps this Holy Man shows all the classical features of elephantiasis and filarial lymphoedema in his right leg. He ignores it; it has never been treated in any way. The Global Alliance for the Elimination of Lymphatic Filariasis intends to abolish this problem.*

Wuchereria bancrofti, with its worldwide distribution, affects 107 million humans; *Brugia malayi* and *Brugia timori* affect some 13 million persons in Asia. Filarial lymphoedema and elephantiasis (the term used to describe the skin changes that arise from lymphatic failure) occur in approximately 44 million of the world's population and are the world's second largest cause of permanent disability after blindness.

Clinical presentation

Only a small proportion of infected individuals exhibit clinical signs, but some have a response to the microfilariae that is known as tropical eosinophilia, and there is also a response to the antigen produced by the microfilariae that can cause a form of glomerular nephritis. Asymptomatic disease is as important a reservoir of infection as the symptomatic.

The lymphatic sequelae of an infection with filariasis are caused by the development of large worms in the lymphatic system. When and if, after a number of years, the worms reach a size that impedes the flow of lymph through the larger lymphatic trunks, complications such as lymphoedema of the limbs and external genitalia, hydrocele, breast oedema and chyluria appear (see later). The swollen limbs are susceptible to the same complications that afflict all forms of lymphoedema – recurrent cellulitis and, rarely, malignant change.

Epidemiological assessment

At one time, the detection of active disease depended upon the laborious and unpopular procedure of taking blood from patients in the middle of the night and then, with a

Box 15.1 *Countries/territories with lymphatic filariasis*

African region

Angola	Kenya
Benin	Liberia
Burkina Faso	Madagascar
Burundi	Malawi
Cameroon	Mali
Cape Verde	Mauritius
Central African Republic	Mozambique
Chad	Niger
Comoros	Nigeria
Congo	Réunion
Democratic Republic of the Congo	Sao Tome and Principe
Equatorial Guinea	Senegal
Ethiopia	Seychelles
Gabon	Sierra Leone
Gambia	Togo
Ghana	Uganda
Guinea	United Republic of Tanzania
Guinea-Bissau	Zambia
Ivory Coast	Zimbabwe

Region of the Americas

Brazil	Haiti
Costa Rica	Suriname
Dominican Republic	Trinidad and Tobago
Guyana	

Eastern Mediterranean region

Egypt	Somalia
Oman	Sudan

South-East Asia region

Bangladesh	Myanmar
India	Nepal
Indonesia	Sri Lanka
Maldives	Thailand

Western Pacific region

American Samoa	Papua New Guinea
China	Philippines
Cook Islands	Republic of Korea
Federated States of Micronesia	Samoa
	Tonga
Fiji	Tuvalu
French Polynesia[a]	Vanuatu
Kiribati	Vietnam
Malaysia	

[a]Windward Islands, Leeward Islands, Tuamotu Archipelago, Austral or Tabuai Islands, Marquesas Islands.

microscope, examining a blood smear for the microfilariae. Today, because all infected persons have antigen in their blood during both the day and the night, the diagnosis can be confirmed with a spot of blood from a single needle prick applied to a card containing antibody to the antigen; it is now therefore a relatively simple process to carry out a population survey. The presence of the antigen indicates current infection. The antigen comes primarily from the adult worm and disappears after destruction of the worm and the microfilariae. Whole populations in whom filarial lymphoedema is endemic can become antigen negative if the worm is eliminated.

Medical treatment of populations

The treatment of filariasis in whole populations has been approached on two fronts: first, by eliminating the filariae by administering effective drugs to the whole population and, second, by morbidity control (discussed in the following sections), teaching individuals how best to look after their large swollen limbs.

For over 50 years, diethylcarbamazine has been used to treat lymphatic filariasis. It is cheap and can be added to salt for daily intake. At the end of the twentieth century, two more effective drugs, ivermectin and albendazole, not only became available, but were also donated by their manufacturers. As a consequence, the World Health Organization organized a Global Alliance for the Elimination of Lymphatic Filariasis,[4,5] which began the massive exercise of sampling whole populations to detect active disease and then delivering two drugs to those populations once a year for 4 years. The Merck Foundation has given two drugs, the original diethylcarbamazine and ivermectin (which has been especially effective in the control of onchocerciasis) to countries and governmental organizations, and SmithKline Beecham has recently given albendazole to the Global Alliance.

The extraordinary potential effectiveness of the elimination programme is based on the fact that it is now realized that *a single intake of two drugs in combination, once a year for 2 years*, usually in the form of a pill, can lead to the public health control of the disease. Experience in India with the use of dimethylcarbamazine over many decades has shown that a 12 day course, or addition of the drug to table salt for 6–12 months, controls the disease by killing the worm that is the source of the microfilaria. This breaks the life cycle by preventing transmission to the mosquito.

In practice, the choice of which of the two drugs to use is determined by their side-effects, which depend upon whether onchocerciasis or lymphatic filariasis is being treated. The rapid death of the microfilariae of *Onchocerca volvulus* or Loa Loa produced by diethylcarbamazine can cause an inflammatory reaction (pruritus, rash, lymphadenopathy, arthralgia, headache and hypotension),[6] which can precipitate disastrous consequences such as blindness.[7] The death of the microfilariae of lymphatic filariasis produced by the use of diethylcarbamazine may precipitate a mild general reaction (fever, dizziness, nausea)[8] but may also evoke a local reaction caused by the death of the worms. Consequently, in countries where onchocerciasis is not prevalent, albendazole and ivermectin should be prescribed.

Dosage

For use throughout the world, except in the loiasis or onchocerciasis zones of sub-Saharan Africa, either of the following two regimens can be used:[1,4]

1 A once-a-year 'single-dose' treatment for 4–6 years with either:
   a) two drugs (optimal): ivermectin (200 μg/kg body weight) together with either diethylcarbamazine (6 mg/kg) or albendazole (400 mg) or
   b) one drug: diethylcarbamazine (6 mg/kg) alone.
   In addition, diethylcarbamazine-fortified salt (0.2–0.4 per cent w/w) should be substituted for regular table/cooking salt for 6–12 months.

2 For the endemic zones of sub-Saharan Africa where onchocerciasis or loiasis may co-exist with bancroftian filariasis (and where it is therefore unsafe to use diethylcarbamazine), the recommended treatment is a once-a-year, single-dose administration for 4–6 years of either:
   a) two drugs (optimal): ivermectin (200 μg/kg) plus albendazole (400 mg) or
   b) one drug: ivermectin (400 μg/kg) alone.
   A 2 week course of the same drugs is used for the treatment of individuals who present with filarial lymphatic problems.

LYMPHATIC COMPLICATIONS OF FILARIASIS

Whereas everyone who has lymphatic filariasis has been bitten by a mosquito, most probably in their childhood, it often takes years before the infection manifests itself as a swollen limb because it takes a number of years for the worms to grow to a size sufficient to obstruct the flow of lymph through the lymphatics. It is sometimes possible to see the worms moving around in the lymphatics during lymphography[9] and with ultrasound. The 'filarial dance sign' was first seen in the ferret model by Case et al.[10,11] The most common sites for worm growth are the main collecting lymphatics that lead up to the lymph nodes of the groin. Worms may also be found in the lymphatics of the genitalia, particularly the scrotum, and more rarely in the collecting lymphatics of the upper limb and breast that drain into the axillary glands.

Large worms impede the flow of lymph, reduce the flow through the draining glands and cause gross dilatation of the upstream lymphatics. These changes do not necessarily lead to a swollen limb. The variations in the clinical effect of worm obstruction has parallels with the variable degree of lymphoedema caused by blockage of the axillary lymph glands by cancer of the breast, the removal of the lymph nodes by surgery or their fibrosis by radiotherapy (*see* Chapter 13). The relationship between worm infestation and limb swelling is unpredictable and often delayed in onset.

The reasons why a prolonged period of time may pass before lymphoedema is manifest are not known. Is it solely a mechanical obstruction related to the size of the worm, or are there other variable reactions in the wall of the lymphatics adjacent to the worms contributing to the obstruction, reactions that may be related to the individual's lymphocyte or immune responsiveness?

Pathology of filarial lymphoedema of the lower limb (*see also* Chapter 4)

Subcutaneous tissues

Persons with lymphatic filariasis are often immobile, their stiffened tissues acting like a plaster cast on joint movement. The lymphatics in normal tissues respond to movement, so that tissue fluid is squeezed and manipulated along elastin fibres into the initial lymphatics, whose valves steer the fluid into the collecting trunks, where distension stimulates a contractile response. When the lymphatic trunks are impaired, as they are in lymphatic filariasis, the large lymphatics are no longer the pathways with the lowest resistance. Lymph has then to be propelled through the tissue planes or through the most distal vessels of a gradually expanding subdermal lymphatic plexus.

When a dye or radioactive material is injected intradermally into normal healthy tissues, it is instantly removed from the site of injection by lymph flow into the main lymphatic trunks – provided there is movement of the tissues. In lymphoedema, however, the dye or radioactive material spreads laterally through the lymphatic plexus and, with much delay, eventually finds itself permeating along tissue planes and into dilated distal lymphatics, which, if the tissues are subjected to movement, conduct it into healthy areas and ultimately into the venous system. In lymphoedema, fibrosis results in an inability of the tissues to expand any further, and the build-up of tissue fluid leads to tissue pressures that in themselves aid the transport of fluid into new low-resistance pathways.

Expansion of the tissues and mechanical distortion of the fibroblasts results in the deposition of collagen, as it replaces the elastin network. Tissue elasticity is replaced by an uneven tissue firmness or brawny oedema rather than pitting. It is a characteristic of lymphoedema that the normal, somewhat homogeneous distribution of tissue components – including an elastin pathway into the lymphatics – is replaced by a heterogeneous and uneven proliferation and local gigantism, which can at times be grotesque. In such tissues, the low-resistance pathways

for the flow of lymph take multiple routes into blind alleys.

Skin

A feature of lymphoedema is that the epithelium may be so changed that it is easily penetrated. The heterogeneity of expansion of the tissues, as mentioned above, and the grotesque unevenness of proliferation of the tissue components, leads to deep crevices and very variable surface barrier function. The epithelium may, in some parts, be atrophic, but it is more often hypertrophic and turning over quickly, with an inadequate ability to create a barrier to irritants and bacteria. The tissues, having lost their elasticity and pliability, crack very easily, and the surface may become infected by organisms such as *Candida* and other fungal infections – all of which break up the surface of the epidermis.

Experimental studies, as well as clinical studies, have shown that all elements of the skin other than elastin tend to increase when it expands, and, as a consequence of the accumulation of cytokines and growth factors, there are more blood vessels and more lymphatics. In particular, there is more collagen and fibroblasts. Even fat cells increase in number. The increased contribution of the epithelium as a rich factory of cytokines, many of which act on receptors in the vascular endothelium and are part of the process whereby injury is followed by an inflammatory response and repair, may contribute to the onset of the lymphoedema.

Venous system

Disease of the venous system cannot be ignored as a factor in the causation of the oedema in patients affected by endemic lymphatic filariasis. Most children and young adults have a healthy and effective venous system, but the venous system may fail in adult life as a result of gravity, injury and inflammation, especially in the immobile. Any resulting rise in capillary filtration (transudation or exudation) increases the load on the lymphatics.

In poor countries, venous insufficiency, injury and inflammation are common and frequently not treated. When they occur in the presence of a lymphatic system containing enlarging, obstructing filarial worms, the rate of appearance and the severity of the filarial lymphoedema are certain to be exacerbated. The excess interstitial fluid and inflammation exacerbate the expansion and thickening of the subcutaneous tissues and the skin, as well as all the changes described above.

Recurrent inflammatory episodes/acute cellulitis

A characteristic feature of lymphoedema is the development of recurrent inflammatory episodes in the subcutaneous tissues (*see* Chapter 6).[12] The skin of the leg, especially pretibially, suddenly becomes red, hot, more swollen and tender. Fever may be of rapid onset with rigors. Such episodes may occur almost weekly. The cause of these episodes is a significant and usually permanent abnormality of the regional lymphatic drainage.[13] The frequency and effect of these attacks has perhaps been best illustrated in the literature on lymphatic filariasis, probably because the environments in which lymphatic filariasis is found and the opportunities for insect bites, trauma, irritants and many forms of infection to penetrate the skin are that much greater. In the Western world, however, the greatly increased incidence of postmastectomy lymphoedema has drawn attention to similar inflammatory episodes.

It was at one time thought that the inflammatory episodes were caused by the filariasis itself, and certainly the death of the worm can in itself lead to an inflammatory episode of 'filarial fever', but it is now clear that most inflammatory episodes are of bacterial, usually streptococcal, origin. The success of treating the inflammatory episodes with antibiotics led to the assumption that all inflammatory episodes were caused by bacteria.[14] In recent years, however, lymphoedema therapists have observed that such attacks can be precipitated merely by the process of massage. This observation plus an understanding of the inflammatory process and of what is happening when there is lymphatic failure, has led to belief that an accumulation in the tissues of the cytokines and immune proteins[15] that are normally taken away by the lymphatics can precipitate an inflammatory episode if they are abruptly and artificially dispersed from one part of the tissues, which has adapted to them, to another part that has not yet done so.

Consequently, even in the field of lymphatic filariasis, there is no longer a rush to treat inflammatory episodes with antibiotics. A preliminary study in which the effect on the inflammatory episodes of antibiotics was compared with doing nothing other than local cleansing of the damaged skin surface[16] has shown that many patients do quite well without the immediate prescription of antibiotics. This has led to a rethinking of management. Attention is gradually moving to a consideration of the health of the epithelium itself and has returned to the older concept of 'barrier function'.

Recurrent inflammatory episodes may therefore sometimes be a consequence of the ease with which bacteria, irritants and the products of the epithelium pass into the tissues and, instead of being effectively cleared through the low-resistance lymphatic pathways, remain in pockets of static fluid. In the case of bacteria, particularly anaerobes, this is an ideal location. There is an increasing awareness in the field of wound healing that bacteria in the depths of a wound – such as a leg ulcer – are often a mixture of anaerobes and aerobes, and that their effect on healing, or on the chronicity of non-healing, is considerable. It has also been realized that a wound surface without the sanctuary for these bacteria of a fibrinous exudate or biofilm, but with healthy granulation tissue or especially an intact epithelium, prevents the penetration of bacteria, and that inflammatory agents can be of many different kinds.

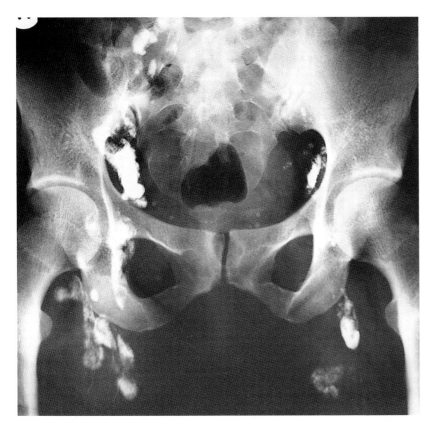

Figure 15.2 *An X-ray lymphograph of a patient with filarial lymphoedema affecting mainly the right leg, showing generalized enlargment of the lymph glands and dilated lymphatics on the right side of the pelvis. The vessels in the upper thigh are not dilated but thin and irregular, and showing signs of secondary obliteration (die-back). Three months after treatment of the filariasis with diethylcarbamazine, much of the oedema had regressed and was easily controlled with elastic stockings.*

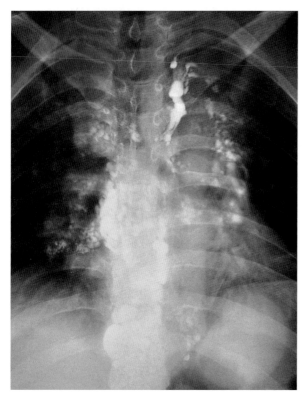

Figure 15.3 *Filarial obstruction at the top of the thoracic duct. The duct and all the mediastinal lymphatics are dilated, tortuous and incompetent, but there is no reflux into the lung substance. In spite of these gross abnormalities, the patient did not have chyluria or a protein-losing enteropathy, which suggests that the lymphatics of the bowel and kidney were unaffected and competent.*

Bacteria are clearly the most important, but irritants of one kind or another – some from the soil – may also feature, as may cytokines released from a damaged epithelium.

Lymphatic valvular incompetence

When the lymphatics below an obstruction caused by adult worms dilate, their valves become incompetent, and lymph may then reflux back into the peripheral lymphatics (Fig. 15.2). In the pelvis, genitalia and lower limbs, reflux is manifest by the appearance of vesicles on the skin, which frequently rupture and leak copious amounts of lymph. When the obstruction is above the point at which the lacteals enter the pre-aortic lymphatics, chyle will leak into and from the vesicles. The thoracic duct is a common place for a filarial obstruction (Fig. 15.3). Chyluria is the most common chylous reflux syndrome to complicate filariasis, but chylous ascites and chylothorax may occur. These conditions are discussed in detail in Chapters 12 and 16.

Investigation

No investigations other than a blood antigen test to confirm that the patient has active filariasis are usually needed when a teenager or adult living in an area in which filariasis is endemic presents with a swollen leg, scrotum or breast, or chyluria. Even when the test is negative, the filariasis having been treated with antifilarial drugs, it is still most likely that the patient has a filarial lymphoedema.

Other secondary causes of lymphoedema (other than filariasis) can usually be detected from the history and general physical examination. Complex investigations, which in a poor country are often not available, are rarely needed. When the oedema is bilateral, other general causes of oedema should be excluded by clinical examination and basic haematological and biochemical tests. The chances of the swelling being caused by a primary lymphatic abnormality are extremely small but this should be suspected if the swelling presents at or soon after birth.

The investigations described in Chapter 6 may, when available, be helpful if the pharmacological treatment of the filariasis followed by conservative care of the limb fails. Lymphangiography is necessary if complex surgical procedures such as lymphovenous anastomoses are being considered (*see* Chapters 12 and 16) but is not necessary before performing a reducing operation or other anti-reflux procedures. In the latter case, the abnormal lymphatics that have to be ligated can be easily visualized during the operation by the subcutaneous injection of Patent Blue Violet.

Treatment

After the treatment of the infection itself and the accompanying control of the further transmission of filariasis by the use of drugs (see above), treatment should be directed towards morbidity control and reduction of the swelling. The most important principle is that the treatment should be of low cost and self-administered. Fortunately, many of the manoeuvres that help to control lymphoedema – movement, elevation and skin hygiene – cost nothing. It is always advisable to wait for a few months before embarking upon anything more than the simple no-cost measures outlined below because mild oedema may resolve completely once the drugs kill the worms.

Skin hygiene

The emphasis is on barrier function. It does not make good sense in the developing world to think that one can make the skin free of bacteria and irritants, but the barrier function of the epithelium can be improved. This is why emollients have to be added to the system of washing.

The effect on the epidermis of various constituents of soaps, the various benefits of cold versus hot water and the degree of vigour used in manipulating the surface of the skin while washing are all debatable, but if the end-point is the health of the epidermal cell, gentle washing with emollients and the removal of excess debris and sanctuary sites for bacteria (e.g. using biofilm), are what is required.

The case for using water at body temperature, or just above, as opposed to cold water relates to the fact that washing and evaporation (which often accompanies wetting) leads to cooling of the tissues, and this has a mixed effect.[17] It may have a variable effect on blood flow, especially when the flow is already sluggish – as in the post-capillary circulation of the adipose tissue – and where there is an increased exudation from the venous system, which also increases the viscosity of the blood. Cooling may also reduce the myotonic response to filling of the lymphatics and have an effect on the easy flow of protein through the tissues and the solidity of the fat globules in the adipose tissue. Cold adipose tissue is very difficult to empty of excess fluid. Manual lymphatic drainage may be more effective in tissues that are pliable, and pliability is helped by warmth. Finally, collagenases need to be activated to help to disperse the excessive fibrosis. Most collagenases are inhibited by being cooled.

Studies of wound healing suggest that the exposure of a leg ulcer during a re-dressing can cause prolonged cooling of the tissues, which can lead to a failure of cell function for many hours. In the field of lymphatic filariasis, limbs are currently usually washed with cold water, but studies are needed to see whether this is appropriate. In the developed world, warming is being increasingly advocated as a potentiator of the effects of vibration or massage.[18] In the management of lymphoedema, simple processes such as washing and removing the daily accumulation of bacteria and irritants from the surface of the skin may reduce the quantity of inflammatory agents penetrating the skin and activating inflammation in the depths of the tissues.

Movement

Movement has three important effects.[17] First, the movement of the peripheral tissues is the means by which fluid and macromolecules are moved into the lymphatics.

Second, the passage of fluid into the lymphatics encouraged by movement stimulates a myotonic response (rhythmical contractions) in the collecting lymphatics, which promotes emptying and forward flow through the lymphatics of the abdomen, thorax and thoracic duct into the venous system. When these central lymphatics are not being emptied, flow from the periphery is impaired.

The third aspect of movement to be considered is breathing. Deep breathing helps to empty the major lymph trunks of the abdomen and thorax into the venous system.[19,20] It is a natural process seen in the yawn of the wakening animal and is a process used for health promotion by many Asian systems of medicine.[21] It has somehow escaped the interest of Western medicine and has not yet been taken up as a valuable manoeuvre in the field of lymphatic filariasis. Breathing lowers venous pressure, enhances the abdomen-to-thorax pressure gradient and stimulates lymphatic wall contraction, all of which enhance emptying of the thoracic duct.

It is especially the immobile patients with dependent, swollen limbs who are likely to have a sluggish lymphatic system in their thorax and abdomen. It has been well demonstrated that attempting to move lymph out of the lower limb without attention to the lymphatic system in the abdomen and thorax may just divert lymph into the genital region.[22] Since the latter is often involved in lymphatic filariasis, attention to a system that might encourage the drainage of the scrotum through the lymphatics of the abdomen deserves more investigation. Most practitioners of manual lymphatic drainage employ breathing exercises at the beginning of treatment. The system they use is identical to the health-promotion effects of breathing postulated by the Asian systems, i.e. inspiring to a count of 5, holding the breath to a count of 5 and expiring to a count of 10. The slow and full expiration of yoga or Chinese traditional medicine known as dragon breathing has a similar effect, but its possible influence in promoting lymph flow has not been promulgated or investigated.

Correct whole-body positioning should be linked with all therapeutic movement regimens. The abdomen and the thoracic region are perhaps best emptied with the patient lying supine while taking deep breaths, the normal attitude of early rising and yawning, with the hands upon the abdomen or the legs flexed to apply a little pressure to the abdomen. The rising pressure within the abdomen as a result of deep breathing encourages emptying into the venous system through the thoracic duct.

Movement of the periphery is often described as 'exercise' and may be interpreted as short periods of vigorous exercise once or twice a day. There is a case for talking about 'movement' rather than 'exercise' and encouraging repetitive, natural movement by telling the patients that they must not allow their tissues to be immobile. Cultural attitudes to exercise determine that promoting 'movement', as opposed to 'exercise', will be more readily accepted by the majority of peoples of the world, of both sexes and all age groups.

Elevation

The whole question of elevation of the limbs should be related not only to the gravitational effects on the lymphatics, but also to the gravitational effects on the veins. An inch of elevation immediately lowers the venous pressure and reduces interstitial fluid production but takes much longer to have an effect on the lymphatics. The main object of elevation, particularly when the lymphatics are of a normal size or partially obliterated, is to reduce the lymph load rather than influence lymphatic drainage. The dilated lymphatics often present in obstructive filarial lymphoedema have, however, been shown, with lymphangiography, to empty quite rapidly when the limb is elevated (S. Jamal, pers. comm.).

Hosiery and elastic bandages, the mainstay of treatment in developed countries, are expensive and often unavailable in the developing world. One should not, however, neglect the fact that there may in any geographical area be a large middle class able to afford hosiery and bandaging. Movement within hosiery and bandaging is more effective in clearing the lymphatics than movement alone, provided the compression is properly applied. The natural, endogenous and to some extent exaggerated 'hose' created by the excessive collagen tissue or fibrosis that characterizes lymphoedema is in fact equivalent to an external stocking. When it comes to examining the effects of movement and the resistance of the tissues provided by hosiery, the containment that is a consequence of fibrosis should not be underestimated; it is, however, very uneven, hosiery providing a more even and higher level of support.

Manual lymphatic drainage

The object of manual lymphatic drainage (*see* Chapter 9) is to promote the movement of lymph within the tissues and assist in the development and diversion of lymph flow through any existing low-resistance pathways into healthy tissues that have an efficient lymphatic system.[23,24]

de Godoy and de Godoy,[25] in Brazil, have shown that manual lymphatic drainage can be simplified so that patients themselves can assist lymph drainage through the skin. The clinician marks the desired direction of flow with a marking pen and provides the patient with a soft roller to move over the skin in the desired direction. Giving patients something they can do for themselves helps to boost their morale and encourages them to take greater care of their limb.

Reducing operations

The reducing operations described in Chapter 10 are used more often in areas in which filarial lymphoedema is endemic than in areas where most of the lymphoedema occurs secondary to medical therapies or is primary in origin. Lymphoedema in endemic areas is often gross, and the skin severely damaged, because the simple conservative measures described above have not been used. When swelling is extreme and the skin unhealthy, Charles's operation is the best option. Dandapats *et al.*[26] have reported results for the Charles's operation in patients with filarial lymphoedema similar to those described in Chapter 11. Sadly, the medical, surgical and anaesthetic expertise required for the successful performance of these operations is often not available to the majority of patients in the poorer developing countries.

Lymphovenous anastomosis

This highly specialized technique is described in Chapter 10. The chance of an anastomosis between a normally sized lymphatic and a vein staying patent in the long term is small, but the lymphatics upstream to a localized worm obstruction in patients with filariasis are usually dilated. Anastomoses between veins and dilated lymphatics or lymph glands that have an increased flow of refluxing lymph passing through them are much more

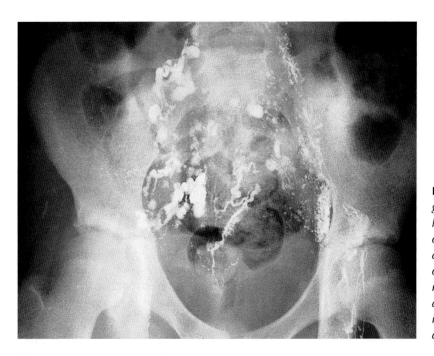

Figure 15.4 *A lymphograph of the grossly dilated retroperitoneal lymphatics of a patient with a filarial obstruction in the thoracic duct and chyluria. The anastomosis of vessels of this size carrying a large flow of refluxing lymph and chyle to an adjacent vein in the groin or abdomen is likely to stay patent and stop the chyluria.*

likely to stay patent and have been shown to provide considerable symptomatic relief,[26] especially when used to treat chyluria (Fig. 15.4) (*see* Chapters 12 and 16).

Microvascular surgery requires considerable surgical expertise and special equipment that is rarely available in developing countries. Whereas limb swelling can be helped with conservative measures and simple reducing operations, conditions such as chyluria, chylous ascites and chylothorax cannot. Even complex special diets do not cure these conditions so until advanced surgical techniques become available in the poorer developing countries, patients with these serious complications of filariasis will suffer and in some cases die.

COMMENT

Lymphatic filariasis is a disease of poverty and the world's second greatest cause of permanent disability. Its management must be of low cost, and indeed the anti-filarial drugs are available free. Systems of no-cost self-help, i.e. skin hygiene, and the avoidance of limb dependency and immobility (which are helpful for many other disease processes also affecting the poor) must be encouraged.[27,28]

Hosiery, support bandaging, antibiotics and surgery are inevitably expensive and consequently second-line therapies. Although they are often first-line therapies in the developed world and have an important role in management, more studies of the self-help measures proposed for affected disadvantaged communities need to be carried out to ascertain just how effective such therapies really are in those who fully comply with the guidelines.

REFERENCES

1. Nutman TB. *Lymphatic filariasis*. London: Imperial College Press, 2000.
2. Leading article. The lymphatic filariases. *Lancet* 1985; **1:** 1135–6.
3. World Health Organization. *Building partnerships for lymphatic filariasis. Strategic Plan September 1999*. Geneva: World Health Organization, 1999.
4. Ottesen EA, Duke BOL, Karam M, *et al.* Strategies and tools for the control/elimination of lymphatic filariasis. *Bulletin of the World Health Organization* 1997; **75:** 491–503.
5. Ottesen EA. Editorial: The global programme for the elimination of lymphatic filariasis. *Tropical Medicine and International Health* 2000; **5:** 591–4.
6. Francis H, Awadzi K, Ottensen EA. The Mazzotti reaction following treatment of onchocerciasis with diethylcarbamazine: clinical severity as a function of infection intensity. *American Journal of Medical Hygiene* 1985; **34:** 529–36.
7. Bird AC, El-Sheih H, Anderson J, Fuglsang H. Changes in visual function and in the posterior segment of the eye during treatment of onchocerciasis with diethylcarbamazine. *British Journal of Ophthalmology* 1980; **64:** 191–200.
8. Ottesen EA. Mechanism and control of reactions to treatment in human filariasis. In: Evered D, Clark S eds. *Filariasis*. Ciba Foundation Symposium No. 127. Chichester: John Wiley & Sons, 1987: 265–79.
9. Young AE, Kinmonth JB. Filariasis. *Proceedings of the Royal Society of Medicine* 1976; **69:** 708–9.
10. Case T, Leis B, Witte M, *et al.* Vascular abnormalities in experimental and human lymphatic filariasis. *Lymphology* 1991; **24:** 174–83.
11. Witte M, McNeill G, Crandall C, *et al.* Whole body lymphangioscintigraphy in ferrets chronically infected with *Brugia malayi. Lymphology* 1988; **21:** 251–7.
12. Dreyer G, Medeiros Z, Netto MJ, Leal NC, de Castro LG, Piessens WF. Acute attacks in the extremities of persons living in an area endemic for bancroftian filariasis: differentiation of two syndromes. *Transactions of the Royal Society of Tropical Medicine and Hygiene* 1999; **93:** 413–17.
13. de Godoy JM, Godoy MdeF, Valente A, *et al.* Lymphoscintigraphic evaluation in patients after erysipelas. *Lymphology* 2000; **33(4):** 144–89.
14. Olszewski WL, Jamal S, Manokaran G, *et al.* Bacteriological studies of skin, tissue fluid, lymph and lymph nodes in patients with filarial lymphoedema. *American Journal of Tropical Medicine and Hygiene* 1997; **57:** 7–15.
15. Olszewski WL, Jamal S, Lukomska B, *et al.* Immune proteins in peripheral tissue fluid-lymph in patients with filarial lymphoedema of the lower limbs. *Lymphology* 1992; **25:** 166–71.
16. Shenoy RK, Suma TK, Rajan K, Kumaraswami V. Prevention of acute adeno-lymphangitis in brugian filariasis: comparison of the efficacy of ivermectin and diethylcarbamazine, each combined with local treatment of the affected limb. *Annals of Tropical Medicine and Parasitology* 1998; **92:** 587–94.
17. Ryan TJ. The skin and its response to movement. *Lymphology* 2000; **31:** 128–9.
18. Ohkuma M. The skin blood flow change after a new lymphoedema therapy by magnetic fields, vibration and heat. *European Journal of Lymphology* 2001; **9:** 83.
19. Browse NL, Lord RSA, Taylor A. Pressure waves and gradients in the canine thoracic duct. *Journal of Physiology* 1971; **213:** 507–24.
20. Browse NL, Rutt DR, Sizeland D, Taylor A. The velocity of lymph flow in the canine thoracic duct. *Journal of Physiology* 1974; **237:** 401–13.
21. Majumdar A. *Ayurveda: the ancient Indian science of healing*. New Delhi: Wheeler Publishing, 1998.
22. Boris M, Weindorf S, Lasinski BB. The risk of genital edema after external pump compression

for lower limb lymphedema. *Lymphology* 1998; **31:** 15–20.

23. Casley-Smith JR, Casley-Smith JR. *Modern treatment for lymphedema*, 5th edn. Adelaide: Lymphoedema Association of Australia, 1997.

24. Twycross R, Jenns K, Todd J. *Lymphoedema*. Oxford: Radcliffe Medical Press, 2000.

25. de Godoy JM, Batigalia F, Godoy MdeF. Preliminary evaluation of a new, more simplified physiotherapy technique for lymphatic drainage. *Lymphology* 2002; **35**: 91–3.

26. Dandapat MC, Mukherjee LM, Patra SK. Evaluation of different surgical procedures in filarial lymphoedema of lower extremity. *Journal of the Indian Medical Association* 1991; **89:** 127–9.

27. Vaqas B, Ryan TJ. Lymphoedema. Pathophysiology and management in resource poor settings – relevant for lymphatic filariasis control programmes (in preparation).

28. Vaqas B, Ryan TJ. An update on the low cost management of lymphedema in the developing world (in preparation).

16

Management of lymph and chyle reflux

Moellenbroch described the presence of chyle in the urine in 1670.[1] The first description of a patient with chylous ascites, which followed a series of kicks and blows to the abdomen, is probably that found in Ionnes De Diemerbroeck's book, published in 1685 and entitled *Opera omnia anatomica et medica*.[2] In 1689, Morton[3] described a patient with chylothorax caused by a rupture of the thoracic duct below an obstructing mass of lymph glands, and in 1740 Hoffman[4] described a case of chylothorax caused by a stab wound that injured the thoracic duct. Thereafter, the early medical literature abounds with descriptions of every variety of lymph and chyle reflux, all summarized in 1931 by Frankenthal.[5]

Whether the refluxing fluid is lymph, chyle or a mixture of both depends solely on the anatomical position of the incompetent lymphatics and the site and degree of any obstruction to normal lymph flow. Dilated incompetent iliac, inguinal and thigh lymphatics may allow lymph to reflux down into the lower limb, but chyle will only appear if the lymphatic incompetence extends up to the level at which the lacteals join the pre-aortic lymphatics and cisterna chyli. Even then, most of the lymph and chyle will flow up through the thoracic duct unless there is an obstruction to flow. Large, distorted, incompetent megalymphatics do not in themselves always present a physiological resistance to onward flow. Reflux through incompetent valves depends on the resistance of the lymphatics to forward flow, the efficiency of the forward propulsive mechanism in the absence of valves, the quantity of lymph flow and the intralymphatic pressure at the height of the refluxing phase. None of these physiological factors has been measured in man so our current forms of treatment have to be based on an anatomical, rather than physiological, demonstration of the abnormality and a belief that the only effective method of preventing

reflux is ligation of the incompetent vessels or lymphovenous shunting at the bottom of the refluxing segment.

All the lymph/chyle reflux syndromes can be subdivided into two categories: primary and secondary (congenital and acquired). As always, the secondary acquired varieties vastly outnumber the primary congenital ones.

Secondary (acquired) reflux is almost always caused by thoracic duct obstruction, usually by filariasis, malignant disease or iatrogenic injuries received during cardiac or oesophageal surgery.

The two *primary (congenital) abnormalities* that cause reflux are similar to those which cause primary lymphoedema of the lower limb (*see* Chapter 7) – congenital incompetent megalymphatics and congenital hypo- or aplasia. When, in 1964, Kinmonth and Taylor[6] described the lymphographic appearances of these two primary (congenital) abnormalities in 19 patients with chylous reflux, they called them syndrome 1 and syndrome 2, but we find it simpler to use the descriptive terms of congenital incompetent megalymphatics and congenital hypo- or aplasia.

It is easy to understand how congenitally incompetent lymphatics throughout the limbs, abdomen and chest permit reflux and produce all the reflux syndromes, but it is less easy to explain how congenital hypoplasia or aplasia has its effect. There is no doubt that it is not possible to find lymphatics in the limbs of some patients with chylous reflux – 5 out of 19 in Kinmonth's series – but there are usually dilated lymphatics somewhere in the upper abdomen, mesentery or chest, and one must assume that these are vessels that have become dilated and incompetent upstream to proximal congenital hypo- or aplasia in the upper abdomen or thoracic duct, or that hypoplasia can co-exist with megaplasia. In our experience, expanded by more extensive lymphangiography and the modern techniques of lymphoscintgraphy, computed tomography (CT) and nuclear magnetic resonance scanning, a generalized hypoplasia of the major upper intra-abdominal and thoracic lymphatics is very rare.

A warning here about the colour of chyle. The word *chylus* means juice. The whiteness of chyle, which is the juice absorbed from the small intestine via the lacteals, comes from the presence of fat absorbed from the lumen of the small intestine, in its natural form, as chylomicrons (Fig. 16.1 and *see* Fig. 12.5). It is very important to remember that the fluid in the lacteals is only white when the diet contains free fat: patients on a low or non-fat diet have clear fluid in their lacteals. This situation commonly occurs in neonates and very young children before they are weaned, and in adults who have been starved for 12 hours before an abdominal operation. In these circumstances, other criteria, such as the triglyceride concentration and lymphocyte count, must be used to confirm that fluid aspirated from the abdominal or pleural cavity has come from the lacteals. Alternatively, the patient should be given food rich in fat, such as milk, 2 or 3 hours before collecting a sample of the effusion. Peritoneal and pleural effusions may also be made turbid and white by the presence of cellular debris and bacteria, an appearance often called pseudo-chylous and commonly associated with diffuse intra-abdominal or thoracic malignancies. This type of effusion does not contain free fat.

Whatever the lymphatic abnormality, primary or secondary, lymph and chyle escape from the dilated lymphatics by two routes: through a defect in a vessel wall (a lymph fistula) or by transudation through intact vessel walls (*see* Chapter 10). This chapter presents our views of the management of each of the lymph/chyle reflux syndromes based on the information provided by lymphograms and our clinical experience. Chyle may reflux into the lower limbs, genitalia, peritoneal cavity, intestine, urinary and genital tracts, pleural cavity and other potential spaces, such as synovial joints and pericardium. Each is described in the following sections.

Chylous reflux syndromes are rare, misdiagnosed and often inadequately treated. They require careful investigation and management, a full understanding by patients of their problem, meticulous surgical technique, sometimes repeated operations and a lifetime of follow-up.

LYMPH/CHYLE REFLUX INTO THE LOWER LIMBS

Lymph and/or chyle may appear in and leak from vesicles on any part of the lower limb, from the groin to the toes (Fig. 16.2).[7] Chyle is usually but not necessarily white (see above), opalescent and sticky; lymph is clear and watery. The leakage is sometimes intermittent and from different sites, sometimes continuous, copious and from a single site.

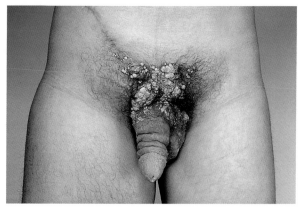

(a)

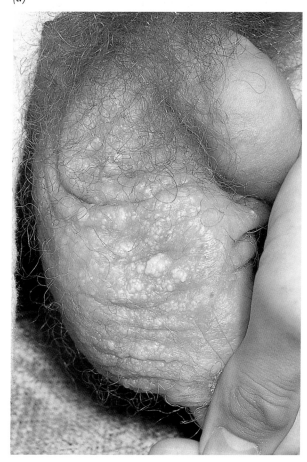

(b)

Figure 16.1 *The colour of chyle. (a) Lymphatic vesicles on the mons veneris and external genitalia filled with thick, white, inspissated chyle. The colour is diagnostic of chyle.
(b) Lymphatic vesicles on the scrotum, some filled with a pale, pearly opalescent fluid, others with dear fluid, whose colour varied with the patient's fat ingestion. It is important to remember that chyle is only white when it contains free fat.*

Clinical presentation

The lymph/chyle leak associated with a primary lymphatic abnormality usually comes from vesicles that appear

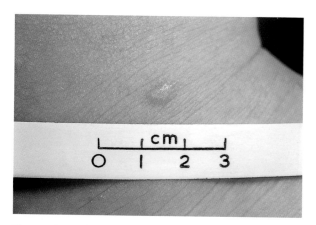

Figure 16.2 *A lymphatic vesicle on the ankle of a young man. This vesicle and others between his toes intermittently leaked copious amounts of lymph. The limb was moderately swollen. The lymphatics throughout the limb were dilated and incompetent.*

on the lymphoedematous limb of a child or adolescent and, rarely, in an adult. Vesicles rarely appear before the lymphoedema. The oedema and the leakage are usually unilateral. Both sexes are equally affected. Although the causative lymphatic abnormality – megalymphatics – is congenital, this is not an inherited condition so there is no family history. Many patients have very pale pink, single or multiple cutaneous angiomata on the affected limb, called by Kinmonth a 'vin rosé' or 'megalymph' patch.[7] Attacks of acute cellulitis in the affected limb are not uncommon.

In addition to lymph/chyle reflux into the lower limb, the patient may have leaking vesicles on the perineum and external genitalia, and other reflux syndromes such as chylous ascites or intestinal reflux with protein-losing enteropathy. If the lymphatic incompetence does not extend up to the level of the cisterna chyli, the leakage will be pure lymph.

The symptoms and signs of reflux steadily worsen as the years pass. There is sometimes a sudden exacerbation of the leakage caused by further vessel dilatation and subsequent valvular incompetence, occasionally being caused by collections of semisolid, inspissated lymph obstructing the duct. Patients with secondary lymph/chyle reflux into a limb have similar symptoms in addition to those attributable to the underlying cause, for example filariasis or neoplastic disease.

Investigation

As there is no condition other than a lymphatic abnormality that produces a small vesicle on the skin of a limb that leaks a clear or milky fluid, the diagnosis is usually obvious, but some of the leaking fluid should nevertheless be collected and examined for chylomicrons and lipid content. The patient's general nutritional state should be assessed. A steady loss of chyle, especially if there is also a chyle leak into the intesine, can cause weight loss and protein and vitamin deficiencies. As secondary reflux is more common than primary reflux, the possible causes should be sought by a full medical investigation.

Lymphoscintigraphy

Although lymphoscintigraphy is a most helpful diagnostic aid when first investigating a swollen limb (*see* Chapter 6),[8] lymphoscintographs do not give sufficient definition of dilated incompetent lymphatics for management decisions.[9]

Lymphangiography

A bipedal lymphangiogram, including if possible a lymphangiogram via a cutaneous vesicle, is an essential investigation (Fig. 16.3).[10,11] Both injections are easy as all the lymphatics in the limb are dilatated and the megalymphatics on the dorsum of the foot, visualized by the interdigital injection of Patent Blue Violet, easy to find even when the foot is very swollen. Patent Blue Violet injected subcutaneously at any site on a limb containing megalymphatics or into a vesicle will rapidly spread into all the adjacent dilated lymphatics (Fig. 16.4).

The standard maximum injection of 7 mL Lipiodol per leg is often insufficient to fill all the lymphatics and may break up within the dilated lymphatics into globules. The injection of more Lipiodol must be avoided because of the dangers of oil embolism, so the Lipiodol must be supplemented with a non-ionic, low osmolar contrast medium, which must be injected quickly through a large needle because these media are water soluble and quickly diffuse out of the lymphatics.

It is usually possible to fill most of the abnormal vessels in the limb, including those which are running towards the leaking vesicles, but it is more important to display the vessels above the leaking area, up through the inguinal, iliac and aortic vessels and to the thoracic duct. The Lipiodol injected into the normal leg often reaches the iliac and aortic regions first and displays these areas much more clearly than that injected into the abnormal leg. The upper abdominal lymphatics must be displayed because chyle can reach the limbs only if the vessels at and below the entry of the mesenteric lymphatics that are carrying the chyle from the intestine into the preaortic lymphatics are incompetent. Without a detailed knowledge of the position and extent of the incompetent vessels above the leaking area, it is impossible to plan an effective operation.

It is not possible to deduce a physiological abnormality from an anatomical appearance. It may be difficult to decide whether the thoracic duct is the site of an obstruction even when there appears to be a complete barrier to the flow of contrast medium. Multiple convoluted channels may resist flow or have a lower than normal resistance to flow.

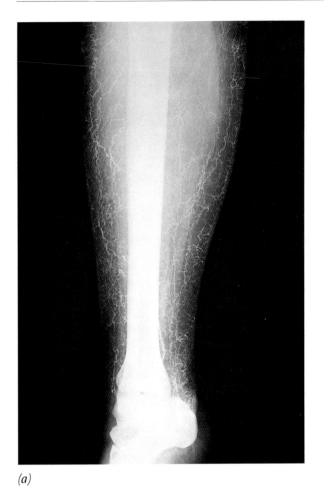

(a)

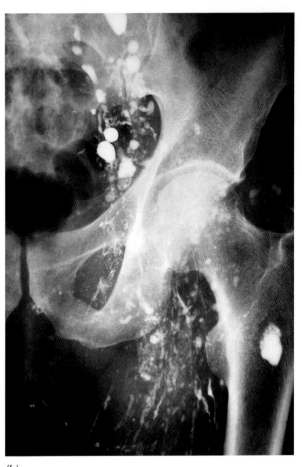

(b)

Figure 16.3 *A typical lymphangiogram of a patient with reflux throughout the left leg. (a) Megalymphatics below the knee. (b) Megalymphatics in the inguinal and iliac regions with a pooling of Lipiodol in large lymphatic lacunae.*

Computed tomography and magnetic resonance imaging

CT and magnetic resonance imaging scans will show dilated lymphatics throughout the subcutaneous tissues (Fig. 16.5) but are seldom helpful when planning management.[12]

Treatment

Any underlying cause, such as lymphoma, should be treated vigorously because a favourable response to treatment may alleviate the reflux. The fat content of the chyle may be reduced by giving the patient a no-fat, medium chain triglyceride supplemented diet, but this seldom reduces the quantity of fluid that refluxes and does not affect the quantity of lymph produced in the leg. Chyle production can be completely stopped by total parenteral nutrition. Lymph production in the leg may be significantly reduced by prolonged bed rest and elevation but only while these treatments are being administered. As they do not cure the patient, they are seldom worth trying except in the preoperative period when any nutritional deficiency is being corrected.

The most effective surgical treatment is ligation and resection of the incompetent vessels through which the reflux is occurring. The ligation stops the reflux, the resection reduces the chance of recurrence through collateral formation. The effectivness of diverting the reflux and reducing the intralymphatic pressure by lymphovenous anastomoses requires further evaluation.

Radical division, ligation and resection of all incompetent lymphatics on the posterior abdominal wall and in the pelvis[6,7,13–15]

The patient should be given two or three pints of milk on the morning of the operation to fill the lymphatics with white chyle, thus making them easier to see (Fig. 16.6a). The operating table should have the facility for obtaining an intraoperative abdominal lymphograph (*see* Chapter 6). Before opening the abdomen, 2 mL Patent Blue Violet should be injected into the subcutaneous tissues of the thigh, the injected area massaged and the limb moved about to encourage the dye to flow up to the iliac and aortic lymphatics (Fig. 16.6b).

The abdomen is then opened through a full-length midline incision or an oblique incision above the

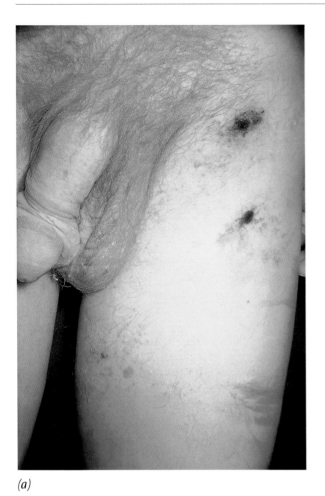 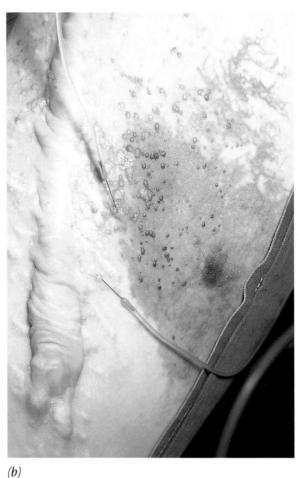

(a)   (b)

Figure 16.4 *(a) Patent Blue Violet injected into the subcutaneous tissue of the thigh has rapidly spread into megalymphatics just beneath the skin of the scrotum. (b) Patent Blue Violet injected directly into a vesicle on the lateral aspect of the thigh filling all the surrounding megalymphatics.*

inguinal ligament on the affected side, depending upon whether the intention is to ligate the lymphatics of the leg and the pelvic organs, perineum and external genitalia or just the lymphatics of the leg. For chylous reflux confined to a limb, we use the oblique extraperitoneal approach and then open the peritoneum to reach the peri-aortic lymphatics. For chylous reflux into a limb and/or into any of the pelvic organs that requires the ligation and excision of lymphatics on both sides of the pelvis, we use the midline intraperitoneal approach (*see* Chapter 12 and below).

If a full midline incision is used, the pre- and peri-aortic vessels are exposed by dividing the retroperitoneum to the left of the small bowel mesentery and peeling it back in either direction to expose the retroperitoneal tissues. When an oblique incision is used, the iliac lymphatics can be exposed and dissected extraperitoneally from the inguinal ligament up to the common iliac artery, but it is then often necessary to open the peritoneum, pack the small bowel away and incise the peritoneum over the common iliac arteries and lower aorta to expose the lymphatics up to the level of the origin of the renal arteries.

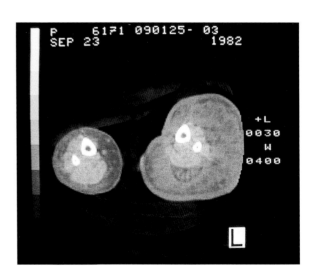

Figure 16.5 *A computed tomography scan of the lower legs of a patient with megalymphatics throughout the left leg. This investigation provides a rapid simple means of diagnosis but is of no value in planning management.*

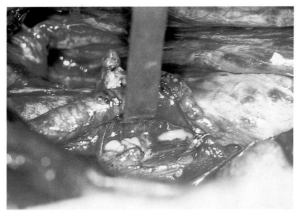

(a)

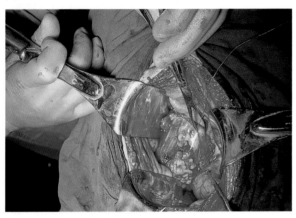

(b)

Figure 16.6 *(a) White, chyle-filled megalymphatics behind the left common iliac artery. This patient drank two pints of milk early on the morning of his operation, the operation being performed through a midline abdominal incision. The peritoneum over the aorta, which has yet to be incised (to the right of the figure), can be seen to be covering masses of white, chyle-filled lymphatics. (b) Megalymphatics around the iliac artery coloured blue by the injection of Patent Blue Violet into the subcutaneous tissues of the thigh. This operation began as an extraperitoneal oblique iliac fossa procedure, but the peritoneum had to be opened to reach the internal iliac lymphatics. The ureter is held up to protect it during the dissection.*

All dissection must be done with great care as the abdominal lymphatics are extremely thin and friable. If a lymphatic is torn or punctured unknowingly and not ligated, it may leak and cause a recurrence of the chylous ascites. This risk is greater at second and third operations when the peritoneum and retroperitoneal tissues are thickened and adherent to nearby tissues.

It is easier to begin by identifying the lymphatics of the pelvis at the level of division of the common iliac arteries and then work upwards. All three chains of lymphatics around the common iliac arteries, on the front of the sacrum, the aorta and vena cava (especially those behind the vessels) and around the ureters must be ligated and

excised. The nervi erigentes should, if possible, be preserved. The clearance of the lymphatics should extend up to the level of the left renal vein.

When all the visible lymphatics have been ligated and excised, a lymphatic adjacent to one or both external iliac arteries should be cannulated and injected with Lipiodol. An intraoperative lymphograph should then be taken to see whether there are any channels passing through or around the area of resection that have not been ligated. If there are any such vessels, the Lipiodol should be replaced with Patent Blue Violet to help visualize the missed vessels because the fact that they have not been ligated implies that they are difficult to see or in an unusual position.

Lymphatic ligation at lower levels

Ligations and excisions just below the groin, or even lower down in the leg, have a very short-lived effect as incompetent collaterals quickly form. These operations should be used only when the patient is not fit enough for a major abdominal procedure.

The overall results of radical ligation and excision are good: reflux is usually stopped for 5 or more years, although some recurrence is inevitable. Surprisingly, ligating all the inguinal and iliac lymphatics rarely makes the swelling of the leg any worse, but the patient should be warned of this possibility. The limb lymph probably returns via competent collateral lymphatics around the trunk. As most patients with reflux already have an oedematous limb, they are rarely worried by the possibility of it getting a little larger.

Lymphovenous anastomosis

Lymphovenous anastomoses have been performed for all varieties of chylous reflux, although the main indication is reflux into the intrapelvic organs[16,17] and kidney secondary to filariasis. Provided there is sufficient flow to keep the anastomoses patent, they may reduce the intralymphatic pressure in the vessels above the anastomoses and thus prevent the progression of dilatation and valvular incompetence down the limb.

Anastomoses between the inguinal lymphatics and the saphenous vein have been reported to cure chylorrhoea and chyluria (see below) but not to effectively reduce reflux into the lower limb. This is not surprising as there will still be reflux from the abdomen into the limb and a high intralymphatic pressure in the vessels not anastomosed to veins. The thoracic duct-to-azygos vein, and pre-aortic lymphatic-to-mesenteric vein, anastomoses that we have performed have not had a worthwhile clinical effect, but we have successfully treated two patients with mild occasional reflux by lymphatic-to-saphenous vein anastomosis.

The few published results suggest that lymphovenous anastomosis is more effective in secondary reflux caused by filariasis than in patients with a primary lymphatic abnormality.

Reducing operations

It is worthwhile adding a reducing operation to the anti-reflux procedure if the lymphoedema accompanying the reflux is severe. This eliminates some of the incompetent vessels as well as reducing the size of the limb, but the anti-reflux operation must be carried out first.

Amputation

We have seen a number of patients who have had progressive amputations for severe reflux, one ending with a disarticulation of the hip. Each time, after removing the leaking segment of the limb, new leaking vesicles have appeared on the amputation stump. One patient had a forefoot, a below-knee and two thigh-level amputations over a 15 year period yet still leaked chyle from his stump! The message is clear – do not perform an amputation for chylous reflux into the lower limb; try to stop the reflux.

CHYLOUS ARTHRITIS

Whenever lymph or chyle refluxes into a limb, the abundant lymphatic plexus beneath the synovium of the joints is likely to be involved. The pressures and movements within the joint may split the thin layer of synovium overlying the bulging lymphatics, rupture some lymphatics and thus cause a chylous effusion.

Clinical presentation

Chylous arthritis is well recognized in areas where filaria is endemic and thoracic duct obstruction and chylous reflux are common.[18] Patients complain of a swollen painful joint, usually the knee, and often have a mild pyrexia. Joint movement is restricted by pain and muscle spasm. Each acute episode subsides in 7–10 days, but episodes may recur a number of times each year. In between the attacks, the joint movements are at first full and painless, but if the attacks continue the joint becomes stiff and painful.

The pyrexia that accompanies the first attack does not usually accompany further attacks, and these, albeit associated with the same degree of swelling, are less painful. This is difficult to understand as it is believed that the pyrexia is caused by the chylomicrons setting up an allergic reaction within the synovium, with a subsequent inflammatory response.[19] It may be that the thickening of the synovium caused by each attack reduces the chances of this form of tissue response. The patient may have other signs of filarial lymphatic disease, such as lymphoedema and leaking vesicles.

We have seen only one case, and Servelle et al.[20] have also described a single case caused by non-filarial congenital megalymphatics.

Investigation

Aspiration of the joint produces a thick, opaque, yellowish-white fluid that looks like pus. Septic arthritis is therefore the main differential diagnosis, and culture of the fluid is essential. Biochemical and microscopic examination will reveal that the fluid has a high lipid content and contains chylomicrons. Filariasis should be confirmed or excluded with the standard antibody tests (see Chapter 15).

A plain radiograph of the joint may show widening of the joint space and synovial thickening. A bilateral pedal lymphogram is helpful if there are other lymphatic symptoms and signs in the limb that are likely to require treatment. It will show dilated lymphatics around the joint, and the 24 hour films may, very rarely, show Lipiodol within the joint. Arthroscopy will reveal the dilated subsynovial lymphatics, but any procedure that pierces the synovium and its underlying lymphatics may worsen the chyle leak.

Treatment

Each episode should be treated by aspiration, rest, immobility, a firm pressure bandage and suitable analgesia. Recurrent attacks cause thickening of the synovium which reduces the chances of further chyle leakage but also causes joint stiffness and pain. Those with clinical experience of this condition find that conservative treatment with prompt aspiration, compression and bed rest as soon as an attack begins keeps the affected joint in good working condition, and that the attacks eventually stop.

Surgical treatment is rarely required. Ligation and excision of the incompetent lymphatics above and around the joint, including synovectomy, may reduce the frequency of the attacks. Local lymphovenous anastomoses may, if they stay patent, also help. Thickening the synovium by irradiation – radiosynovectomy – has been claimed to help.[21]

CHYLOUS REFLUX INTO THE EXTERNAL GENITALIA

Most cases of acquired (secondary) penoscrotal and labial lymphoedema in filarial areas are caused by the reflux of chyle down incompetent abdominal lymphatics below a filarial thoracic duct obstruction.

Most cases of secondary lymphoedema of the genitalia in non-filarial areas are caused by secondary malignant disease and chronic infection in the inguinal lymph glands, but there is a group of patients who develop an obstruction of the lymphatics draining the scrotum (see Fig. 12.10b) following an attack of acute scrotal cellulitis.

These patients and those with primary genital lymph-oedema do not have chylous reflux into the scrotum or labia because their iliac and abdominal lymphatics are normal. They are mentioned here because the lymph-filled vesicles that develop on their skin are transparent and colourless, and must not be mistakenly interpreted as indicating chylous reflux.

The causes of primary (congenital) genital lymph-oedema in both non-filarial and filarial areas are similar to the causes of primary lymphoedema of the lower limb – absence or obliteration/obstruction, congenital or acquired (80 per cent), and incompetent megalymph-atics (20 per cent). Only those patients with incompetent, dilated retroperitoneal aortic and iliac lymphatics develop chylous reflux. Patients with a primary occlusion or absence of the lymphatics draining the scrotum often have lymph-filled vesicles on the skin of their genitalia, which should not be mistakenly diagnosed as chylous reflux.

Thus, as with reflux into the lower limb, there are only two common causes of chylous reflux into the genitalia – secondary lymphatic incompetence usually caused by filariasis, and congenitally incompetent megalymphatics. The treatment of the reflux into the labial, penile or scro-tal skin is therefore the same as that of reflux into the lower limb, with one helpful addition. Reducing the size of the penis, scotum or labia is a far more effective way of excising all or most of the incompetent vessels than is reducing the size of the thigh and leg. It is therefore sometimes worthwhile in elderly, less fit patients per-forming the excisional operation first and keeping the more major procedure of ligation of the abdominal and iliac lymphatics in reserve should troublesome reflux persist or recur, although we prefer whenever possible to perform the ligation/excision procedure first followed by the genital reduction 6–8 weeks later. The treatment of all forms of lymphoedema of the genitalia is discussed fully in Chapter 12, and the treatment of reflux into the perineum and limbs, and therefore of the external geni-talia, in the previous section.

Chyle may also reflux into and leak through vesicles in the vagina and uterus (colporrhoea and metrorrhoea), and through vesicles in the male and female urethra, to cause a chylous urethral discharge often associated with and sometimes misinterpreted as chyluria. Chylous colporrhoea and metrorrhoea are discussed in the next section, and chyluria and chylous urethral discharge on pp. 278–81.

CHYLOUS COLPORRHOEA AND CHYLOUS METRORRHOEA

When chyle refluxes into the cavity of the uterus or through the surface of the cervix or the walls of the vagina, it runs out of the vagina and the patient complains of a thin, white, milky vaginal discharge. The correct medical term for a chylous vaginal discharge is chylous colporrhoea or chylocolporrhoea. Only when it is known that the discharge is definitely coming from the uterus, a fact unknown to the patient at presentation and only revealed by investigation, is it correct to call it chyl-ous metrorrhoea. The chylous discharge should not be called chylous metrorrhagia because the word 'metror-rhagia' means intermenstrual bleeding and chyle is not blood.

Clinical presentation[22–25]

The continuous leakage of a white, sticky, slightly greasy fluid from the vagina is a rare but most distressing symptom. The discharge usually begins in early life when the child begins to eat a normal adult diet and become physically active. In the three cases we have seen, the discharge began between the ages of 3 and 5 (Fig. 16.7). The patients had to wear some form of sanitary pad at all times, and the skin of the vulva and perineum became red and sore.

In adult life, the discharge makes intercourse distaste-ful, although the lymphatic vesicles in the vagina are not tender and the vaginal epithelium between the vesicles is healthy. Patients with chylocolporrhoea often

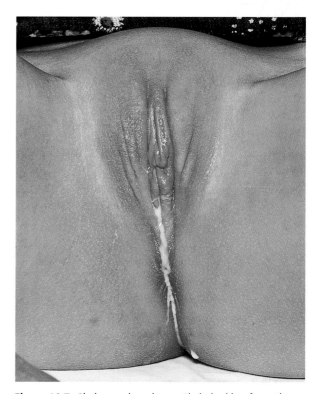

Figure 16.7 *Chylous colporrhoea. Chyle leaking from the vagina of a 10-year-old girl, and running down over the perineum.*

have lymphoedema of the lower limbs with evidence of lymph reflux, such as leaking cutaneous vesicles, and chylous ascites.

Investigation

The extent of the lymphatic abnormality and the site or sites of leakage are best determined by a careful clinical

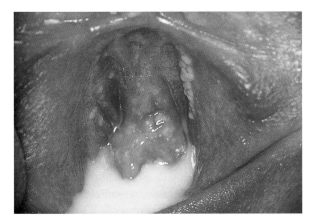

Figure 16.8 *Chylous colporrhoea caused by leaking vesicles on the wall of the vagina.*

examination and lymphangiography. Culposcopy often reveals chyle-filled vesicles on the walls of the vagina, usually high up in the fornices, and on the cervix (Fig. 16.8). Chyle may also be seen exuding from the os cervix. Bimanual examination reveals a normal or slightly bulky uterus. The lymphatic malformation on the floor of the pelvis is soft and impalpable.

A bipedal lymphangiogram will delineate the extent of the megalymphatic abnormality (Fig. 16.9) and may show Lipiodol leaking into the body of the uterus and/or the vagina. This leak may also be displayed by lymphoscintigraphy.

Chylometrorrhoea – chyle leaking from the uterus – arises from incompetent pelvic lymphatics, whereas chyle leaking from low vaginal vesicles may come from either incompetent pelvic or perineal/inguinal lymphatics. In the latter case, it may be necessary to perform a lymphangiogram by injecting Lipiodol directly into a low vaginal vesicle to identify which set of lymphatics is incompetent, an essential piece of information for planning surgical treatment.

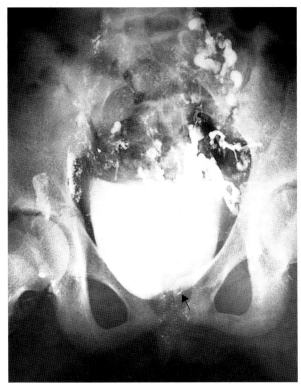

(a)

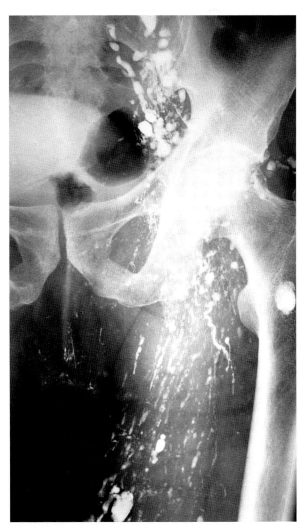

(b)

Figure 16.9 *Chylous colporrhoea caused by incompetent megalymphatics allowing reflux to the vaginal wall from (a) the iliac lymphatics (site of leak arrowed) and (b) the medial inguinal lymphatics.*

Routine haematological and biochemical tests should be performed at regular intervals to monitor the patient's nutritional state.

Treatment

The discharge of chyle can be stopped by ligating the incompetent lymphatics around the uterus and vault of the vagina.[7,26] This involves an extensive and meticulous dissection, ligation and excision of *all* the lymphatics on the sides and floor of the pelvis after visualizing them by injecting Patent Blue Violet into the subcutaneous tissues of the upper thigh and groin. Care should be taken to preserve the autonomic nerve fibres running to the uterus across the floor of the pelvis. Any vessels left open or accidentally pricked by a needle may continue to leak and cause a chylous ascites.

It is sometimes necessary to perform a total hysterectomy in order to obliterate all the lymphatics on the pelvic floor. As most women with chylous colporrhoea are of child-bearing age, hysterectomy is an operation of last resort and should be used only when one or two attempts at ligation have failed.

The medial inguinal lymphatics must also be exposed, ligated and excised if the preoperative investigations indicate that some of the chyle is reaching the vaginal wall through these vessels. All patients should be warned that however radical the surgical clearance of the lymphatics in the pelvis, the colporrhoea is likely to recur 5–10 years later.

In view of the reports of the successful treatment of chyluria by lymphaticovenous anastomoses in the groin (*see* p. 278), such a procedure may be worth attempting before embarking upon a major abdominal operation, particularly if there are low vaginal vesicles draining to incompetent medial inguinal lymphatics.

CHYLOUS ASCITES

A case of chylous ascites following abdominal trauma was described by de Diemerbroeck in 1685.[2] Four years later, Morton[3] described a patient with chylothorax and chylous ascites caused by tuberculous lymph nodes obstructing the thoracic duct. Many cases have subsequently been described and have been incorporated into a recent detailed review by Aalami *et al.*[27]

Chylous ascites is uncommon, probably accounting for approximately 1 in every 50 000 hospital admissions. The recorded incidence is thought to be increasing as methods of investigation improve and more aggressive forms of treatment for secondary malignant disease in the lymph glands, such as irradiation and surgical lymphadenectomy, develop.[28–30] The prognosis for those whose ascites is caused by malignant disease is poor.[31] Those with primary lymphatic problems do better but still have a significant mortality rate.[32]

Pathology

The causes of chylous ascites may be divided into primary and secondary, the latter being by far the most common. In both groups, the chyle refluxes down primarily or secondarily dilated incompetent lymphatics at and below the cisterna chyli, and enters the peritoneal cavity by transuding either though the walls of the lymphatics and their peritoneal covering or though a hole in a lymphatic and the overlying peritoneum, a lymphatic–peritoneal cavity fistula (Fig. 16.10).

Secondary chylous ascites

In filarial areas of the world, the most common cause of secondary chylous ascites is filarial obstruction of the thoracic duct. The next most common cause is tuberculosis (Fig. 16.10a) because many of the filarial areas are areas of poverty and poor nutrition.

In non-filarial areas, secondary chylous ascites is usually caused by malignant disease in the upper abdominal and thoracic lymph glands, usually lymphoma[31] and sometimes secondary carcinoma. Any form of external trauma to the abdomen can damage the retroperitoneal lymphatics.[33] Chylous ascites is a recognized feature of the 'battered baby' syndrome.[34,35] Postoperative chylous ascites may follow vascular operations that involve dissection around the aorta and root of the mesentery[36] and aortic lymphadenectomy for malignant disease.[37]

There is also a multitude of occasional causes of secondary chylous ascites, such as pericarditis, pancreatitis, retroperitoneal fibrosis and sarcoidosis, designed to test the clinician's diagnostic acumen. A very thorough investigation of each patient is essential before concluding, by exclusion, that a chylous ascites is caused by a primary abnormality of the lymphatics.[27] Whatever the underlying cause, all cases of secondary chylous ascites follow some form of thoracic duct obstruction or direct injury.

Primary chylous ascites

There are three intrinsic (primary) abnormalities of the lymphatics that may cause chylous ascites.

First, congenitally incompetent megalymphatics affecting all the intra-abdominal retroperitoneal lymphatics (and usually the lymphatics of one or both lower limbs), with or without involvement of the lacteals, which allows chyle to reflux down the aortic lymphatics and enter the peritoneal space via a hole in the wall of a lymphatic (a fistula), or by a generalized transudation through the walls of the retroperitoneal lymphatics and

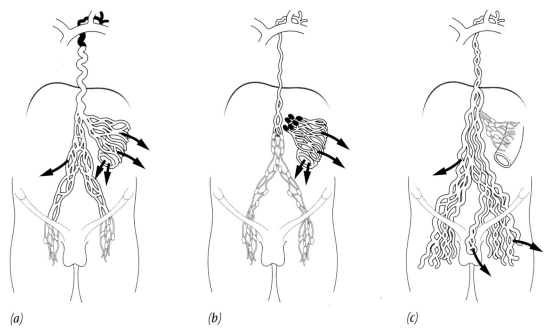

(a)   *(b)*   *(c)*

Figure 16.10 *The non-traumatic causes of chylous ascites. There are three mechanisms (other than direct trauma) that, by causing upstream lymphatic dilatation and incompetence, predispose, first, to the transudation of chyle through the walls of the intra-abdominal lymphatics and/or lacteals, and second, to the rupture of a lymphatic and the formation of a lymphatic–peritoneal cavity fistula. (a) Thoracic duct obstruction (secondary or primary), which may cause a fistula and/or transudation from the retroperitoneal and intestinal lymphatics. (b) Mesenteric lymph gland obstruction (invariably secondary) causing the transudation of chyle from the lacteals into the abdominal cavity and the lumen of the bowel. (c) Congenitally dilated incompetent megalymphatics, but no anatomical obstruction, which may transude chyle or rupture and fistulate, often with normal lacteals and mesenteric lymph glands.*

their covering of peritoneum and the intestinal serosa (Fig. 16.10c).

Second, a congenital physiological obstruction of the thoracic duct caused by an aplasia or malformation leading to upstream dilatation and incompetence of the lymphatic tributaries. This allows reflux of chyle down throughout the aortic and iliac lymphatics and sometimes the lacteals, permitting the chyle to transude into the peritoneal cavity or flow into it via a fistula (Fig. 16.10a). Some of these patients have a distal or proximal obliteration of the lymphatics of their lower limbs.

Third, an obstruction within the mesenteric lymph glands that prevents chyle reaching the cisterna chyli. This leads to dilatation of the lacteals throughout the wall of the small bowel, including those in the intestinal villi, with transudation of chyle through the serosal surface of the bowel into the peritoneal cavity and through the villi into the lumen of the intestine, with a subsequent protein-losing enteropathy (Fig. 16.10b) (see below). We do not know the cause of the obstruction within the mesenteric lymph glands. It may be a congenital abnormality as some of these patients also have obliterated leg lymphatics or a fibrosis similar to that seen in the iliac and inguinal lymph glands in patients with

proximal obstructive lymphoedema of the lower limb (*see* p. 274). The glands themselves are full of chyle, and their histology is uninterpretable.

Clinical presentation

Most patients present with a painless, progressive abdominal distension. As the swelling increases, the rising diaphragm impedes respiration, causing breathlessness and respiratory embarrassment. Sensations of abdominal fullness and vomiting are common in children. In our own collection of 45 patients,[38] 60 per cent showed malnutrition and weight loss, 46 per cent complained of breathing difficulties, and 46 per cent had steatorrhoea, causing an increased frequency of defecation and pale stools. If chylous ascites develops suddenly, it may cause severe abdominal pain and tenderness. Sometimes misnamed 'acute chylous peritonitis', the pain is caused by the distension; chyle does not irritate the peritoneum.

Many patients have the symptoms and signs of the underlying cause of the chylous ascites, for example of filariasis, tuberculosis, lymphoma or recent trauma, and some will have signs of other lymphatic abnormalities, such as chylous reflux to the kidneys, urinary tract, genitalia and limbs, and lower limb lymphoedema. The only physical signs attributable to the ascites are the abdominal distension, shifting dullness on percussion, and sometimes striae gravidarum. All the other causes of abdominal distension (fetus, fat, fluid, faeces, fibroids, etc.) must be excluded.

Investigation

If physical examination and an ultrasound scan confirm the presence of free fluid within the peritoneal cavity, it is essential to perform a paracentesis and determine the nature of the fluid.

Paracentesis

A turbid yellowish-white fluid does not necessarily contain chyle. 'Pseudochylous' ascites occurs in association with some intra-abdominal malignancies and peritonitis, the turbidity being caused by degenerating epithelial cells and/or bacteria. The milky colour of true chylous ascites is caused by the presence of chylomicrons. These can be identified by microscopy, by staining with Sudan Red and by lipoprotein analysis. Chyle contains less protein than plasma, 1–4 per cent fat and up to eight times more triglycerides than plasma.[39–41]

Computed tomography and nuclear magnetic resonance scans

These sometimes help to define the nature of the fluid before paracentesis and may show dilated retroperitoneal lymphatics. If the patient lies still for some time before the scan, the fat and water may separate and become visible as a fatty/non-fatty fluid/fluid level.[42–48] Small bowel affected with intestinal reflux has a thickened wall.

CT scans may show the presence of coeliac or pelvic lymph gland malignant disease or other unsuspected causes of the patient's abdominal distension.

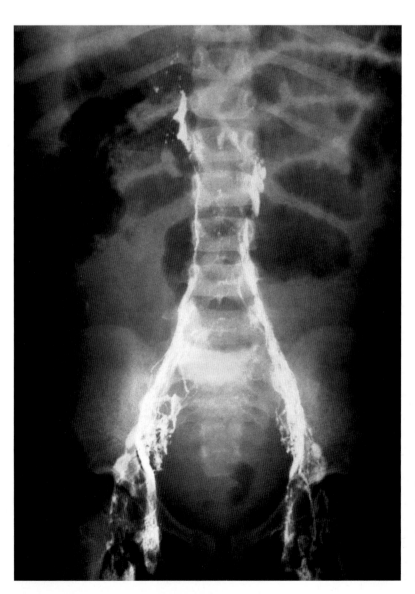

Figure 16.11a *Lymphangiographs of the lymphatic–peritoneal cavity fistulae shown in Fig. 16.13. The retroperitoneal lymphatics do not appear to be dilated, as they were in the limbs, because they have been decompressed by the fistula. Lipiodol is just beginning to appear in the peritoneal cavity to the right side of the first lumbar vertebra.*

Lymphoscintigraphy

A bipedal lymphoscintigram should reveal the presence of any dilated lymphatics in the limbs and abdomen. It may also reveal the site of a lymphatic–peritoneal fistula.[45,46] Late scans may show the presence and level of a thoracic duct obstruction. The anatomical definition of the lymphatics on lymphoscintography is not, however, sufficient for surgical planning: a standard bipedal lymphogram is essential.

Lymphography

Bipedal lymphograms with Lipiodol, supplemented with a non-ionic, water-soluble contrast medium if the early radiographs show a large capacious system of megalymphatics, is an essential diagnostic and presurgical investigation. Knowing the site where the chyle is leaking into the peritoneum is of great assistance during laparotomy (Figs 16.11 and 16.12).

We have not experienced any of the serious side-effects claimed by some to be a contraindication to lymphography (*see* Chapter 6).[47,48]

Laparoscopy/laparotomy

Laparoscopy can be used to diagnose the presence of chylous ascites and assess the state of the small bowel, but in many cases the final diagnosis cannot be made until a full diagnostic laparotomy has been performed.[49] Before doing this, it is wise to perform all the preoperative investigations so that the laparotomy can be used for the administration of treatment rather than just for confirming the diagnosis.

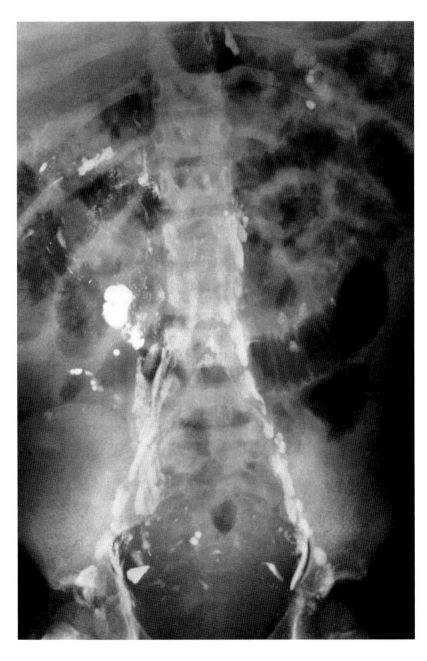

Figure 16.11b *Lymphadenograph of the same patient obtained 24 hours after performing the lymphangiogram, showing large collections of Lipiodol within the peritoneal cavity and a mass of partially filled congenital megalymphatics to the right of the vertebral column.*

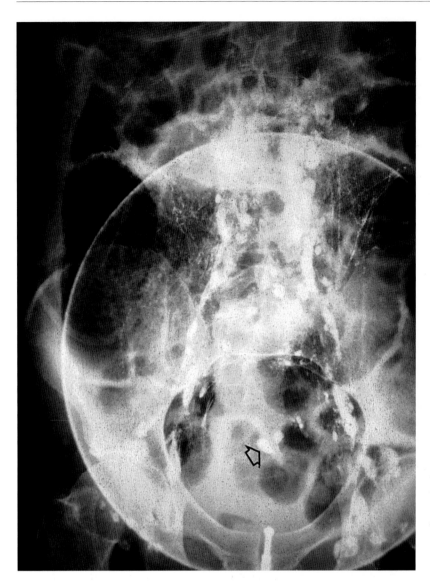

Figure 16.12 *The 24 hour lymphadenograph of a patient with chylous ascites and a large mass of pre-aortic lymphomatous lymph glands. The site of leakage was not detected because chyle was exuding from the whole surface of the mass of lymph glands, but free intraperitoneal Lipiodol is visible lying in the rectovesical pouch (arrowed).*

Treatment

Management should begin with the treatment of any underlying causative disease assisted by dietary measures to reduce the production of chyle.

Chylous ascites caused by malignant disease in the upper abdominal or thoracic lymph glands, especially lymphoma, may resolve when the disease is treated by radio- or chemotherapy. Similarly, ascites caused by intra-abdominal tuberculous lymphadenitis may resolve with appropriate antibiotic treatment. Unfortunately, chylous ascites caused by filariasis is a late complication of the disease process and develops when fibrosis and dead worms begin to obstruct the lymphatics, so the pharmacological treatment of the filariasis, which must be given, rarely affects the ascites.

Diet

Any pre-existing malnutrition should be corrected and the patient monitored while on dietary treatment to ensure that a good nutritive state is maintained. Whether there is an underlying treatable disease or a primary lymphatic abnormality, it is always worthwhile reducing chyle production by giving the patient a strict no-fat diet supplemented with medium chain triglycerides and extra vitamins.[48] This diet may not affect a large, tense abdomen but will reduce the rate of refilling after paracentesis and sometimes stops it recurring altogether.[35,37,49,50]

Diuretics

Diuretics are a valuable adjunct to dietary control. The Mayo Clinic has reported successful control with diuretics (spironolactone) alone in 86 per cent of a group of patients with chylous ascites that followed abdominal irradiation.[51] The effect of dietary control plus diuretics has not been extensively studied, but a 67 per cent response rate has been reported in 12 patients with primary intestinal reflux and protein-losing enteropathy.

Total parenteral nutrition

Total parenteral nutrition should be considered if dietary restrictions fail or give only slight relief. As this is a major procedure with significant complications, its possible benefits must be carefully weighed against its disadvantages. It appears to be more effective in children than adults[52–54] and has been used more often for paediatric chylothorax than chylous ascites (see below).

Total parenteral nutrition should be given for at least 3 weeks to assess its effectiveness and may have to be continued for many months. This makes it unsuitable for patients with an underlying malignant disease of poor prognosis. Children and adolescents do not tolerate dietary control or total parenteral nutrition well and are unlikely to accept it as a lifelong therapy. Unless there is a dramatic response to dietary measures and no recurrence after stopping them, an attempt at a surgical cure should be considered.

Paracentesis

Paracentesis relieves the distension and discomfort but has no effect on the basic problem. It should be used in conjunction with the dietary and diuretic regimen described above. The repeated aspiration of large volumes of a protein- and fat-rich fluid can lead to malnutrition and should be avoided except when other treatments have failed and the distension is painful and the prognosis poor.

Peritoneovenous shunts

Returning the chyle to the bloodstream through a valved peritoneovenous shunt is a logical form of treatment that should abolish the ascites and maintain nutrition. Unfortunately, these shunts sometimes occlude because chyle is viscid and sticky. In our experience, and that of others,[28,31,55–57] many LeVeen[56] and Denver Shunts function well for a few weeks or months but hardly ever stay patent for longer than a year. Occluded shunts can be replaced but repeated operations for shunt replacement increase the risk of complications such as infection, peritonitis and coagulopathies.

Surgery

Much can be learnt from the investigations described above, especially if they reveal a single leaking fistula, but whether effective treatment is possible ultimately depends on a careful examination of all the abdominal contents at an exploratory laparotomy.

A full-length midline incision is required to allow the abdomen to be explored from the diaphragm to the pelvis. On opening the abdomen, all the chyle should be sucked out and the peritoneum washed clean. Exploration will usually reveal one or more of three abnormalities:

1 A definite single or localized area of lymph fistulae. The orifice of a fistula may be sharply defined and chyle seen to leak through it (Fig. 16.13).

2 A boggy, greyish-white patch of ectactic lymphatics covered with a thin layer of peritoneum but without any obvious fistula, which, if watched for a few minutes, will be seen to have chyle oozing through its surface. Such areas usually lie beneath the posterior or pelvic peritoneum, may be 5–20 cm across and may extend forwards into the root of the mesentery (Fig. 16.14).

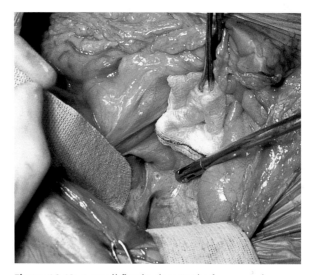

Figure 16.13 *A small fistula close to the foramen of Winslow that was the cause of gross chylous ascites. The lymphangiograph (see Fig. 16.11a) accurately identifed the site of the leak. This fistula was easy to close with a few non-absorbable sutures, and the patient was cured.*

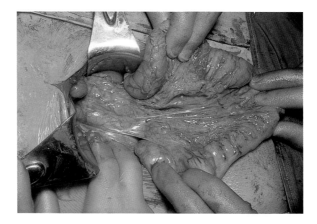

Figure 16.14 *Dilated megalymphatics at the root of the mesentery extending down through the mesentery and on to the surface of the bowel, all exuding chyle. This patient had congenital retroperitoneal megalymphatics and megalacteals (see Fig. 16.10c) but did not have protein-losing enteropathy.*

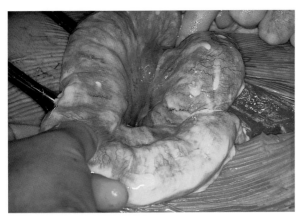

Figure 16.15 *Thickened oedematous small bowel and mesentery partially obscuring grossly dilated lacteals, exuding chyle and causing severe chylous ascites.*

3 Dilated, chyle-filled lymphatics in the mesentery and over the serosal surface of the small intestine. Although this lymphatic abnormality affects the whole of the small intestine, there is often a segment of 1–2 m of bowel that looks much worse than the remainder (Fig. 16.15).

The surgical treatment of these three abnormalities is as follows:

1 A single fistula can be closed with deep, non-absorbable, occluding sutures, taking care not to puncture other lymphatics, which might then leak into the peritoneum along the course of the suture. It is also important not to include or damage nearby structures such as the ureter or major vessels within these sutures.
2 Large patches of leaking lymphatics should be over-sewn and compressed (imbrication) by incorporating the omentum into the stitches and positioning it so that it covers and adheres to the leaking area. This procedure can be difficult if tissues cannot be found that are strong enough to hold the large stitches needed to compress the lesion and when the omentum cannot be pulled over the abnormal area. Smaller patches not involving or close to important structures can be excised, taking care not to leave any unligated open lymphatics at the edges of the excision that could become fistulae. A full block dissection of the retroperitoneal lymph glands with ligation and over-sewing of all the afferent and efferent lymph vessels can occasionally be performed, but most patches are too big to excise safely.
3 The management of chyle leaking from the surface of the small bowel is dealt with in detail below. The only surgical treatment is resection of as much of the affected bowel as possible, consistent with leaving enough bowel to ensure adequate nutrition. If the affected area is well demarcated, its resection will cure the ascites. Even when there is not a localized area,

resection of the worst area often has a worthwhile effect. Lacteal-to-mesenteric vein anastomoses have not, in our experience, been successful.

The results of these procedures are unpredictable.[27] In our own series of 45 patients,[38] conservative management related to diet and medium chain triglycerides (rather than total parenteral nutrition) was successful in only 34 per cent of cases. Six out of the 12 patients who had a localized single or patch of fistulae closable by oversewing were cured, and a quarter improved. Two out of the 12 patients who had a bowel resection were cured, and six improved. All nine of the peritoneovenous shunts inserted became blocked within 3–6 months, but one patient's ascites remained cured and two were improved. In this particular series of patients, we saw none with leaking patches of retroperitoneal megalymphatics, but the two cases we have seen and treated by oversewing were improved.

Aalami *et al.*,[27] from a review the world literature, reported the results of the treatment of 156 patients. The ascites resolved in 43 per cent of the 105 who were treated conservatively. Of the 51 patients treated surgically, 41 per cent were successfully treated by the ligation of a fistula and 37 per cent with a peritoneovenous shunt. Little can be learnt from these figures as the numbers are small, most are single case reports, the underlying lymphatic abnormalities are extremely variable and often poorly defined, and the follow-up periods varied from weeks to years.

INTESTINAL CHYLOUS REFLUX (PROTEIN-LOSING ENTEROPATHY)

When chyle cannot pass through the lacteals, cisterna chyli and thoracic duct into the bloodstream, it refluxes back into the villi and diffuses back through the intestinal mucosa into the lumen of the bowel. A steady loss of protein, fat, minerals such as calcium and fat-soluble vitamins causes weight loss, steatorrhoea and diarrhoea, tetany and a hypoproteinaemic oedema. This condition is known as 'protein-losing enteropathy', but as other important nutrients are also lost and because some of the chyle leaks into the peritoneal cavity, it might better be called an 'exudative enteropathy'.[58]

Pathology

Waldmann *et al.*[59] have described over 70 causes of protein loss from the intestine. The lymphatic causes can be divided into secondary and primary. The secondary causes are conditions that obstruct the flow of chyle through the mesenteric lymph glands, cisterna chyli or thoracic duct, the majority being various primary and secondary malignant diseases in the lymph glands. The degree of protein loss they produce is not severe, and treatment should be directed towards the underlying primary pathology. If the underlying disease, for example a lymphoma, can be treated, the protein-losing enteropathy may subside. When it cannot be treated, the protein loss continues but is not usually a major clinical problem if the patient has an incurable malignant disease and a short prognosis.

There are two primary lymphatic abnormalities that cause protein-losing enteropathy: intrinsic mesenteric lymph gland obstruction/fibrosis and mesenteric/aortic incompetent megalymphatics (see Fig. 16.10b and c). The pathology of the former group appears to be hypoplasia or fibrotic obstruction of the small bowel lymph glands similar to the abnormality that causes proximal obstructive lymphoedema of the lower limb (see Chapter 7). The majority of these patients also have an obstructive lymphoedema of one limb that has appeared some years before the symptoms of the protein loss. A few have chylous ascites and genital lymphoedema, although some have no other lymphatic abnormality. The limb swelling is not always caused by a lymphatic abnormality: it may be caused by the hypoproteinaemia.

A study of the small bowel protein loss of 55 patients with primary lymphoedema of the lower limb[60,61] showed 12 to have protein losses of between 2.5 and 18 per cent, significantly greater than the upper limit of normal of 1.5 per cent. Eight of the 12 patients had hypocalcaemia. These findings are not surprising as the two abnormalities causing protein-losing enteropathy are similar to the two main causes of lymphoedema of the lower limb.

Clinical presentation

Protein-losing enteropathy may present at any age, but most of the patients with a primary lymphatic abnormality present in adolescence or early adult life.

Tiredness, weakness and abdominal distension are the most common presenting symptoms. These are often accompanied by the appearance of a mild, bilateral lower limb oedema or a worsening of any existing lymphoedema. Diarrhoea and steatorrhoea are common, the latter causing pale faeces. Patients may not realize that their faeces are abnormal because their faeces may have been pale for many years.

Patients may complain of paraesthesiae and carpopedal spasms if their serum calcium falls significantly. The abdomen may be distended with a chylous ascites, but the volume of ascitic fluid is sometimes small and not clinically detectable.

Investigation

Tiredness and weakness are extremely common symptoms of many diseases, but if they occur in a patient with a lymphatic abnormality, the possibility of a protein-losing enteropathy caused by a primary lymphatic abnormality should be considered.

Chromium chloride test for intestinal protein loss

In this test,[61,62] 30 μCi of $^{51}CrCl_3$, which binds tightly to the plasma proteins, is injected intravenously, 1 mL solution being kept for a baseline radioactivity count. All the faeces passed over the next 5 days must be collected and the radioactivity of the whole sample measured. The excretion of more than 2 per cent of the administered dose of chromium chloride is considered abnormal. Care must be taken not to contaminate the stool sample with urine, especially in children, as 30 per cent of the isotope is excreted in the urine.

Biochemistry

A full biochemical study of the plasma levels of protein and calcium must be obtained. In the first 12 patients studied at St Thomas' Hospital, London,[60] 10 had a total protein level below the lower level of the normal range – on average 78 per cent, the lowest being 60 per cent, of normal. Eight patients had a serum calcium level below normal (on average 83 per cent of normal), of which the lowest was 54 per cent of normal.

Small bowel enema

A barium study of the small bowel may demonstrate prominent valvulae conniventes, swelling of the bowel wall and submucosa, and enlarged villi (Fig. 16.16).

Small bowel endoscopy and mucosal biopsy

A biopsy of the mucosa via an endoscope or with a Crosby capsule will show villi with dilated central lacteals often containing inspissated chyle. Chyle-filled lacteals distending the villi will be seen if the endoscope can be passed well down the jejunum (Fig. 16.17).

^{99m}Tc-labelled albumin scintigraphy

When 740 MBq fresh ^{99m}Tc-labelled human albumin is injected intravenously, some may leak into the lumen of the bowel (if the mesenteric lymphatics are abnormal) and be visible on scans taken 1–24 hours later. Chiu et al.[63] tested 26 patients suspected of having protein-losing enteropathy in this way and found 25 to have a positive result for the test. The route from the blood stream to the lumen of the bowel is not, however, necessarily via incompetent lymphatics so lymphography is still required to confirm that the cause of the protein loss is an underlying lymphatic abnormality.

Lymphoscintigraphy

Lymphoscintigraphy with ^{99m}Tc-labelled human serum albumin may show dilated or obstructed lymphatics and, if sufficient isotope gets into the bloodstream, may demonstrate a leak into the lumen of the bowel as occurs after an intravenous injection (see above), this being visible on an abdominal scintigraph.[63,64]

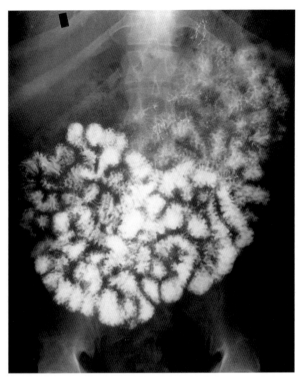

Figure 16.16 *The small bowel meal of a patient with protein-losing enteropathy. The villi in the upper jejunum are enlarged, being almost globular in shape. The villi in the lower part of the small bowel are not so prominent, but the space between the loops of bowel is widened by bowel wall oedema.*

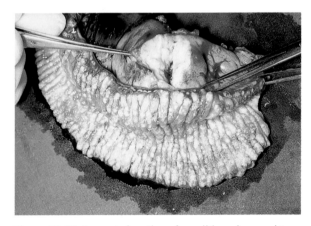

Figure 16.17 *A resected section of small bowel opened to show the intestinal villi distended with chyle. The lymph gland draining this area has been opened to show that it is also oedematous and packed with chyle.*

Pedal lymphangiography

A bipedal lymphangiogram is essential to ascertain the state of the abdominal lymphatics. If the abdominal peri-aortic lymphatics are normal, it is likely that there is mesenteric gland fibrosis or lymphatic hypoplasia. If there are dilated megalymphatics, the Lipiodol may

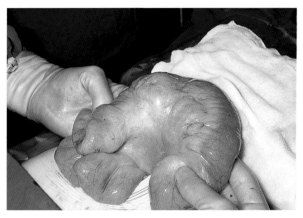

Figure 16.18 *The typical appearance of a loop of small bowel affected by chylous obstruction and reflux. The mesentery is thickened, the bowel wall oedematous and the lacteals on the surface of the bowel full of chyle. This is the external appearance of the loop of bowel illustrated in Fig. 16.17.*

be seen refluxing down the lacteals, even into the intestinal villi.

Laparotomy

The extent of the intestinal abnormality can only be properly assessed by laparotomy. There is always some free chyle in the peritoneal cavity. The affected bowel is oedematous, thickened and covered with dilated, chyle-filled lymphatics. The mesentery is swollen and thickened, often obscuring the dilated lacteals within it. The lymph glands at the base of the mesentery are usually enlarged and full of chyle (Fig. 16.18). The pre-aortic retroperitoneal tissues need not be exposed to assess the state of the peri-aortic lymphatics as they should have been defined by the preoperative lymphogram. Exploring this area carries the risk of unknowingly damaging the lymphatics and exacerbating any associated chylous ascites.

Mesenteric lymphangiography

The best way to determine whether the lacteal dilatation is caused by an obstruction in the mesenteric lymph glands or is part of a generalized abdominal lymphangiectasia is to perform a mesenteric lymphangiogram.[58] Patent Blue Violet is not needed as the white, chyle-filled lymphatics on the serosal surface of the bowel are easy to see (Fig. 16.19a).

After placing the bowel over an X-ray cassette, a fine lymphangiogram needle is inserted into a serosal lymphatic and Lipiodol slowly injected. The radiographs may show the Lipiodol passing up the lacteals, stopping at the lymph glands and then refluxing back into the bowel wall and intestinal villi (Fig. 16.19b) or running through the glands into dilated pre-aortic lymphatics. A full-sized abdominal radiograph will then display the distended

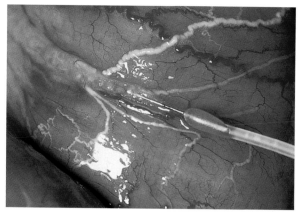

(a)

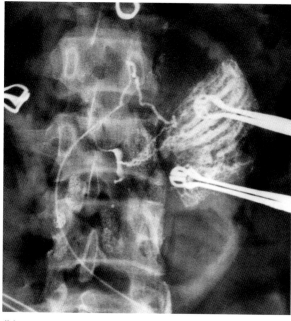

(b)

Figure 16.19 *Mesenteric lymphangiography. (a) When the subserosal lymphatics are dilated and white, they are easy to see and cannulate with a fine lymphangiogram needle. (b) The mesenteric lymphangiograph of the bowel illustrated in Figs 16.17 and 16.18. The Lipiodol does not run cephalad into the cisterna chyli but refluxes into the dilated lacteals in the intestinal villi.*

mesenteric glands' efferent lymphatics, the cisterna chyli and reflux down towards the pelvis.

Treatment

The conservative treatment for chylous ascites described in the previous section should be tried first. A non-fat diet supplemented with medium chain triglycerides will often significantly reduce the chyle leak and help to restore the patient's protein and electrolyte balance. Two thirds of patients have a favourable response to this treatment.[65,66] If the treatment does not succeed, and if the

patient consents, it is worth trying total parenteral nutrition for 3–6 months, but this cannot be continued indefinitely and is theoretically more likely to help those with a generalized lymphangiectasis than those with obstruction within the mesenteric glands.

Octreotide, which reduces mesenteric blood flow and the production of intestinal lymph, has been reported to be of value.[67,68] Dietary control is essential even after resecting the worst affected segment of bowel because the remaining bowel is abnormal and will continue to leak.

Laparotomy and small bowel resection

If conservative treatment fails after diligent application, it is worth performing a laparotomy, first to be quite certain of the diagnosis, and second to decide whether a small bowel resection would be helpful. The diagnostic appearance of affected bowel has been described above. Three degrees of severity may be apparent:

1 A segment of the small intestine, 2–3 m in length, may be abnormal, but the remainder of the small bowel looks and feels normal.
2 A segment of small intestine may be grossly abnormal, the remainder being thickened and oedematous but less severely affected.
3 The whole of the small intestine may be severely affected – swollen, oedematous and covered with dilated, chyle-filled subserosal lymphatics.

The treatment of disease sharply localized to a single segment of bowel (degree 1 above) is resection and anastomosis.[49,58,69]

The treatment of the second category above – widespread disease that is severe in a localized segment – is also resection and anastomosis. In these circumstances, the bowel at the anastomotic suture line is abnormal, but it heals well and we have seen no complications in the patients we have treated in this way.

There is no satisfactory treatment for widespread, severe involvement of the whole bowel. A massive, near-total small bowel resection is unlikely to help because life with a very short bowel is probably worse than life with protein-losing enteropathy. If an extensive resection is a likely option, it should be fully discussed with the patient before the operation, especially if he or she may have to face the prospect of a lifetime on total parenteral nutrition.

Small bowel transplantation

Small bowel transplantation may perhaps become the treatment of choice for these patients. It is interesting to note that although no lymphatic anastomoses are made when the small bowel is transplanted, patients do not, in the short term, develop a clinically significant lymphatic obstruction and protein-losing enteropathy; they may, however, do so in the long term.

Lymphovenous anastomosis

When there is a generalized lymphangiectasis, lymphovenous anastomoses have the potential to divert the chyle into the bloodstream and reduce the protein loss. Cases have been reported of these anastomoses relieving chylous reflux into the abdomen and limbs, but there is little information about their effect on the protein-losing enteropathy.[70]

The only procedure that might help, if the peri-aortic lymphatics are normal, is an anastomosis between the lacteals or a mesenteric lymph gland and a nearby mesenteric vein. The lymph gland-to-vein anastomoses that we have performed in primary non-filarial cases have not stayed patent, and we have never attempted lymphatic-to-mesenteric vein anastomoses because the lacteals are single, straight vessels, rather than arcades like the veins and arteries, so decompressing one, two or even three lacteals is unlikely to have a significant effect on a long length of bowel.

CHYLURIA

The fact that fat may appear in the urine has been recognized since the time of Hippocrates. In 1670, Moellenbroch[1] suggested that chyluria might be caused by an abnormal connection between the lymphatics and the urinary system. In the nineteenth century, Prout[71] suggested that chyluria was caused by a lymphatic obstruction between the kidney and thoracic duct. It is now realized that chyle can get into the urine when dilated, incompetent abdominal and renal lymphatics and an incompetent thoracic duct allow chyle to flow from the region of the cisterna chyli, retrogradely, into the kidneys or down incompetent pre-aortic lymphatics to the lymphatics of the bladder and ureters. This abnormality may be congenital (primary) or acquired (secondary).

Acquired obstruction of the thoracic duct is by far the most common cause of chyluria because thoracic duct obstruction is a common complication of filariasis. As a result of filariasis being by far the most usual cause of chyluria, some classifications of the aetiology of chyluria are divided into parasitic and non-parasitic. In non-filarial areas, acquired thoracic duct obstruction may be caused by malignant disease and trauma.

Congenital (primary) thoracic duct abnormalities are rare. The thoracic duct and all the retroperitoneal lymphatics may be deformed, dilated and incompetent or partially absent, with secondary dilatation and incompetence of the upstream lymphatics, including those from the small bowel and kidneys. Whether the localized, congenital abnormality of the thoracic duct is caused by the same genetic abnormality that causes the abnormality of the limb lymphatics in some of these patients is not known. Over the past 30 years, the only primary lymphatic abnormality to cause chyluria that we have seen is congenitally incompetent megalymphatics.

Clinical features

Chyluria occurs in 2 per cent of patients with filariasis,[72] when it usually presents in the second and third decades of life. It is otherwise very rare. The patient complains of passing thick, milky-white urine, especially when physically active, but the act of micturition is not painful (Fig. 16.20). The milkiness is less in the morning after a night's rest and during periods of bed rest. There may be occasional episodes of haematuria.

The chyluria may persist for days, weeks or months and then stop suddenly, only to recur months or years later. When the loss of chyle is persistent, patients often lose weight and feel debilitated. There are no physical signs apart from weight loss and sometimes anaemia, but there may be symptoms and signs caused by the underlying filariasis (*see* Chapter 15) or causative malignant disease in the abdomen or chest.

Leakage into the bladder caused by pelvic megalymphatics is sometimes associated with lymphoedema of the limbs and external genitalia with leaking cutaneous vesicles.

If a patient dribbles milky fluid from the penis or urethra at times unrelated to micturition, he or she probably does not have chyluria but is leaking chyle directly into the urethra. Such patients are likely to have

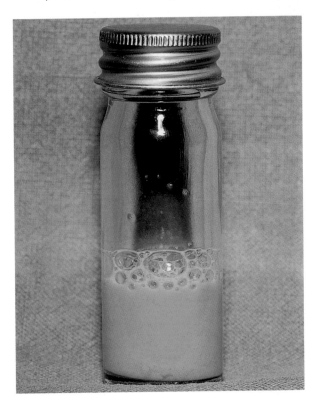

Figure 16.20 *Chyluria. A specimen of the thick, milky urine passed by a patient with a filaritic obstruction of his thoracic duct.*

chyle-filled vesicles on the surface of the penis or in the vagina that also leak chyle (Fig. 16.21).

Investigation

It is important to confirm by biochemical tests and microscopic examination that the discoloration of the urine is caused by the presence of chyle. The detection of chylomicrons and a high level of fat in the urine is diagnostic. It is then very important to establish whether the lymphatic abnormality has arisen secondary to another disease. Filariasis can be confirmed with filarial IgG antibody tests[73] and if necessary by examining a smear of blood taken at night for microfilariae. Intra-abdominal and intrathoracic malignant disease should be excluded by the relevant investigations.

CT and NMR scans may reveal masses of dilated megalymphatics in the retroperitoneal, peri-renal and pelvic areas, thus indicating the most probable area of chyle leak, but neither can detect the direction of lymph flow or the exact site of the leak.[74,75]

Lymphoscintigraphy, although not providing the precise anatomical images of a lymphograph, may sometimes be better at revealing the site of the chyle leak.[76,77]

During *lymphography*,[7] it is essential to examine the whole of the intra-abdominal lymph system with bipedal lymphograms, taking films at frequent intervals as the Lipiodol passes up the iliac and aortic lymphatics in order to display incompetent megalymphatics and any retrograde flow away from the main vessels towards the bladder, ureters or kidney (Fig. 16.22). Lipiodol is often seen leaking into the calyces of the kidney, and droplets of Lipiodol may be detected in the bladder. The lymphogram should be continued until the cisterna chyli and thoracic duct have been visualized. In patients with filariasis, the most common cause of chyluria is obstruction of the thoracic duct.

Observation of the ureteric orifices during *cystoscopy* is a helpful investigation if the lymphogram suggests that the reflux is occurring through only one kidney. The milky urine may be seen to be coming from one ureteric orifice. Cystoscopy with panendoscopy is necessary to exclude or confirm the presence of lymphatic vesicles and areas of chyle leakage on the epithelium of the urethra and bladder.

Direct inspection of the lining of the ureter by *ureteroscopy* may identify the site or sites of the chyle leak.

Treatment

Mild symptoms need no treatment provided the patient's nutrition and body weight are maintained; active treatment is indicated if the patient is losing weight and the chyluria heavy. A low- or no-fat diet supplemented with medium chain triglycerides will reduce the quantity of chyle absorbed by the small bowel and thus reduce the quantity of chyle that is leaking into the urine. This form of severe dietary control is expensive and impractical in many of the countries where filariasis is endemic. It may

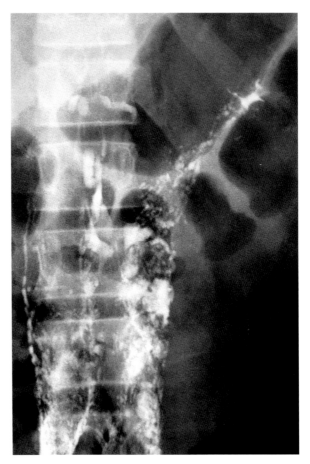

Figure 16.22a *Lymphangiograph showing Lipiodol refluxing from dilated, incompetent, pre-aortic lymphatics into the lymphatics of the renal pedicle and then into one of the calyces of the kidney. This patient's chyluria was cured by ligating and excising all the lymphatics in the renal pedicle.*

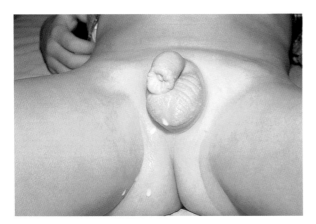

Figure 16.21 *Milky-white fluid draining from the penis of a young boy. This was not chyluria but a leak of chyle from vesicles in the urethra (see text). Vesicles containing chyle can be seen on the prepuce and scrotal skin. This patient had congenital aortic and pelvic incompetent megalymphatics.*

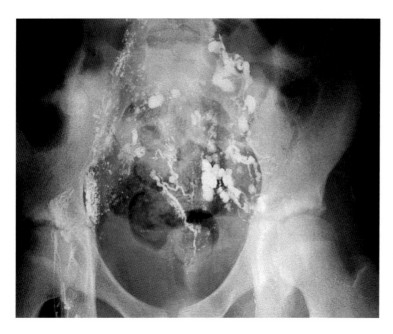

Figure 16.22b *Chyluria caused by chyle refluxing into vesicles beneath the epithelium of the bladder. This lymphangiograph shows incompetent megalymphatics throughout the pelvis with Lipiodol running downwards towards the bladder. This patient's chyluria was cured by ligating all the lymphatics crossing the floor of the pelvis running towards the bladder.*

also cause confusion because if the fat is removed from the chyle, the urine becomes colourless. Therefore, to avoid unecessary dieting, it is wise to return to a normal diet and to check whether the leak is still present, recommencing the no-fat diet only if the chyluria returns. It is important to monitor patients' blood lipid levels and weight when they are taking a no-fat medium chain triglyceride supplemented diet.

The reflux of chyle into the urinary tract may be prevented by two methods:

- The dilated, incompetent lymphatics through which the reflux is occurring can be ligated and excised. Attempts to occlude incompetent lymphatics by the direct injection of sclerosants[78] or retrogradely injecting the leaking sites via the renal pelvis[7] have not been successful: collaterals form rapidly and the chyluria soon returns.
- The refluxing chyle can be diverted away from the urinary tract and into the bloodstream by lymphovenous anastomoses.

Ligation and excision of the dilated lymphatics

This is a major operation. When the leakage is occurring into the kidney, the kidney must be exposed via a retroperitoneal approach and all the lymphatics in and around the renal pedicle between the kidney and the periaortic lymphatics ligated and excised. Great care must be taken to ensure that the ligation is thorough lest a lymphocele develop postoperatively around the kidney. A sufficient length of the incompetent vessels must be excised to ensure that reconnections cannot develop and reflux recur. This is a major procedure in which damage to the renal artery, vein or ureter can lead to the loss of the kidney, and it should be performed by a surgeon skilled in vascular surgical techniques. There are reports of this procedure being successfully performed laparoscopically.

Leakage into the ureter or bladder is treated by excising all the lymphatics around these organs and on the inner wall and floor of the pelvis, as described on p. 262.

Diverting the chyle away from the kidney

This is achieved by anastomosing the dilated lymphatics to adjacent veins. It is a difficult technique that became feasible with the development of vascular microsurgical techniques. It has been mainly practised in China. Zhao and colleagues[79] have reported 95 males treated by lymphaticovenous anastomoses between megalymphatics and the spermatic cord veins in the inguinal region, and 30 females treated by anastomoses between lymphatics and veins in the foot, lower leg and thigh. All these patients had widespread lymphatic dilatation and incompetence. The effect of these anastomoses was to produce a gradual general reduction in the high pressure throughout the system, a hypothesis supported by the fact that fistulae into the kidney took up to 6 months to close. Nevertheless, the authors claim a 75 per cent success rate, and as this is a 'minor', albeit technically difficult, procedure with few serious complications and little postoperative morbidity it is clearly worth trying in patients with generalized megalymphatics. It is not suitable when the reflux is confined to dilated lymphatics in the renal pedicle and upper abdomen.

Hou *et al.*[80] and others[81] have reported a similar 75 per cent abolition of chyluria in 30 patients with the same type of widespread lymphangiectasis treated by anastomosing a hollowed out inguinal lymph gland to the saphenous vein. This operation is easier to perform than a direct lymphatic-to-vein anastomosis.

Both forms of anastomosis probably remain patent only because there is a high rate of lymph/chyle flow. We have not found any form of lymphovenous anastomosis to remain patent when the flow of lymph is normal and/or intermittent.

CHYLOUS URETHRAL DISCHARGE

Whereas chyle that leaks into the urine collecting and conducting systems of the kidneys, ureters and bladder immediately becomes mixed with the urine and is noticed only during micturition, chyle that leaks into the urethra may constantly dribble out of the external meatus (see Fig. 16.21, p. 279). Patients consequently often complain of a urethral discharge. When there are no leaking vesicles in the bladder wall, the urine will be clear except for the first few millilitres that wash out the urethra at the beginning of micturition. Patients are often first investigated for the common causes of a urethral discharge if the milkiness of the discharge is not noticed. It is therefore important to remember this rare condition when a patient has any other stigmata of lymphatic disease. The diagnosis is confirmed by finding chylomicrons in the discharge.

The investigation and treatment are similar to those of all forms of chylous reflux – careful lymphographic delineation of the site and extent of the incompetent vessels followed by ligation and excision of the incompetent vessels that are carrying chyle to the urethral wall, which may lie on the inner walls of the pelvis or among the medial inguinal lymphatics.

CHYLOTHORAX

The true prevalence of chylothorax is not known, and it may occur at any age. The abnormalities which allow chyle to collect in the pleural cavity are similar to those which cause chylous ascites, with the addition of one major acquired cause – intrathoracic cardiac, thoracic and oesophageal surgery. Secondary (acquired) chylothorax is far more common than the primary (congenital) variety. All secondary chylothoraces, except those resulting from trauma, are caused by an obstruction to the flow of chyle that causes upstream duct and lymphatic dilatation, valvular incompetence and leakage of chyle through a fistula or by transudation into the pleural cavity.

Pathology

Acquired (secondary) chylothorax

Acquired (secondary) chylothorax may follow a direct injury to the thoracic duct or thoracic duct obstruction.

Thoracic duct injury

Thoracic duct injury, once rare, is now one of the most common causes of secondary chylothorax because it is not an infrequent complication of cardiothoracic surgery on neonates and young children. All the extra-cardiac cardiothoracic procedures, for example the Blalock operation, the repair of an aortic coarctation, the closure of a ductus arteriosus, the Fontan and Senning operations (cardiac operations performed in the presence of a high central venous pressure) and the repair of a tracheobronchial fistula, may be followed by a unilateral chylothorax. The reported incidence of this complication after cardiothoracic surgery varies from 0.25 to 2.5 per cent.[82,83] The iatrogenic injury leaves a defect in the duct through which chyle leaks into the pleural space, this continuing until the defect heals spontaneously or is closed surgically. There is also a high incidence (2 per cent) of chylothorax after oesophageal surgery, especially when the oesophagus is removed without a thoracotomy.

Thoracic duct obstruction

Filariasis is the most common cause of thoracic duct obstruction in adults from filarial areas. In non-filarial areas, the most probable cause of obstruction of the thoracic duct is enlarged malignant mediastinal lymph glands (Fig. 16.23a). Lymphoma is the most frequent malignancy, but secondary carcinomatous deposits in lymph glands adjacent to the thoracic duct from intra-abdominal, pulmonary and head and neck carcinomata are not uncommon.[84]

Thoracic duct obstruction may also be caused by thrombosis of the subclavian vein, usually caused by the presence of a long-standing central venous catheter.[85] Obstruction at the termination of a normal thoracic duct by venous thrombosis alone rarely causes the duct to rupture and leak, but if there is a concomitant minor non-penetrating injury during cardiothoracic surgery, leakage is more likely. Some of the chylothoraces of neonates and children are caused by this combination.

Thoracic duct obstruction may cause a chyle leak in three ways:

- Duct distension may progress to rupture and the formation of a fistula between a mediastinal lymphatic and the pleural space.
- Chyle may transude through the dilated mediastinal lymphatics and the overlying pleura.
- The lymphatic dilatation and valvular incompetence may extend into the lungs, allowing chyle to reflux throughout the substance of the lung and ooze out into the pleural space through the lymphatics beneath the visceral pleura. When this occurs, the chyle may also leak into the alveoli and bronchioles and be coughed up, a condition known as bronchorrhoea.

Primary (congenital) chylothorax

Several congenital lymphatic abnormalities may cause a chylothorax. First, an obstruction or deformity of the upper part of the duct can obstruct the flow of chyle and cause upstream dilatation and incompetence with fistula

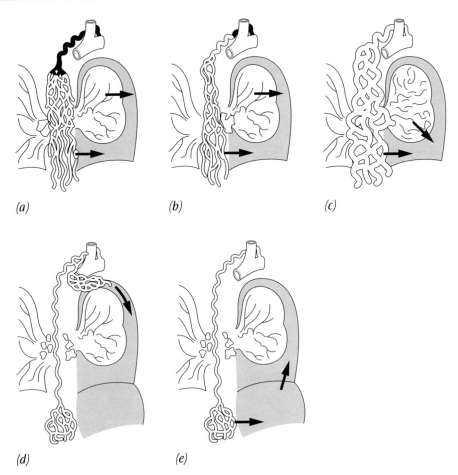

Figure 16.23 *Non-traumatic causes of chylothorax. There are three mechanisms (other than trauma) that, by causing upstream lymphatic dilatation and incompetence, predispose towards, first, the transudation of chyle through the walls of the mediastinal and/or lung lymphatics, and second, the rupture of a lymphatic and the formation of a lymphatic–pleural cavity fistula. (a) Acquired mediastinal thoracic duct and/or lung lymphatic obstruction (usually filariasis or malignant disease) causing an upstream fistula or the reflux of chyle into the lung and its transudation through the visceral pleura. (b) Terminal thoracic duct obstruction (acquired or congenital) causing an upstream fistula or transudation from the mediastinal and/or lung lymphatics. (c) Congenital lymphangiectatic deformity of the thoracic duct with reflux into the pleural cavity via a fistula or into the lung substance and transudation through the visceral pleura. There are also two mechanisms by which chyle may reach the pleural cavity in the presence of an unobstructed thoracic duct. (d) Leakage of a lymphangiomatous malformation connected with the thoracic duct, and thus containing chyle, through a fistula or by transudation. Such lymphangiomata usually lie in the upper part of the chest and are associated with other congenital abnormalities (see text). (e) Leakage of chylous ascites into the pleural cavity through a patent foramen in the diaphragm.*

formation or transudation between the mediastinal lymphatics and the pleural space (Fig. 16.23b).

Second, there may be a diffuse congenital megalymphatic deformity of the duct and all the mediastinal lymphatics (a true congenital lymphangiectasis) with valvular incompetence and reflux through the mediastinal lymphatics, and fistula formation or transudation into the pleural space (Fig. 16.23c). When the lymphatics in the lung are similarly abnormal, the chyle will leak through to and exude from the surface of the lung. The megalymphatic abnormality rarely affects only the lungs, and chyle does not usually reflux into the lungs unless there is some thoracic duct obstruction, functional or mechanical, above the entry of the pulmonary lymphatics into the thoracic duct.

Third, lymphangiomata or patches of gross lymphangiomatosis beneath the parietal pleura may leak chyle and lymph into the pleural cavity (Fig. 16.23d). Such abnormalities are more frequent in patients with other congenital abnormalities such as Turner's, Down's or Noonan's syndrome or disappearing bone disease.

Finally, chylous ascites may leak from the abdomen into the chest through patent foraminae in the diaphragm. Chyle may also leak into the pleural cavity from lymphatics on the diaphragm and chest wall that are acting as collaterals around a low thoracic or upper abdominal duct occlusion that is itself causing chylous ascites (Fig. 16.23e). In these circumstances, the classification of the cause of the chylothorax – acquired or congenital – depends upon the cause of the chylous ascites.

Clinical presentation

Many minor degrees of chylothorax are symptomless and discovered by chance on a chest radiograph performed as part of the investigation of a chest injury or illness or following cardiothoracic surgery.[86]

Seventy per cent of our own series of 20 patients,[87] none of whom had had cardiothoracic surgery, complained of breathlessness sometimes accompanied by recurrent chest infections. Those with severe bilateral effusions were breathless at rest and showed early heart failure. Two of our 20 patients had bronchorrhoea. Symptoms and signs arising from the prime cause, for example cardiothoracic surgery, lymphoma, secondary carcinoma, filariasis or subclavian vein thrombosis, are common.

Chylothorax should be considered in any patient found to have dyspnoea and a pleural effusion after cardiac or oesophageal surgery even though a haemothorax or leaking anastomosis is more likely. There may be other lymphatic associated abnormalities such as chylous ascites, lymphoedema of a limb or stigmata of other congenital deformities.

Investigation

A *chest X-ray* will confirm the presence and extent of the pleural effusion (Fig. 16.24) and sometimes reveal its cause within the superior mediastinum (Fig. 16.25).

A full biochemical and pathological analysis of the pleural effusion, obtained by *thoracocentesis*, is essential to confirm that it is chyle. The criteria for this diagnosis if chylomicrons are not present have been enumerated by Staats *et al.*[40] and Straaten *et al.*[88] The triglyceride level must be greater than 1.2 mmol/L and the total number of white blood cells greater than 1000 cells/mL with a predominance of mononuclear cells. Although a milky-white appearance suggests that the fluid is chyle, the same appearance can be produced by cellular debris so a biochemical confirmation of the nature of the fluid is essential.

Cholesterol pleural effusions are thick and cloudy and look chyliferous, but, in contrast to chyle and in common with most other pleural effusions, have a high cholesterol content.

CT and NMR scans provide extra information about the extent of the effusion and the presence of abnormalities in the mediastinum, such as enlarged lymph glands and dilated lymphatics. They may also reveal other asymptomatic collections of chyle in the pericardial sac and abdomen.

Lymphoscintigraphy may show the isotope lying in dilated mediastinal lymphatics below the obstruction and isotope in the effusion within the pleural cavity. It rarely shows the exact site of a fistula.

Lymphangiography is the only method that clearly delineates the anatomy of the mediastinal lymphatics

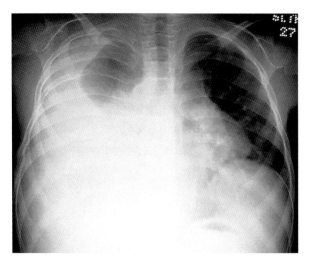

Figure 16.24 *A massive right-sided chylothorax in a young boy with a total lymphangiectatic congenital deformation of his thoracic duct.*

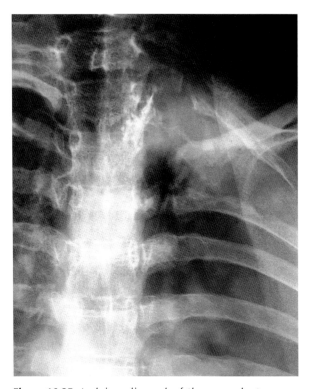

Figure 16.25 *A plain radiograph of the upper chest that revealed the probable cause of the patient's chylothorax – a lymphangiomatous malformation associated with disappearing bone disease. There is a little Lipiodol in the lymphangioma close to the end of the thoracic duct.*

(Fig. 16.26).[7,87,89,90] If the transit of Lipiodol is watched carefully with X-ray screening and repeated check films, the exact site of a fistula may be found. The reflux of chyle into the lungs is rarely seen beyond the central portion of the lungs, but its presence suggests that there is

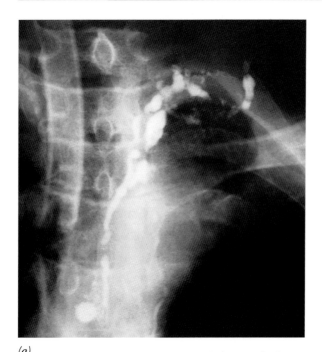

(a)

reflux throughout the lung and transudation through the visceral pleura.

Thoracoscopy may be used to confirm the diagnosis. It is more helpful when the effusion is unilateral because it may reveal the site of the chyle leak

Phlebography of the great veins may be necessary if a subclavian/jugular vein thrombosis is suspected to be the cause of the thoracic duct obstruction or if the insertion of a pleurovenous shunt is being considered.

General investigations to detect an underlying cause of the chylothorax and assess the state of the patient's nutrition are an essential precursor to the investigations described above.

Treatment

As the majority of cases of chylothorax, except those following trauma and filariasis, are secondary to disease in

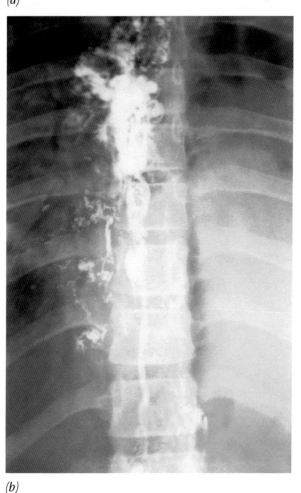

(b)

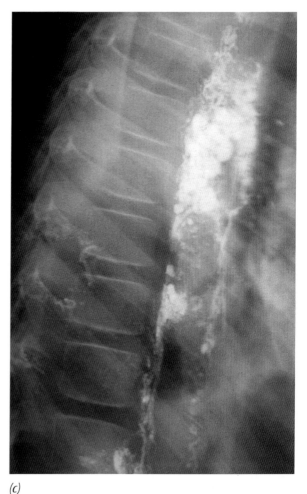

(c)

Figure 16.26 *Lymphangiographs of five patients illustrating some of the abnormalities that may cause a chylothorax. (a) Congenital abnormality of the terminal few centimetres of the thoracic duct. (b) Ectatic malformation of the upper third of the thoracic duct with reflux into the right lung and around the chest wall. The duct below the abnormality is normal. (c) Ectatic malformation of the whole of the thoracic duct, which also extended into the abdomen, causing a chylothorax and chylous ascites. It is not possible to say whether the thoracic duct never developed or whether it occluded during fetal life.*

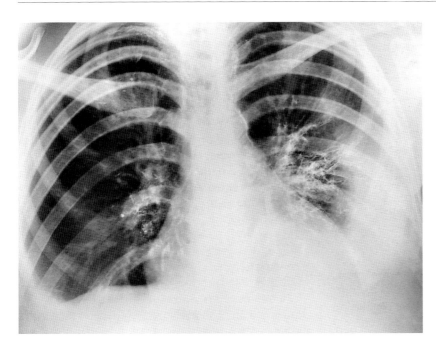

Figure 16.26d *Reflux into both lungs caused by a mass of malignant lymph glands in the mediastinum.*

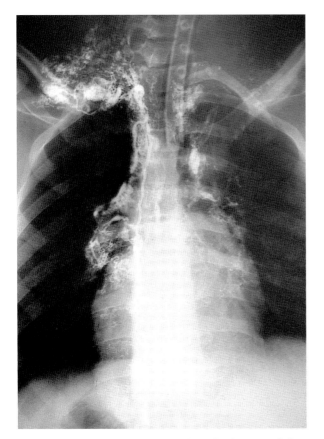

Figure 16.26e *Extensive lymphangioma in the apex of the right pleural cavity connected to the thorax duct and associated with disappearing bone disease.*

the lymph glands of the mediastinum, this disease must, if present, be treated first. During this treatment, the symptoms caused by the effusion should be managed conservatively by thoracocentesis and diet.

Diet

Chyle production should be reduced by giving the patient a no-fat diet supplemented with medium chain triglycerides, or if necessary total parenteral nutrition.[83,86,91,92]

Somastatin

Somastatin reduces the rate of intestinal lymph production and reduces chyle absorption by reducing mesenteric blood flow.[93] There are a number of reports of its successfully reducing chyle absorption in children after cardiothoracic surgery to a degree that allows a fistula to heal.

Thoracocentesis

This should initially be carried out to confirm the diagnosis. As much of the effusion as possible should be aspirated and the rate of re-collection monitored with daily radiographs. Rapid re-formation producing respiratory embarrassment should be treated by *continuous pleural drainage*. The amount of the leak should be carefully measured daily.

The combination of the above conservative measures can be expected to result in the closure of 30–40 per cent of post-paediatric cardiothoracic surgery chylous fistulae within 14 days. Another 40 per cent of fistulae are likely to close if the treatment is continued for another 4 weeks, but this should only be done if the daily volume of the chyle leak is reducing and the treatment is not causing any nutritive or other complications.[83,91] These forms of conservative treatment should also be used during the treatment of any underlying cause of the chylothorax as the combination of treatment of a thoracic duct obstruction caused by malignant lymph glands with pleural drainage and diet may stop the leak.

The failure of conservative treatment, as judged by a chyle leak of more than 1.5 L per day in adults and 100 mL per year of age per day in children is an indication for surgical intervention.[83,91,92]

Thoracotomy

Exploration of the thoracic cavity may be the only way of reaching a definitive diagnosis, but it is advisable to have investigated the patient fully so that logical therapeutic measures may be performed at the same time.

Fistula closure

A single fistula following trauma, after cardiothoracic surgery or non-specific in nature may be closed by simple suturing. This is likely to block the duct completely, but providing the lymphatics of the mediastinum and abdomen are normal, this does not cause any problems. Chyle will reach the venous system by collateral routes. Small fistulae can be blocked with fibrin glue, and the procedure can be attempted through a thoracoscope.

Thoracic duct ligation[83–86,91,94]

Adhesions, oedema and inflammation often make it difficult to find the site of the thoracic duct injury after cardiothoracic surgery. In such cases, it is easier to ligate the thoracic duct via a thoracotomy or by video-assisted thoracoscopy[95,96] just above the diaphragm where it lies on the right side of the aorta. When the duct is not visible, the mass of tissues on the right of the aorta between it and the azygos vein should be ligated. This operation was first performed by Lampson in 1948[97] and is considered by paediatric surgeons to be the treatment of choice for the surgical correction of post-cardiothoracic chylothorax in neonates and children.

It must be stressed that thoracic duct ligation should not be performed if the lymphatics in the mediastinum and abdomen are abnormal and that this treatment should be used only for an acquired duct injury. Ligating a leaking duct with congenitally abnormal upstream lymphatics will cause chylous ascites and not stop the chylothorax.

Excision and/or imbrication of clusters of leaking lymphatics

Circumscribed leaking lymphangiomata may be excised if they are not intertwined with other vital structures. Leaks from large lymphangiomata and from patches of lymphangiectatic vessels can sometimes be suppressed by imbricating stitches through their substance to compress them and by sewing adjacent normal tissue over them, but this is difficult and often fails. The chest does not contain a structure similar to the omentum that can be used for this purpose, although the omentum can be brought up through or behind the diaphragm to help to compress leaking vessels that are lying low down in the chest.

Pleurodesis

Obliteration of the pleural space will prevent the accumulation of chyle within it. The usual methods of pleurodesis employed to prevent recurrent pneumothorax, such as the installation of talc or fibrin glue, do not work because the flow of chyle through the mediastinum and lungs is usually so great that it dilutes the sclerosant and keeps the parietal and visceral pleura apart. The only effective way of achieving pleurodesis in patients with otherwise surgically irremediable lymphatic abnormalities is by parietal pleurectomy followed by pleural suction drainage until the visceral pleura sticks to the denuded inner surface of the thoracic cage.[87]

The whole of the parietal pleura can be stripped off through a sixth rib thoracotomy. The edges of the parietal pleura are freed from the edges of the thoracotomy and held away from the ribs with forceps so that the fingers can be pushed beneath the pleura. The whole of the parietal pleura can then be stripped off by blunt finger dissection; the stripping process is easy because the pleura tends to be thicker than normal. There is little bleeding, and there are few lymphatics beneath it. The diaphragmatic pleura does not strip easily and is best abraded. The mediastinal pleura covers many important structures and many dilated, thin-walled lymphatics. It can be stripped off, but damaging the underlying lymphatics increases the chance of chyle leaking into the chest and preventing adhesion formation. It is often safer to abrade the mediastinal pleura with a nylon abrasive pad.

Two chest drains, apical and basal, with low-pressure suction are inserted and tethered to the chest wall. Suction must be continued, often for 2–3 weeks, until the chyle leak stops.

Decortication

Some patients who have had a chylous effusion for many years, often congenital in origin, develop a thick layer of fibrin over the lung surface (Fig. 16.27a) that stops the lung expanding when the effusion is removed. This complication can be predicted from the thickness of the visceral pleura on a CT scan and by the failure of the lung to expand fully after the initial thoracocentesis. In such patients, simple removal of the effusion does not cure the respiratory embarrassment: the layer of fibrin must also be removed. Decortication is a delicate procedure. Special care must be taken to avoid damaging the underlying lung and causing an alveolar–pleural fistula because the free passage of air into the pleural space makes it far more difficult to suck the lungs right out to the chest wall. Any air leak visible during positive-pressure ventilation before closing the thoracotomy should be carefully oversewn with a very fine suture or blocked with fibrin glue.

46. Pui MH, Yueh TC. Lymphoscintigraphy in chyluria, chyloperitoneum and chylothorax. *Journal of Nuclear Medicine* 1998; **39:** 1292–6.

47. Nubie M. Lymphoedema and chylo-ascites: an unusual complication of lymphangiography. *Netherlands Journal of Medicine* 1977; **20:** 18–22.

48. Weinstein LD, Scanlon GT, Hersh T. Chylous ascites. Management with medium-chain triglycerides and exacerbation by lymphangiography. *American Journal of Digestive Diseases* 1969; **14:** 500–9.

49. Fox U, Lucani G. Disorders of the intestinal mesenteric lymphatic system. *Lymphology* 1993; **26:** 61–6.

50. Viswanathan U, Putnam T. Therapeutic intravenous alimentation for traumatic chylous ascites in a child. *Journal of Pediatric Surgery* 1974; **9:** 405–6.

51. Lenz S, Schray M, Wilson T. Chylous ascites after whole abdomen irradiation for gynaecological malignancy. *International Journal of Radiation Oncology, Biology and Physics* 1990; **19:** 435–8.

52. Asch MJ, Sherman NJ. Management of refractory chylous ascites by total parenteral nutrition. *Journal of Pediatrics* 1979; **94:** 260–2.

53. Dillard RP, Stewart AG. Total parenteral nutrition in the management of traumatic chylous ascites in infancy. *Clinical Pediatrics (Philadelphia)* 1985; **24:** 290–2.

54. Alliet P, Young C, Lebenthal E. Chylous ascites: total parenteral nutrition as a primary therapeutic modality. *European Journal of Pediatrics* 1992; **151:** 213–4.

55. Kerr RS, Powis SJ, Ross JR, Wynne-Williams CJ. Peritoneovenous shunt in the management of paediatric chylous ascites. *British Journal of Surgery* 1985; **72:** 443–4.

56. LeVeen HH, Wapnick S, Grosberg S, Kinney MJ. Further experience with peritoneo-venous shunt for ascites. *Annals of Surgery* 1976; **184:** 574–81.

57. Guttman FM, Montupet P, Bloss RS. Experience with peritoneo-venous shunting for congenital chylous ascites in infants and children. *Journal of Pediatric Surgery* 1982; **17:** 368–72.

58. Kinmonth JB, Cox SJ. Protein-losing enteropathy in primary lymphoedema: mesenteric lymphography and gut resection. *British Journal of Surgery* 1974; **61:** 589–93.

59. Waldmann TA, Steinfeld J, Dutcher TF, Davidson JD, Gordon RS. The role of gastrointestinal system in idiopathic hypoproteinaemia. *Gastroenterology* 1961; **41:** 197–207.

60. Kinmonth JB, Eustace PW. Gut protein loss in lymphoedema. *Proceedings of the Royal Society of Medicine* 1975; **68:** 673–5.

61. Eustace PW, Gaunt JI, Croft DN. Incidence of protein-losing enteropathy in primary lymphoedema using chromium-51 chloride technique. *British Medical Journal* 1975; **2:** 737.

62. Walker-Smith JA, Skyring AP, Mistilis SP. Use of 51CrCl3 in the diagnosis of protein-losing enteropathy. *Gut* 1967; **8:** 166–8.

63. Chiu NT, Lee BF, Hwang SJ, Chang JM, Liu GC, Yu HS. Protein-losing enteropathy; diagnosis with (99m)Tc-labelled human serum albumin scintigraphy. *Radiology* 2001; **219:** 86–90.

64. Wang SJ, Tsai SC, Lau JL. Tc-99m albumin scintigraphy to monitor the effect of treatment in protein-losing enteropathy. *Clinical Nuclear Medicine* 2000; **25:** 197–9.

65. Jeffries GH, Chapman A, Sleisenger M. Low fat diet in intestinal lymphangiectasis. *New England Journal of Medicine* 1964; **270:** 761–7.

66. Stoelinga GBA, Van Munster EJ, Sloof JP. Chylous effusions into the intestines in patients with protein-losing enteropathy. *Pediatrics* 1963; **31:** 1011–16.

67. Kuroiwa G, Takayama T, Sato Y, *et al.* Primary intestinal lymphangiectasia successfully treated with octreotide. *Journal of Gastroenterology* 2001; **36:** 129–32.

68. Ballinger AB, Farthing MJ. Octreotide in the treatment of intestinal lymphangiectasis. *European Journal of Gastroenterology and Hepatology* 1998; **10:** 699–702.

69. Persic M, Browse NL, Prpic I. Intestinal lymphangiectasia and protein-losing enteropathy responding to small bowel resection. *Archives of Disease in Childhood* 1998; **78:** 194–7.

70. Mistilis SP, Skyring AP. Intestinal lymphangiectasia. *American Journal of Medicine* 1996; **40:** 634–41.

71. Prout W. *On the nature and treatment of stomach and renal diseases.* London: Churchill, 1841.

72. Ray PW, Rao SS. Chyluria of filarial origin. *British Journal of Urology* 1939; **11:** 48–64.

73. Mehta VK, Lohar H, Banerjee GK, Reddy MV, Harinath BC. Surgical filariasis: immunoscreening for filarial IgG antibodies using *Wuchereria bancrofti* microfilarial excretory-secretory antigen. *Journal of Community Diseases* 1999; **31:** 35–40.

74. Haynes JW, Miller PR, Zingas AP. Computed tomography and lymphangiography in chyluria. *Journal of Computer Assisted Tomography* 1984; **8:** 341–2.

75. Wadsworth DE, Glazer HS, McClennan BL. Chyluria. *Urological Radiology* 1983; **5:** 117–19.

76. Nishiyama Y, Yamamoto Y, Mori Y, *et al.* Usefulness of technetium-99m human serum albumin lymphoscintigraphy in chyluria. *Clinical Nuclear Medicine* 1998; **23:** 429–31.

77. Pui MH, Yueh TC. Lymphoscintigraphy in chyluria, chyloperitoneum and chylothorax. *Journal of Nuclear Medicine* 1998; **39:** 1292–6.

78. Shanmugam TV, Prakash JV, Sivashankar G. Povidone iodine used as a sclerosing agent in the treatment of chyluria. *British Journal of Urology* 1998; **82:** 587.

79. Zhao WP, Hou LQ, Shen JL. Summary and prospects of 14 years experience with treatment of chyluria by microsurgery. *European Urology* 1988; **15:** 219–22.

80. Hou LQ, Liu QY, Kong QY, *et al.* Lymphonodovenous anastomosis in the treatment of chyluria. *Chinese Medical Journal* 1991; **104:** 392–4.

81. Ji YZ, Zheng JH, Chen JN, Wu ZD. Microsurgery in the treatment of chyluria and scrotal lymphangial fistula. *British Journal of Urology* 1993; **72:** 952–4.

82. Higgins CB, Mulder DG. Chylothorax after surgery for congenital heart disease. *Journal of Thoracic and Cardiovascular Surgery* 1971; **61:** 411–18.

83. Beghetti M, LaScala G, Belli D, Bugman P, Kalangos A, LeCoultre C. Etiology and management of pediatric chylothorax. *Journal of Pediatrics* 2000; **136:** 653–8.

84. Merrigan BA, Winter DC, O'Sullivan GC. Chylothorax. *British Journal of Surgery* 1997; **84:** 15–20.

85. Milsom JW, Kron IL, Rheuban KS, Rodgers BM. Chylothorax: an assessment of current surgical management. *Journal of Thoracic and Cardiovascular Surgery* 1985; **89:** 221–7.

86. Paes ML, Powell H. Chylothorax: an update. *British Journal of Hospital Medicine* 1994; **51:** 482–90.

87. Browse NL, Allen DR, Wilson NM. Management of chylothorax. *British Journal of Surgery* 1997; **84:** 1711–16.

88. Straaten HL, Gerards LJ, Krediet TG. Chylothorax in the neonatal period. *European Journal of Pediatrics* 1993; **152:** 2–5.

89. Freundlich IM. The role of lymphangiography in chylothorax. A report of six nontraumatic cases. *American Journal of Roentgenology, Radium Therapy and Nuclear Medicine* 1975; **125:** 617–27.

90. Miller JI. Diagnosis and management of chylothorax. *Chest Surgery Clinics of North America* 1996; **6:** 139–48.

91. Buttiker V, Fanconi S, Burger R. Chylothorax in children. *Chest* 1999; **116:** 682–7.

92. Selle JG, Snyder WH, Schreiber JT. Chylothorax: indications for surgery. *Annals of Surgery* 1973; **177:** 245–9.

93. Ullibarri JI, Sanz Y, Fuentz C, Mancha A, Aramendra M, Sanchez C. Reduction of lymphorrhagia from ruptured thoracic duct by somastatin. *Lancet* 1990; **2:** 258.

94. Hopkins RL, Akingbola OA, Frieberg EM. Chylothorax. *Annals of Thoracic Surgery* 1998; **66:** 1845–6.

95. Kent RP, Pinson RW. Thoracoscopic ligation of the thoracic duct. *Surgical Endoscopy* 1993; **7:** 52–3.

96. Wurnig PN, Hollaus PH, Ohtsuka T, Flege JB, Wolf RK. Thoracoscopic direct clipping of the thoracic duct for chylopericardium and chylothorax. *Annals of Thoracic Surgery* 2000; **70:** 1662–5.

97. Lampson RS. Traumatic chylothorax. A review of the literature and report of a case treated by mediastinal ligation of the thoracic duct. *Journal of Thoracic Surgery* 1948; **17:** 778–91.

98. Azizkhan RG, Canfield J, Alford BA, Rodgers BM. Pleuroperitoneal shunts in the management of neonatal chylothorax. *Journal of Pediatric Surgery* 1983; **18:** 842–50.

99. Engum SA, Rescorla FJ, West KW, Scherer LR, Grosfeld JL. The use of pleuroperitoneal shunts in the management of persistent chylothorax in infants. *Journal of Pediatric Surgery* 1999; **34:** 286–90.

100. Podevin G, Levard G, Larroquet M, Gruner M. Pleuroperitoneal shunt in the management of chylothorax caused by thoracic lymphatic dysplasia. *Journal of Pediatric Surgery* 1999; **34:** 1420–2.

101. Hasebrok K. Analyse einer chylosen pericardialen Flussigkeit (Chylopericardium). *Zeitschrift für Physiologie und Chemie* 1888; **12:** 289.

102. Dunn RP. Primary chylopericardium, a review of the literature and an illustrated case. *American Heart Journal* 1975; **89:** 369–77.

103. Gallant TE, Hunziker RJ, Gibson TC. Primary pericardium. The role of lymphangiography. *American Journal of Roentgenology* 1977; **129:** 1043–5.

104. Rao PS, Whisennand HH. Chylopericardium. *Annals of Thoracic Surgery* 1983; **36:** 499–52.

105. Lopez-Castilla JD, Soult JA, Falcon JM, *et al.* Primary idiopathic chylopericardium in a 2 month old successfully treated without surgery. *Journal of Pediatric Surgery* 2000; **35:** 646–8.

106. Chan BB, Murphy MC, Rodgers BM. Management of chylopericardium. *Journal of Pediatric Surgery* 1990; **25:** 1185–9.

107. Backer CL. Thoracic duct ligation for chylopericardium. *Journal of Thoracic and Cardiovascular Surgery* 1998; **115:** 734.

108. Hartnell GG. Laparoscopic pericardial fenestration. *Lancet* 1992; **340:** 737.

109. Sakata S, Yoshida I, Otani Y, Ishikawa S, Morishita Y. Thoracoscopic treatment of primary chylopericardium. *Annals of Thoracic Surgery* 2000; **69:** 1581–2.

110. Furrer M, Hopf M, Ris HB. Isolated primary chylopericardium: treatment by thoracoscopic thoracic duct ligation and pericardial fenestration. *Journal of Thoracic and Cardiovascular Surgery* 1996; **112:** 1120–1.

17

The relationship between the lymphatics and chronic venous disease

Veins and lymphatics are inextricably linked. Their endothelial parentage is probably identical as lymphatics and veins have a common origin. They have synergistic functions, the lymphatics clearing the tissues of what the cardiovascular system, particularly the veins, leaves behind. Both venous and lymph flow depend in part upon peripheral skeletal muscle pumping, and consequently the principles underlying compression therapy for chronic venous disease and lymphoedema are similar.

VENOUS AND LYMPHATIC DEVELOPMENT

Vasculogenesis is the development of vascular endothelium from mesoderm-derived precursors called angioblasts. Angiogenesis is the sprouting or splitting of capillaries from existing vessels once the primary vascular plexus has formed. Whereas angiogenesis continues throughout life, vasculogenesis is restricted to embryonic development.

Pro-angiogenesis factors exert their effects via specific cell surface receptor tyrosine kinases. One receptor, vascular endothelial growth factor receptor-3 (VEGFR-3, originally called FLT4), for which the ligands are VEGF-C and VEGF-D, has been found, on day 12 of mouse embryogenesis, to be present on venous and presumptive lymphatic endothelium but not arterial endothelium. At a later stage of development, VEGFR-3 becomes restricted to the endothelium of the lymphatics and the post-capillary venules of adult tissues.[1] The gene for

VEGFR-3 is now known to be responsible for lymph-angiogenesis, mutations in this gene being the cause of Milroy's disease.[2] This recent molecular work therefore supports the widely accepted theory of Sabin, who, in 1908, suggested that lymphatics developed from veins.[3,4]

GENETIC DISORDERS AFFECTING BOTH VEINS AND LYMPHATICS

Developmental malformations in which anomalies of the veins and lymphatics co-exist are well described. Such conditions tend to be sporadic, implying that the fault is caused by a somatic, rather than a germline, genetic mutation. In Klippel–Trenaunay syndrome, for example (see Chapter 18), the presenting problem may be lymphoedema caused by lymphatic hypoplasia even though the condition's main features are venous abnormalities (varicosities and deep vein aplasia), elongated bone growth and soft tissue hypertrophy.

Inherited forms of lymphoedema may also have associated venous abnormalities. In lymphoedema–distichiasis syndrome, for which the underlying gene is now known,[5] childhood-onset varicose veins are a frequent finding. In a four-generation, 70-member family with lymphoedema–distichiasis syndrome, all those with definite lymphoedema (confirmed by lymphoscinti-graphy) had both clinical and functional evidence of venous disease.[6]

PHYSIOLOGY OF OEDEMA IN VENOUS DISEASE

Oedema is a frequent finding in patients with moderate-to-advanced venous disease,[7] in whom it is often considered to be solely caused by increased capillary filtration ('venous' oedema). Chronic venous hypertension increases the time-averaged capillary pressure and consequently the average filtration rate. In normal circumstances, lymph flow increases to compensate, and this mechanism presumably operates satisfactorily in those patients with venous disease who exhibit no oedema. By inference, oedema associated with venous disease must be caused by either capillary filtration overwhelming lymph drainage or a failure of the lymph-collecting system in its own right (lymphoedema). Studies of the epidemiology and clinical features of oedema in venous disease suggest the latter hypothesis. In a study of 58 patients with chronic venous ulcers, Prasad et al.[8] found that 55 per cent of individuals exhibited pitting oedema and that, when clinical criteria were used to judge the presence of lymphatic insufficiency, 22 per cent (13 out of 58) of ulcerated limbs showed skin changes typical of lymphoedema, namely a positive Kaposi–Stemmer sign and features of elephantiasis.

INITIAL LYMPHATIC NETWORK IN THE SKIN IN VENOUS DISEASE

Gravity generates high intravascular pressures in dependent regions such as the lower leg, causing high levels of capillary filtration even without venous disease. A desirable adaptation to cope with the high fluid load and limit oedema would be a high lymph drainage capacity. There is in fact a more extensive dermal lymphatic network in the leg than the arm, this creating a greater surface area for tissue fluid absorption. Stanton et al., using fluorescence microlymphography, stereologically analysed a mosaic of the dermal lymphatic network and found both the radial lymphatic length density and the maximum lymphatic density to be significantly greater in the leg than the arm (Fig. 17.1).[9]

Chronic ambulatory venous hypertension caused by venous reflux means that high capillary pressure and filtration persist even during walking, leading to a chronic fluid overload on the lymph-collecting system. Fluorescence microlymphography using FITC-dextran as a tracer has revealed morphological abnormalities of the dermal lymphatic capillaries in the gaiter skin of patients with incipient venous ulceration[10] and an increasing obliteration of the lymphatic network accompanying the advance in trophic skin changes. There is also an increased leakage of FITC-dextran from the initial lymphatics in trophic skin compared with that of normal skin, indicating an increased lymphatic permeability. Studies

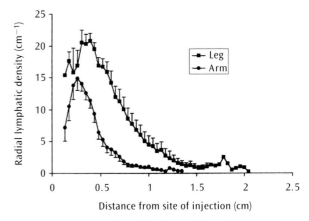

Figure 17.1 The density of the dermal lymphatics in the forearm and lower leg of 16 men aged between 19 and 25 years, measured at increasing distances from the centre of an injected upper-dermal depot of FITC-dextran. The distance of spread (the radial lymphatic density) and the maximum lymphatic density are significantly greater in the leg than the arm. Adapted from reference 9.

using indirect lymphography have also confirmed structural damage to the lymphatic network in venous disease.[11]

LOWER LIMB LYMPH DRAINAGE IN VENOUS DISEASE

Studies using direct lymphography have demonstrated the main limb lymphatic trunks to be largely intact in chronic venous disease. Nevertheless, the occasional reflux of injected contrast material from the main lymph trunks into the dermal lymphatic network (dermal backflow) some distance from the injection site suggests a fault within the lymph drainage pathways. In a quantitative lymphoscintigraphic study of patients with venous ulcers, lymphatic function, as measured by the ilio-inguinal lymph gland uptake of isotopic tracer lymph drainage, has been demonstrated to be significantly impaired in ulcerated legs (Fig. 17.2).[12]

Lymphoscintigraphy measures all three stages of lymph flow:

- the bulk flow of escaped plasma proteins and fluid through the interstitial matrix towards the initial lymphatics;
- the entry into and passage of lymph along the initial lymphatics;
- the active propulsion of lymph within the contractile lymphatic collectors to the regional lymph glands.

Lymph gland uptake measurements (unlike direct lymphography) therefore reflect initial lymphatic as well as collector lymphatic function. There are no abnormalities of the main collecting lymphatics in limbs with post-thrombotic syndrome following an iliofemoral

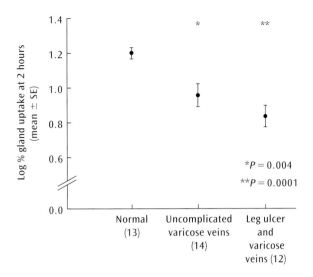

Figure 17.2 *The inguinal lymph gland uptake of ^{99m}Tc-labelled antimony sulphur colloid, injected subcutaneously into the first web space of the foot, of 26 patients with chronic venous hypertension and of 13 normal subjects. There is significantly reduced lymph transport in the patients with uncomplicated varicose veins and a still greater reduction in those with venous ulceration. Adapted from reference 12.*

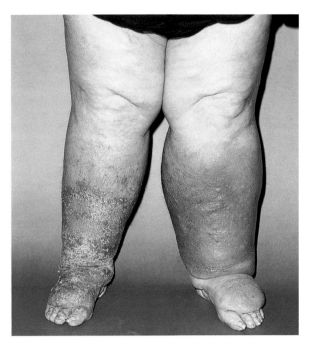

Figure 17.3 *Lymphoedema resulting from long-standing venous disease. Venous eczema and some venous oedema are present in the right leg, but the swelling on the patient's left is worse and caused by secondary lymphatic insufficiency. Bilateral long saphenous vein incompetence is evident.*

thrombosis,[13] and we have not found any abnormalities of the collecting lymphatics of legs in chronic venous disease and ulceration.[14] It is therefore likely that the impaired lymph drainage that has been demonstrated in ulcerated limbs, in non-ulcerated limbs with venous trophic changes, in legs with deep vein incompetence and with increasing age in normal limbs[12] in the presence of what other studies[13,14] have shown to be anatomically normal-looking collecting lymphatics on X-ray lymphography indicates a deficiency of interstitial matrix lymph flow and initial lymphatic absorption.

The significance of a study of subfascial lower limb lymph drainage in patients with post-thrombotic syndrome following an intramuscular injection of tracer into a calf muscle,[11] which demonstrated reduced subfascial lymph transport, is uncertain.

IMPLICATIONS FOR TREATMENT

The lymph-collecting system appears to be able to cope with the increased lymph production that accompanies uncomplicated venous disease, but damage to the initial lymphatics by local inflammation and the chronic fluid overload as the venous disease progresses seems, in some instances, to lead to lymph drainage failure. To what extent deep vein thrombosis compromises subfascial lymph drainage is not known. The variable and unpredictable collateral lymph drainage via the epifascial, subcutaneous and skin vessels that develops when the normal routes are damaged, just as it does with the veins, probably accounts for the considerable variability of the clinical picture.[15]

Lymphoedema is not a cause of skin ulceration, but any form of oedema is certainly a discouragement to wound healing, and treatment directed towards its elimination is essential if the tissue destruction (lipodermatosclerosis) and ulceration are to be prevented or delayed. The presence of oedema in limbs exhibiting post-thrombotic syndrome and/or venous ulcers indicates that treatment is suboptimal (Fig. 17.3).

Infection, particularly recurrent lymphangitis/cellulitis, is a known complication of lymphoedema but not venous disease. Its recurrence in venous ulcer patients should alert the clinician to the likelihood of lymphatic insufficiency and prompt a review of the adequacy of compression therapy. It may not be a coincidence that the optimal compression therapy for venous ulcers, for example the four-layer bandage method,[16] is little different in principle from and has a similar effect to multilayer lymphoedema bandaging techniques. Treatments designed to improve lymph as well as venous drainage are ideal for advanced venous disease (*see* Chapter 9).

There has been a tendency over recent years to discount the role of the lymphatics in the production of the tissue damage caused by chronic venous insufficiency. This appears to be derived from the false assumption that the presence of normal collecting lymphatics implies that the microlymphatics are also normal, and has perhaps been perversely encouraged by our inability to treat any damaged initial and microcollecting lymphatics. The microlymphatic circulation in venous insufficiency needs further investigation, but in the meantime the reduction of oedema by proper adequate compression therapy must be pursued, with the understanding that it is not only the veins that are causing the oedema.

REFERENCES

1. Kaipainen A, Korhonen J, Mostonen T, et al. Expression of the fms-like tyrosine kinase 4 gene becomes restricted to lymphatic endothelium during development. *Proceedings of the National Academy of Sciences of the USA* 1995; **92:** 3566–70.

2. Karkkainen MJ, Ferrell RE, Lawrence EC, et al. Missense mutations interfere with VEGFR-3 signalling in primary lymphoedema. *Nature Genetics* 2000; **25:** 153–9.

3. Sabin FR. On the origin of the lymphatic system from the veins. *American Journal of Anatomy* 1902; **1:** 367.

4. Sabin FR. Further evidence on the origin of the lymphatic endothelium from the endothelium of the blood vascular system. *Anatomical Record* 1908; **2:** 46–55.

5. Fang J, Dagenais SL, Erickson RP, et al. Mutations in FOXC2 (MFH-1), a forkhead family transcription factor, are responsible for the hereditary lymphoedema distichiasis syndrome. *American Journal of Human Genetics* 2000; **67:** 1382–88.

6. Rosbotham JL, Brice GW, Child AH, et al. Distichiasis lymphoedema: clinical features, venous function and lymphoscintigraphy. *British Journal of Dermatology* 2000; **142:** 148–52.

7. Mortimer PS. Implications of the lymphatic system in CVI-associated edema. *Angiology* 2000; **51:** 3–7.

8. Prasad A, Ali-Khan A, Mortimer PS. Leg ulcers and oedema: a study exploring the prevalence, aetiology and possible significance of oedema in venous ulcers. *Phlebology* 1990; **5:** 181–7.

9. Stanton AWB, Patel HS, Levick JR, Mortimer PS. Increased dermal lymphatic density in the human leg compared with the forearm. *Microvascular Research* 1999; **57:** 320–8.

10. Bollinger A, Senring G, Franzeck UK. Lymphatic microangiopathy, a complication of severe chronic venous incompetence. *Lympnology* 1982; **15:** 60–5.

11. Partsch H, Urbanek A, Wenzel-Hora B. Dermal lymphangiography in chronic venous incompetence. In: Bollinger A, Partsch H, Wolfe JHN eds. *The initial lymphatics*. Stuttgart: Thieme, 1985: 178–87.

12. Bull RH, Gane JN, Evans JEC, Joseph AE, Mortimer PS. Abnormal lymph drainage in patients with chronic venous leg ulcers. *Journal of the American Academy of Dermatology* 1993; **28:** 585–90.

13. Negus D, Edwards JM, Kinmonth JB. The iliac veins in relation to lymphoedema. *British Journal of Surgery* 1969; **56:** 481–6.

14. Kinmonth JB. *The lymphatics*. London: Arnold, 1982.

15. Tiedjen KU, Knorz S, Heimann KD. The skin: lymphatic collateral organ? *Scope – On Phlebology and Lymphology* 1994; **1:** 7–12.

16. Blair SD, Wright DDI, Backhouse CM, Riddle E, McCollum CN. Sustained compression and healing of chronic venous ulcers. *British Medical Journal* 1988; **297:** 1159–61.

18

The lymphatics in congenital and mixed arterial abnormalities

There are an almost infinite variety and mixture of congenital arterial and venous abnormalities of the limbs, with an equal number of descriptive titles and eponyms. Because the arterial or venous abnormality is the clinically obvious dominant feature and the main cause of the patient's symptoms, the possibility of a concomitant lymphatic abnormality is usually ignored. There are, however, often lymphatic abnormalities accompanying venous or arterial abnormalities, which may make a significant contribution to the symptoms and signs. A number of investigators have tried to produce an inclusive classification of the peripheral vascular abnormalities, with a small degree of success.[1–6] Kinmonth has argued[7] that it is simpler and of greater clinical value to group them together under the single name of 'mixed vascular deformities' and then subdivide them according to the dominant vascular abnormality – venous, arteriovenous fistulae and angiomata.

The most common congenital venous abnormality affecting a whole limb is the Klippel–Trenaunay syndrome, which comprises congenital varicose veins, a cutaneous naevus and limb hypertrophy.[2] Although these patients may have a slightly increased limb blood flow caused by the increased blood flow through the naevus,[8] they do *not* have arteriovenous fistulae.

The preponderant arterial abnormality affecting a whole limb is the Parkes Weber syndrome,[3] also known as Robertson's giant limb,[9] a syndrome encompassing multiple, congenital, microscopic arteriovenous fistulae causing overgrowth of the limb and sometimes high-output heart failure.

The common localized arterial and/or venous abnormalities are the angiomata, which present as isolated masses of hamartomatous vascular tissue, sometimes purely venous, sometimes purely arteriolar, but often mixed.

This group includes patients with haemangiomata and dyschondroplasia, Maffucci's syndrome.[10,11]

Some patients have clinical features of more than one of these three groups, but they are rare, and one of the three syndromes is usually dominant. This chapter describes the state of the lymphatics as defined by lymphography in these three groups.

LYMPHATICS IN KLIPPEL–TRENAUNAY SYNDROME

The earliest reports of single cases of the Klippel–Trenaunay syndrome (Fig. 18.1) mention abnormalities such as oedema and cutaneous vesicles that were probably lymphatic in origin but not recognized as such at the time.[1,12,13] Beck[12] described oedema in addition to muscle hypertrophy. Freidberg[13] mentioned vesicles, which he called pemphigus. Trelat and Monod's case[1] also had tissue oedema, but, surprisingly, Klippel and Trenaunay, in their important paper,[2] did not mention the presence of oedema. In 1962, Servelle[14] reported eight patients with Klippel–Trenaunay syndrome who had elephantiasis.

In 1971, Pokrovosky et al.[15] performed lymphograms on 19 patients with venous angiodysplasias and found lymphatic hypoplasia in three, but it is not clear how many of his patients had true Klippel–Trenaunay syndrome. In 1973, Biasi et al.[16] studied 12 patients with angiodysplasias, six of whom probably had Klippel–Trenaunay syndrome, and found three of the six to have lymphatic hypoplasia. Hamatake,[17] in 1974, studied six patients with 'haemolymphatic disorders' who appeared to have Klippel–Trenaunay syndrome and found hypoplastic lymphatics in four.

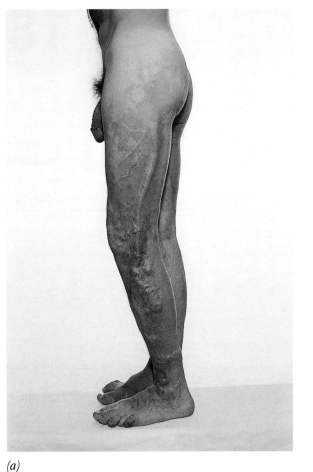

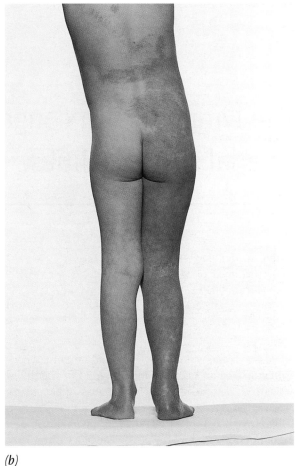

(a)   *(b)*

Figure 18.1 *Klippel–Trenaunay syndrome: varicose veins, cutaneous naevi and limb hypertrophy. (a) Limb hypertrophy and congenital varicose veins. (b) The naevus and its metameric distribution.*

Between 1965 and 1985 we saw, at St Thomas' Hospital, London, more than a hundred patients with Klippel–Trenaunay Syndrome, 49 of whom have been the subject of a special study.[8] The lymphograms that were performed on 14 of this group[7,8,18,19] revealed:

- cutaneous lymph-filled vesicles (that only very rarely connected with the main collecting lymphatics) in 22 per cent;[8]
- clinically apparent lymphoedema in 15 per cent;[8]
- distal aplasia or numerical hypoplasia in 75 per cent (Fig. 18.2).[8,18] The number of lymphatics seen in the thigh was reduced by 50 per cent (from a mean for a normal limb of 11 to 4.5),[20] with a similar 50 per cent reduction in their diameter, in both the calf and the thigh;[20]
- after injection into the groin lymph glands, a reduced number of iliac lymphatics was observed (Fig. 18.3);
- fewer and smaller inguinal and iliac lymph glands (Fig. 18.3).[19] In a comparison between 65 normal lymphographs and eight from patients with Klippel–Trenaunay syndrome, the number of inguinal and iliac lymph glands was reduced from 6 to 2, and 8 to 2, respectively.[20]

Comment

Klippel–Trenaunay syndrome is a congenital but not an inherited disorder. We have seen one family in which two siblings each had the condition in one leg but have never seen a patient with a family history of the condition. In the 49 patients subject to our special review,[8] the abnormality was present at birth in 43 and appeared before the age of 10 in the other six.

The absence of any evidence of an inherited genetic defect, together with the presence of abnormalities in the bones (overgrowth), soft tissues (hypertrophy) and lymphatics (hypoplasia), as well as other conditions such as syndactyly and hypospadias, strongly suggests that Klippel–Trenaunay syndrome is a generalized mesodermal developmental abnormality.[21] A mesodermal defect or event occurring in utero at a very early age primarily affecting angiogenesis could explain all the clinical features, the bony and soft tissue abnormalities being the consequence of the changes in limb haemodynamics following the failure of the veins to develop properly and the persistence of some of the primitive vascular reticular network in the cutaneous naevi.[21]

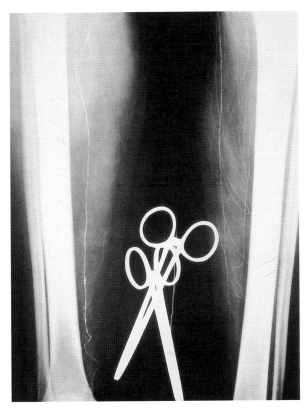

Figure 18.2 *Bilateral lymphograph showing the reduced number of lymphatics opacified in the right leg in Klippel–Trenaunay syndrome compared with the usual number in the normal left leg.*

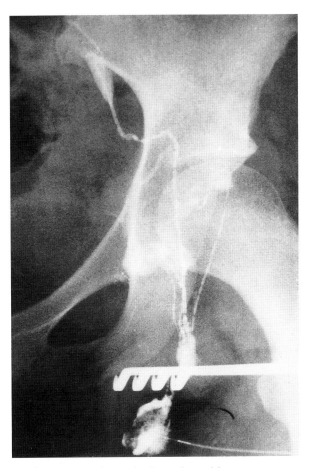

Figure 18.3 *Lymphograph of a patient with Klippel–Trenaunay syndrome who had no detectable lymphatics in the foot, the lymphograph being obtained by injecting the Lipiodol into an inguinal lymph gland. A reduced number of small inguinal and iliac lymphatics and glands are seen.*

As the development of the veins and the lymphatics are closely linked, it is not surprising that there should be a lymphatic abnormality in the majority of cases and that this should be a failure to develop (aplasia or hypoplasia) similar to the failure of the deep veins to develop properly that occurs in 20 per cent of patients with Klippel–Trenaunay syndrome.[8] Two of our patients have undergone two lymphograms performed 4 and 5 years apart. In both cases, the second lymphograph was identical to the first, suggesting that there is not a progressive obliteration of the distal lymphatics but a true congenital deficiency. We therefore believe that the lymphatic abnormality is a true congenital distal aplasia or numerical hypoplasia and that there is currently no evidence to suggest that there is an underlying germline genetic abnormality.

Treatment

The lymphatic abnormalities (the lymphoedema and vesicles) are rarely the principal symptom, but when they are they should be treated in the standard way. Areas of leaky vesicles may be excised. Gross swelling unresponsive to conservative treatment may be surgically excised (*see* Chapters 10 and 11), but special care must be given to the prevention of deep vein thrombosis, which is a common and life-threatening complication of any form of major surgery on patients with Klippel–Trenaunay syndrome,[8] and to the prevention of excessive bleeding from the multitude of subcutaneous varicose veins.

LYMPHATICS IN PARKES WEBER SYNDROME

Although one of the features of the Parkes Weber syndrome (multiple arteriovenous fistulae)[3] (Fig. 18.4) is an overgrown, enlarged limb, none of the original case descriptions suggested that some of the increase in size might have been lymphoedema until Robertson's detailed review in 1956.[9] In his study, Robertson stated that 'a degree of lymphoedema is not infrequently present' and described three patients with 'huge lymphatics in the groin' – presumably dilated, incompetent megalymphatics that were visible to the naked eye. Although, at the time of this report, lymphangiography was in its infancy, some of these cases were studied by Kinmonth and colleagues[7,22,23] and found to have dilated tortuous lymphatics.

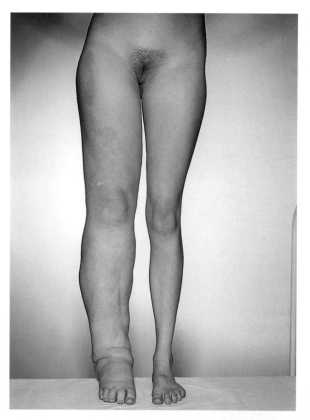

Between 1965 and 1975, we performed lymphograms on 13 patients with Parkes Weber syndrome.[18] Nine of their enlarged limbs had dilated, tortuous, sometimes incompetent megalymphatics (Fig. 18.5a and b). This abnormality was usually worse in the lower half of the limb, the average number and diameter of both calf and thigh lymphatics being increased by 60 per cent and 50 per cent, respectively.[20] The number of inguinal lymph glands lay in the normal range, but in this group of patients the number of iliac glands was reduced (Fig. 18.5c). Two limbs had normal lymphatics. No lymphatics could be found in the dorsum of the foot of two patients, but this is likely to have been caused by an acquired obliteration secondary to recurrent inflammation and ulceration around the ankle rather than being a true aplasia. The lymphatics of the patients' normal limbs were normal.

The effect of the greatly increased blood flow through these limbs would be to increase lymph production. A permanently increased lymph flow would cause

Figure 18.4 *Parkes Weber syndrome. A young woman with overgrowth of the whole limb caused by multiple arteriovenous fistulae.*

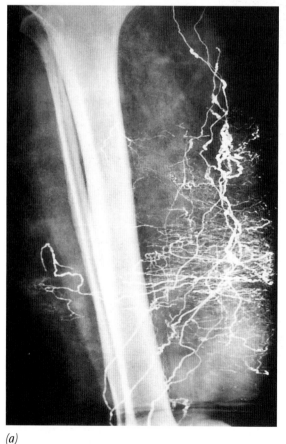

(a)

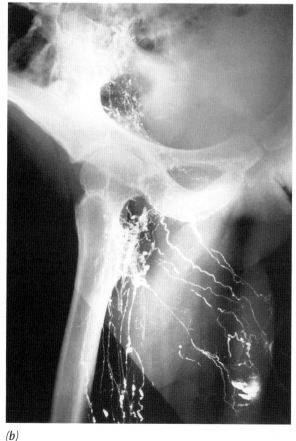

(b)

Figure 18.5 *Lymphatics in the Parkes Weber syndrome. (a) Dilated tortuous lower leg lymphatics. (b) Dilated tortuous upper thigh and iliac lymphatics opacified by a bipedal lymphogram combined with the injection of Lipiodol into a vesicle on the inner side of the thigh.*

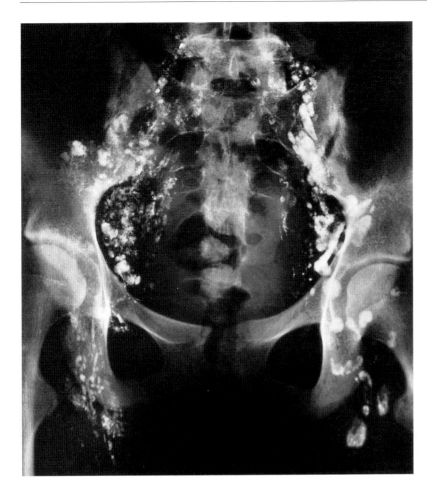

Figure 18.5c *Multiple small right iliac lymph glands situated between the dilated tortuous iliac lymphatics of a patient with Parkes Weber syndrome of the right leg. The dilatation of the lymphatics is beginning to spread to the left side.*

lymphatic dilatation. Thus, the lymphatic abnormality (megalymphatics) may be a secondary, acquired phenomenon rather than part of the congenital arteriovenous abnormality. Although the mean number of inguinal and iliac lymph glands was normal, the range was much greater – three patients had 50 per cent fewer than the normal mean number and four had 50 per cent more. The latter glands were fragmented and lay between dilated iliac lymphatics (Fig. 18.5c). It is likely that these changes resulted from differences in lymph and arterial blood flow and did not reflect a primary congenital abnormality.

The observation by Young[19] that half the patients with megalymphatics had a minor thoracic duct abnormality is unlikely to be relevant because the true incidence of minor variations of thoracic duct anatomy is unknown and it is difficult to envisage why or how multiple arterio-venous fistulae in a limb could affect a short segment of the thoracic duct in the chest. The balance of the evidence points to the conclusion that the lymphatic abnormalities found in limbs with multiple arteriovenous fistulae (dilatation, tortuosity and incompetence) are an acquired phenomenon caused by an increased lymph flow rather than a primary congenital abnormality.

Treatment

The lymphoedema rarely needs surgical reduction and, because of the risk of severe haemorrhage, should be avoided. Lymphatic vesicles caused by lymph reflux may be treated in the standard way (*see* Chapter 10), but to avoid the risk of bleeding complications, it is best to choose the smallest procedure possible, for example a simple superficial excision of the troublesome vesicles, rather than an extensive ligation of deep, incompetent lymphatics.

LYMPHATICS IN LIMBS WITH MULTIPLE OR DIFFUSE ANGIOMATA

In our study of seven patients with scattered mixed angiomata (Fig. 18.6), some of which were venous, others capillary and some haemolymphangiomatous, we found a variety of abnormalities: 2 were normal, 3 had a reduced number of lymphatics, and 2 had numerical hyperplasia.[18] The patients with hypoplastic lymphatics had vessels that were narrower than normal, and possessed fewer inguinal and fewer iliac lymph glands than

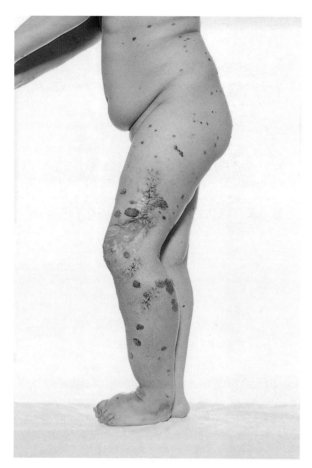

Figure 18.6 *An example of a patient with multiple angiomata. The patients we studied with multiple angiomata showed no specific pattern of lymphatic abnormality.*

usual.[20] None of these patients had lymphoedema or any other stigmata of a lymphatic abnormality.

The small number studied and the diverse nature of the lesions makes it impossible to deduce any clear relationship between the lymphatics and the angiomata. It might be that venous angiomata are associated with hypoplastic lymphatics in a way similar to that observed in Klippel–Trenaunay syndrome. On the other hand, none of the angiomata contained localized arteriovenous fistulae, so the finding of two patients with numerical hyperplasia out of a group of seven must remain unexplained.

Treatment

Angiomata may be excised, but they are sometimes extensive and the advice and assistance of a plastic/reconstructive surgeon is often needed.

MAFFUCCI'S SYNDROME

This syndrome[10,11] consists of diffuse, multiple haemolymphangiomata accompanied by severe deformities of bone and cartilage. The original descriptive title was

'haemangiomata with dyschondroplasia', but bone as well as cartilage is in fact involved, and there are usually lymphangiomata as well as angiomata. The lymphatics of these patients, in the tissues and limbs involved, are abnormal, the vessels and glands usually being hypoplastic.[7]

Treatment

There is no treatment for the basic genetic abnormality, but troublesome angiomata can be excised if indicated. The lymphatic elements of the haemolymphangiomata do not connect with the main collecting trunks but may lie very close to them, an important anatomical relationship to be taken into account if an angioma is to be excised.

REFERENCES

1. Trelat U, Monod A. De l'hypertrophie unilaterale partielle ou totale du corps. *Archives Générale Médicale (Paris)* 1869; **13:** 536–58.
2. Klippel M, Trenaunay P. Du noevus variqueux osteo-hypertrophiques. *Archives Générale Médicale (Paris)* 1900; **185:** 641–72.
3. Parkes Weber F. Angioma formation in connection with hypertrophy of limbs and hemi-hypertrophy. *British Journal of Dermatology* 1907; **19:** 231–5.
4. Malan E. *Vascular malformations.* Milan: Carlo Erba, 1974.
5. Vollmar J. Zur Geschichte und Terminlogie der Syndrome nach F. Parkes Weber und Klippel–Trenaunay. *Vasa* 1974; **3:** 231–41.
6. Mulliken JB, Glowacki J. Hemangiomas and vascular malformations in infants and children: a classification based on endothelial characteristics. *Plastic and Reconstructive Surgery* 1982; **69:** 412–22.
7. Kinmonth JB. *The lymphatics.* London: Arnold; 1972.
8. Baskerville PA, Ackroyd JS, Lea Thomas M, Browse NL. The Klippel–Trenaunay syndrome: clinical, radiological and haemodynamic features and management. *British Journal of Surgery* 1985; **72:** 232–6.
9. Robertson DJ. Congenital arteriovenous fistulae of the extremities. *Annals of the Royal College of Surgeons* 1956; **18:** 73–98.
10. Bean WB. *Vascular spiders and related lesions of the skin.* Springfield, IL: Charles C. Thomas, 1958.
11. Carlton A, Elkington JStC, Greenfield JG, Robb-Smith AHT. Maffucci's syndrome. *Quarterly Journal of Medicine* 1942; **11:** 203–7.
12. Beck G. Hypertrophie congénitale d'un membre. *Archives of General Medicine* 1837; **13:** 99.
13. Freidberg H. Riesenwuchs des rechten Beines. *Virchows Archives* 1867; **40:** 353.
14. Servelle M. *Oedèmes chroniques des membres.* Paris: Masson, 1962.

15. Pokrovosky AV, Moskalenko JD, Tkhor SN. The state of the lymph system in congenital arterial and venous disease. *Vesn. Khir.* 1971; **107:** 74.

16. Biasi G, Sala A, Bigliol R. La linfografia nelle angiodisplasie degli arti. *Angiologia: Minerva Chirurgia* 1973; **28:** 918–25.

17. Hamatake Y. Clinical studies of congenital angiodysplasias in limbs. *Fukuoka Acta Medica* 1974; **65:** 833–63.

18. Kinmonth JB, Young AE, Edwards JM, O'Donnell TF, Thomas ML. Mixed vascular deformities of the lower limbs, with particular reference to lymphography and surgical treatment. *British Journal of Surgery* 1976; **63:** 899–906.

19. Young AE. Mixed Vascular Deformities. MChir thesis, University of Cambridge, 1978.

20. O'Donnell TF Jr, Edwards JM, Kinmonth JB. Lymphography in congenital mixed vascular deformities of the lower extremities. *Journal of Cardiovascular Surgery (Torino)* 1976; **17:** 535–40.

21. Baskerville PA, Ackroyd JS, Browse NL. The aetiology of the Klippel–Trenaunay syndrome. *Annals of Surgery* 1985; **202:** 624–7.

22. Kinmonth JB, Kemp Harper RA, Taylor GW. Lymphangiography by radiological methods. *Journal of Faculty of Radiology* 1955; **6:** 2–8.

23. Kinmonth JB, Taylor GW, Tracy GD, Marsh JD. Primary lymphoedema: clinical and lymphangiographic studies of a series of 107 patients in which the lower limbs were affected. *British Journal of Surgery* 1957; **45:** 1–10.

19

Lymphangiomata, lymph cysts and fistulae, lymphangiomatosis and lymphangiosarcoma

The term 'lymphangioma' is widely used to describe benign neoplastic or hamartomatous conditions of the lymph vessels. There are three forms of lymphangioma. Some consist of a mass of microscopically sized lymphatics within a thin capsule (lymphangioma simplex), others are collections of much larger, macroscopic, dilated lymphatics with muscular walls (lymphangioma cavernosa), and the third form comprises the large lymph cyst(s) (cystic lymphangioma/hygroma).[1-3] These variations in form and the fact that they often occur together make lymphangiomata difficult to classify and have given rise to a variety of confusing descriptive names. The terms 'hygroma' and 'lymphangioma' are synonymous. The addition of the adjective 'cystic' to any of these three varieties should depend solely upon whether or not the lymph-filled cavities are large enough to be seen, felt and, if big enough, demonstrate the physical characteristics of a cyst, namely fluctuation and a transmitted percussion thrill.

The most important feature of all lymphangiomata is the fact that they are *not part of the normal lymph-conducting system*. Even though some, such as the microscopically dilated lymphatics of lymphangioma simplex sometimes connect with normal lymphatics and may be partly filled during an injection into a subcutaneous collecting lymphatic, they do not interfere with or interrupt normal lymph conduction.

To add to the diagnostic confusion, it should be remembered that dilated conducting lymphatics may be as large as those seen in lymphangiomata and collections of them look like lymphangiomata; they are not, however, hamartomata or benign malignancies but simply ectatic conducting vessels. Confusion between *lymphangiectasis* of the conducting vessels and the dilated vessels that form a lymphangioma is a common cause of misdiagnosis.

This chapter discusses the clinical management of five benign lymphangiomatous malformations. Four of these – cystic hygroma, intra-abdominal retroperitonal lymphangioma and mesenteric lymph cysts, intrathoracic lymphangioma and lymphangioma circumscriptum – are clinically distinct and well known to paediatricians, dermatologists and surgeons. The fifth, which we call lymphangiomatosis, occurs in the subcutaneous tissues and bone, is extremely rare and has not previously been well described. There is only one malignant disease of lymphatics: lymphangiosarcoma.

CYSTIC HYGROMA (CYSTIC LYMPHANGIOMA)

Cystic hygroma is the name given to large lymph cysts, usually solitary, often lobulated and loculated and sometimes multiple, that develop in the subcutaneous tissues. They were first described by Redenbacher in 1828.[4] Although most often found in the neck, cystic hygromata can occur in the axilla, groin, mediastinum and retroperitoneum.

It is generally accepted that these cysts are remnants of primitive lymph vessels that, having failed during embryonic life to become part of the developing lymph-conducting system, became isolated enclosed sacs. Why some fill with lymph to a considerable size before birth while others remain empty until adult life is not known.

The mechanism by which lymph-like fluid is secreted into and/or resorbed from them has not been defined.

The name 'hygroma' has been used for almost 200 years, but the more correct pathological name is cystic lymphangioma.

Clinical features

Approximately 50 per cent of cystic hygromata are present at birth, mainly in the neck and superior mediastinum but sometimes in the axilla and groin (Fig. 19.1a–e).[5]

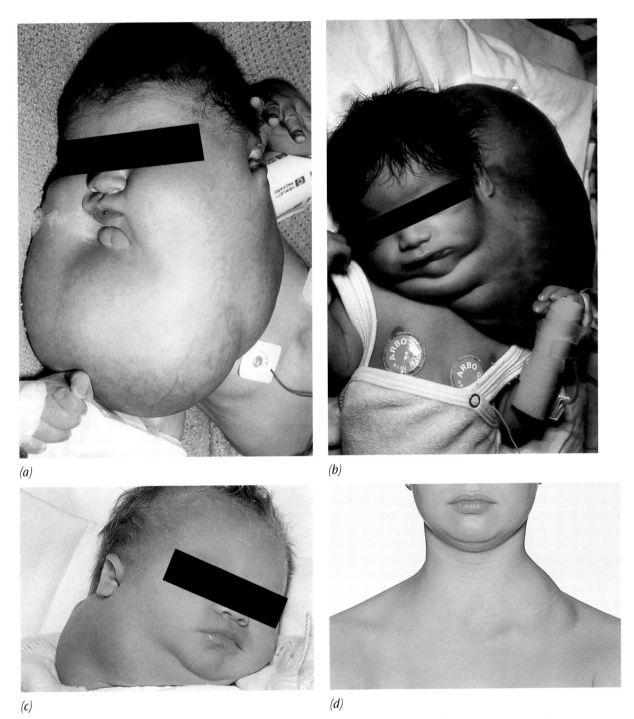

(a)

(b)

(c)

(d)

Figure 19.1a–d *Cystic hygromata (cystic lymphangiomata). (a, b) Examples of the massive cystic hygromata that can cause severe respiratory embarrassment. (a) A lesion that occupies the whole of the anterior aspect of the neck. (b) A lesion on the left posterolateral aspect of the neck that is causing acute lateral flexion of the neck and breathing difficulties. (c) A slightly smaller but more typical neonatal cystic hygroma causing considerable disfigurement but not affecting breathing or swallowing. (d) The majority of cervical cystic hygromata lie at the base of the posterior triangle of the neck just above the clavicle. This patient's cyst was excised when she was a child but reappeared 10 years later.*

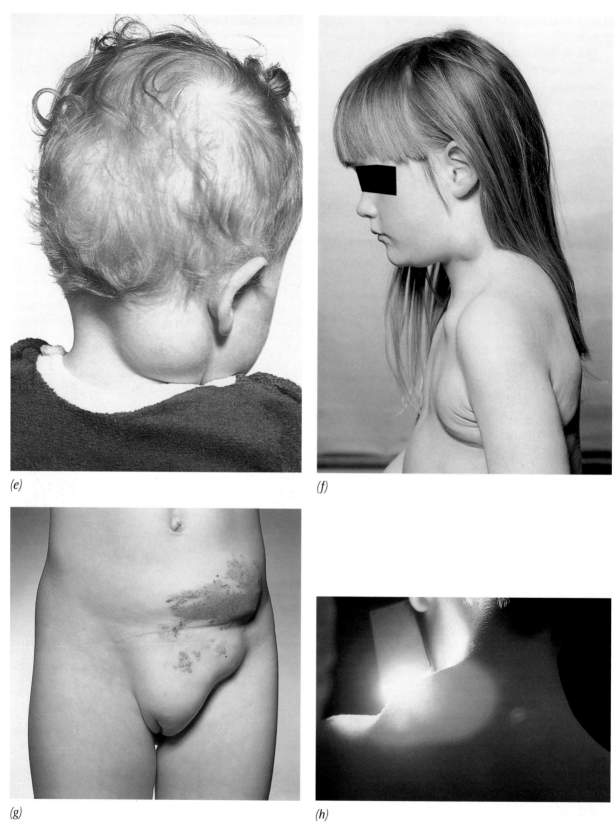

(e)

(f)

(g)

(h)

Figure 19.1e–h *(e) A posterior cervical cystic hygroma. (f) A large cystic hygroma of the axilla and a small hygroma in the upper part of the neck. (g) A cystic hygroma in the groin associated with an overlying lymphangioma circumscriptum. (h) Brilliant translucence, the classical diagnostic feature of a cystic hygroma. Illustrations a, b and f reproduced by kind permission of the Department of Paediatric Surgery, Queen's Medical Centre, Nottingham.*

Most of the remaining 50 per cent present during the first few years of life, but a few lie dormant for many years and present in adult life,[6] often following a stimulus to secretion into the cyst such as a minor injury or an upper respiratory tract infection with cervical lymphadenitis. The fluid occasionally absorbs spontaneously and the swelling disappears. Cystic hygromata are usually lobulated, soft, fluctuant, non-tender swellings. Their diagnostic clinical sign is brilliant translucence.

In the short neck of an infant, the swelling may interfere with swallowing and breathing, impair movement and cause a scoliosis of the cervical spine (Fig. 19.1a and b). If a cyst becomes infected, it enlarges and becomes painful. Episodes of infection occur in 25 per cent of cases.[5] A sudden increase in size may be caused by haemorrhage into the cyst. This occurred in 10 per cent of Broomhead's series, one case having a fatal outcome.[5] Sudden enlargement is more likely to cause swallowing or respiratory problems.

Investigation

It is important to define the extent of a hygroma before choosing treatment because it is often much more extensive than clinical examination suggests.

Plain X-rays, *ultrasound*, *computed tomography* (CT) and *nuclear magnetic resonance* (NMR) scans,[7–10] with and without the injection of a radio-opaque contrast medium into the cyst, are all helpful. Although some cystic swellings are multilobular with open communications between the lobules, others are collections of separate non-communicating cysts that cannot be opacified by a single injection. Ten per cent of cervical cystic hygromata plunge into the mediastinum and insinuate themselves between major vessels and nerves, with their thin wall closely adherent to these structures. This potential surgical hazard is best displayed by a CT or NMR scan (Fig. 19.2). Prenatal ultrasound studies may detect the presence of a cystic hygroma in utero.[11,12]

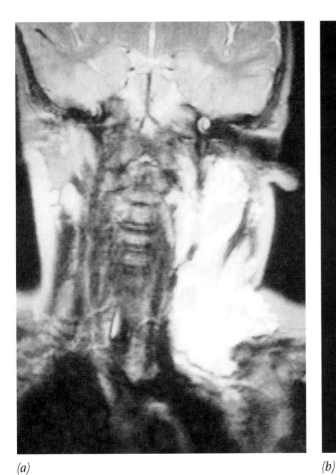

(a)

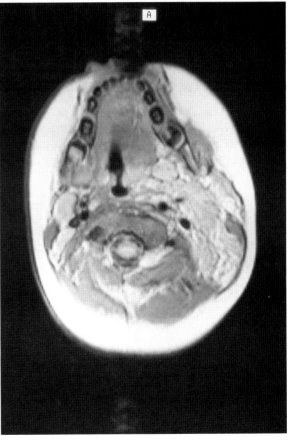

(b)

Figure 19.2 *Nuclear magnetic resonance scans of a large lobulated cystic hygroma in the neck. (a) Axial STIR scan showing the cyst surrounding the major neck vessels and extending down below the clavicle. (b) Coronal STIR scan showing the cyst extending medially deep to the mandible and displacing the pharynx to the right. Reproduced by kind permission of the Department of Paediatric Surgery, Queen's Medical Centre, Nottingham.*

Cystic hygromata on the left side of the neck may lie close to the last few centimetres of the thoracic duct. If it is felt necessary to identify this relationship, the thoracic duct should be opacified by performing a bipedal lymphangiogram. Whereas lymphangiography is rarely helpful in defining the anatomical relationships of cervical cystic hygromata because they do not connect or interfere with the normal lymphatics of the head and neck or arm, it is important to define the normal lymphatic anatomy before excising a cystic hygroma in the groin or axilla in order to avoid damaging adjacent lymphatics and causing lymphoedema.

Treatment

Aspiration

Aspiration to reduce the size of the cyst may be necessary as an emergency procedure if the cyst has suddenly enlarged and is causing problems with swallowing or breathing. Sudden enlargement is sometimes caused by infection so it is important to culture the aspirate and, if indicated, administer an appropriate antibiotic. Very rarely, fluid will not re-collect after aspiration; it is thus always worthwhile trying aspiration before considering other forms of treatment.

Sclerotherapy

The ideal 'minimally invasive' treatment would be an injection that destroyed the cyst's endothelium and obliterated the cystic space, but cystic hygromata unfortunately have three anatomical features that make this difficult to achieve:

- Multicystic lesions are not uncommon and require separate injections into each cyst.
- Lobulated lesions are difficult to fill if the connections between the lobules are narrow.
- Even if all the endothelium is destroyed, the position of the cysts often makes it difficult to compress their walls together and obliterate the space by either external compression or internal suction, especially if the cyst is lying in the superior mediastinum.

Many sclerosants – hypertonic saline, boiling water, quinine, urethane, ethanolamine, talc – have been tried, but none of these has regularly produced long-term success.[13] The injection of bleomycin[14–16] has produced better results but has been discontinued following reports that it may cause the development of pulmonary fibrosis. In 1987, Ogita and colleagues[17] reported the effect of injecting the substance OK-432. OK-432 is produced by culturing the low-virulence Su strain of type III group A *Streptococcus pyogenes* with penicillin G potassium, followed by lyophilization, which results in the disappearance of any streptolysin-S-producing ability.[18]

OK-432 was first used to treat malignant intrapleural and intraperitoneal effusions.[19]

In a series of 9 patients with ages ranging from 4 months to 14 years, aspiration and a single injection of OK-432 'cured' 5, a second injection 'cured' another 3, and 1 patient was improved but not cured.[17] The word 'cured' is presented in inverted commas because the follow-up of this study was very short – 6–12 months – but these results are better than those usually obtained for sclerotherapy, with few side-effects, such as slight tenderness and a temporary increase in size of the cystic hygroma. Thus, although this injectate is clearly not the final answer, this study suggests that methods of injection sclerotherapy should be pursued.

Sclerotherapy can be of some benefit even when it fails as it usually leaves the wall of the cyst thickened, fibrous and much easier to remove surgically than the very thin friable wall of a virgin cyst.

Surgical excision

The complete excision of a cyst or cysts guarantees a permanent cure. Incomplete excision resulting from technical or anatomical difficulties is, however, associated with a recurrence rate of approximately 50 per cent.[5,20]

Surgery should be avoided in the early weeks of life because it is technically difficult and risky. Complications, such as respiratory or alimentary obstruction, infection and haemorrhage, can usually be alleviated by aspiration. If aspiration fails, partial excision of the easily accessible part of the cyst will relieve the symptoms and allow a further attempt at excision years later.

There is no optimum time for attempting excision, but most paediatric surgeons prefer to wait until the child is at least 2 years old, and in cases not associated with symptoms or significant disfigurement, the operation can be delayed into adolescence or adult life. The chance of incomplete excision and recurrence, damage to the recurrent laryngeal and other cervical nerves, even damage to the oesophagus and, in neonates with massive cysts, death must be fully explained to the parents or patient. Modern scanning techniques that display all the anatomical relations of the cyst give the surgeon a far clearer idea of the likelihood of such complications occurring.

The majority of cervical cystic hygromata can be approached through a skin crease incision low in the neck, taking care not to divide more than one or at the most two of the supraclavicular nerves. Splitting the manubrium sterni to reach cysts in the superior mediastinum is rarely justifiable. The wall of a previously untreated cyst consists of a very thin layer of fibrous tissue lined by a layer of flattened endothelial cells. Septae and areas where cysts lie together often consist of little more than two layers of endothelium. The walls of the cyst are extremely fragile and often break when touched, held or pulled by forceps in the course of the dissection. Dissection must therefore be extremely gentle and meticulous. There are few blood vessels in the cyst wall so minor bleeding and oozing is rarely a problem. Previous aspirations or attempts at sclerotherapy that have made the wall of the cyst thicker, stronger and easier to handle may also have made it more adherent to adjacent structures and more vascular.

When faced with a friable area of cyst wall adherent to a vital structure such as a nerve or major blood vessel, it is better to accept an incomplete excision than damage a vital structure because it must always be remembered that cystic hygromata are benign, rarely life-threatening lesions. A small recurrence is preferable to a damaged recurrent laryngeal nerve or a major intraoperative haemorrhage.

The chance of residual pieces of the cyst wall developing into recurrent cysts can be reduced by scraping off their endothelium with a curette, painting the internal surface with a cytotoxic agent, such as diluted ethamoline, hypertonic saline or a cytotoxic wound washout fluid, and placing suction drains to stop fluid collecting and help adjacent cyst walls to adhere together.

INTRA-ABDOMINAL RETROPERITONEAL LYMPHANGIOMATA AND MESENTERIC LYMPH CYSTS

The preceding section discussed the common variety of large, often solitary cystic lesions that develop in the subcutaneous tissues of the neck, axilla, groin and breasts. Similar lesions may occur within the abdomen, but one third of abdominal lymphangiomata are either lymphangioma simplex (masses of microscopically sized lymphatics that often communicate with the adjacent normal lymphatics) or lymphangioma cavernosum (large clusters of macroscopically cavernous lymphatics with muscular walls that only sometimes connect with the adjacent normal lymphatics).[21] Mesenteric lymph cysts and retroperitoneal lymphangiomata are rare conditions estimated to occur in fewer then 1 per 100 000 hospital admissions and accounting for only 5 per cent of all lymphangiomata.[22]

Although the two are of similar pathology and embryological origin, we apply the term 'retroperitoneal lymphangioma' to the multicystic, cavernous lymphangiomata behind the posterior peritoneum that may spread forwards into the root of the mesentery, and reserve the term 'mesenteric cyst' for the large single (or multiple) cysts that are found within the mesentery or sometimes in the omentum. Both varieties may present at any age, but retroperitonal lymphangiomata usually become apparent during childhood whereas mesenteric lymph cysts are more often discovered during adult life.

Although there are two histologically distinct types of retroperitoneal lymphangiomata – lymphangioma simplex and cavernosa – they behave in a similar manner, and some pathologists consider that subdividing them in this way is irrelevant, particularly as different varieties often occur together.[1–3,23,24] On the other hand, mesenteric lymph cysts differ histologically and clinically from the other two types of lymphangiomata. Unlike normal lymphatics, they are often lined by cubical or columnar endothelium, do not have any muscle cells in their wall[25,26] and behave differently. Lymphangiomata are more likely to enlarge and insinuate themselves between adjacent structures[21] whereas mesenteric lymph cysts enlarge slowly and tend to displace adjacent tissues.

Clinical presentation

Both retroperitoneal lymphangiomata and mesenteric lymph cysts invariably present as abdominal distension or an abdominal mass.

Retroperitoneal lymphangioma

Retroperitoneal lymphangioma usually presents in the first 2 years of life[27] as a soft, slowly enlarging mass, sometimes associated with mild abdominal discomfort or a 'dragging' sensation. There is often an associated ascites, sometimes chylous in nature.[21] Acute pain caused by an intralesional haemorrhage or infection is rare[28] and often misdiagnosed as appendicitis.[29] Extensive lesions may be associated with a consumptive coagulopathy.[30] If the lesion enlarges, it may press upon adjacent structures and produce the symptoms of subacute or chronic intestinal obstruction[31] or ureteric obstruction.[32,33] When diffuse, enlarging lesions presenting in adult life are frequently thought to be malignant.[34]

Mesenteric cysts

Mesenteric cysts are usually symptomless and detected by chance during a routine physical examination or laparotomy. If they suddenly enlarge following an intracystic haemorrhage or infection, they may cause acute abdominal pain or intestinal obstruction. Acute pain may also be caused by rupture or torsion.[28,35,36]

Investigation

Ultrasound scans will detect single and multicystic lesions and indicate their relationship to adjacent structures, similar information also being gathered from *CT* and *NMR* scans (Fig. 19.3). Routine *plain X-rays* are of little value but may reveal calcification in the wall of a long-standing cyst. A *barium meal and follow-through* or an *excretory urogram* is indicated if there are symptoms suggestive of intestinal or ureteric obstruction.

It is important to know the relationship between a lymphangioma and the normal lymphatics lest a patch of lymphangiectasis (pathologically dilated lymph-conducting lymphatics, possibly associated with chylous reflux) be misdiagnosed as a lymphangioma (pathologically proliferating, non-conducting, closed lymphatic

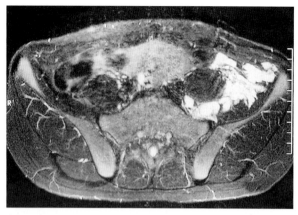

(a)

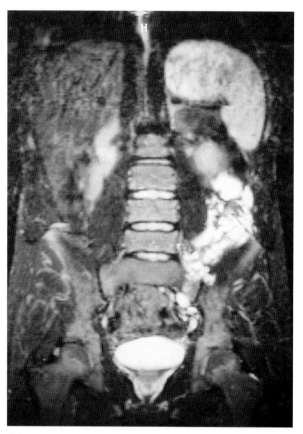

(b)

Figure 19.3 *A nuclear magnetic resonance scan of an extensive retroperitoneal cystic hygroma, consisting of many independent and some interconnecting cysts. (a) Coronal T2-weighted scan showing the lesion extending between the iliacus and psoas muscles. (b) Axial turbo spin-echo scan showing the lesion extending upwards to the lower pole of the left kidney. Reproduced by kind permission of the Department of Paediatric Surgery, Queen's Medical Centre, Nottingham.*

channels without smooth muscle proliferation). For this reason, we perform bilateral ascending *lymphograms* on all patients except those with clearly solitary or multi-locular cysts confined to the mesentery.

Treatment

The treatment of choice is complete excision. This may involve resection of part of any organ involved, such as bowel.[21] When complete excision is not possible, usually because the lesion is diffuse and extensive, the excision of as much of the lesion's walls as possible and internal marsupialization is an acceptable alternative, although it carries a risk of recurrence.[37] Marsupialization should not be performed if there is a significant connection between the lesion and the normal lymphatics or lacteals as this might produce an ascites of lymph or chyle, which might require a further laparotomy to cure it.

INTRATHORACIC LYMPHANGIOMATA

Intrathoracic lymphangiomata are found in all three mediastinal compartments, anterior, superior and posterior, approximately one third occurring in each. They are rare and account for only 1 per cent of all lymphangiomata.[38]

Almost all the lesions in the superior mediastinum are extensions of cystic hygromata in the neck. Most present in children and young people, causing symptoms and giving rise to complications similar to those associated with cervical cystic hygroma, as described above. They do not connect with the normal lymphatics.

The lesions in the anterior and posterior mediastinum usually have a mixed cavernous and cystic structure, present in adult life and are symptomless. They are often first detected on a routine chest radiograph. On rare occasions, they present with complications such as chylothorax, infection causing pain and dyspnoea or skeletal pain from an associated vanishing bone disease (Gorham's syndrome).[39,40]

Investigation

Plain chest radiographs usually reveal the lesion but not its relationship to adjacent structures, this information being best obtained from a *CT* or *NMR* scan.[41]

Any lesion with an associated lymph or chylous pleural effusion and *all* lesions in the posterior mediastinum should be studied with *bipedal lymphograms* to ascertain the relationships between the lesion and the thoracic duct, and the presence of any reflux of lymph into the lesion, lungs or pleural cavity. If reflux is present, a diagnosis of lymphangiectasis (incompetent lymph-conducting megalymphatics) rather than lymphangioma should be considered.

Gorham's syndrome[39,40] is an osteolytic disease of bone caused by angiomatosis within bone that is sometimes associated with lymphangiomatous changes in the adjacent soft tissues. As it most often affects the thoracic vertebrae and ribs, the associated lymphangiomata are invariably intrathoracic. All patients with intrathoracic lymphangiomata should undergo full spinal and rib X-ray studies.[42]

Treatment

Provided the symptoms justify major surgery, the best treatment is complete excision. Lesions in the superior mediastinum may lie between and be closely adherent to the great vessels. Partial excision, curettage and suction drainage to obliterate the space is often a safe option when set against the risks of major vessel or nerve damage, even though partial excision carries an increased risk of recurrence. When excising lesions in the posterior mediastinum, it is important to identify and preserve the thoracic duct. Lymphangiomata associated with Gorham's syndrome may be very vascular and are best treated expectantly rather than surgically.

Lymphangio*leiomyo*matosis, a rare, low-grade neoplasm of the smooth muscle of the lymphatic wall that occurs in women in their reproductive years, may, when it affects the lungs, produce appearances clinically and radiologically similar to those of a diffuse lymphangioma or lymphangiectasis (*see* Chapter 4).

TRAUMATIC LYMPH CYSTS (LYMPHOCELE) AND LYMPH FISTULAE

Lymphatics are divided every time tissues are disrupted by accidental or deliberate surgical trauma. As the flow of lymph through each lymphatic is small, divided lymphatics normally collapse, and their cut ends become blocked with fibrin. The wound then heals normally. This natural closing process may not, however, occur if a collection of lymph glands or large lymphatics, such as those found in the groin and around the iliac arteries and abdominal aorta, are divided. If lymph continues to leak from divided lymphatics, it collects in the tissues in the form of a large pseudo-cyst, usually called a lymphocele.

Lymphoceles are a well-recognized complication of surgery in the groin,[43] especially if a number of inguinal lymph glands are divided, and following renal transplantation if both the iliac artery and vein are widely exposed and manipulated. In both these sites, the leaking lymph can become a large palpable pseudocyst, a lymphocele. Should the lymphocele burst through the overlying wound, a lymph fistula results. Damage to the lymphatics around the abdominal aorta during vascular surgery or aortic lymphadenectomy[44,45] may likewise leave lymphatics leaking lymph and chyle into the abdominal cavity to produce a chylous ascites. A similar complication may follow blunt trauma.[46] Extensive excision of the axillary glands may also be complicated by a postoperative axillary lymphocele.

The diagnosis and differentiation from a haematoma can easily be made with an ultrasound scan or by aspirating some of the contents of the swelling. Its extent can be determined by the direct injection of a radio-opaque contrast medium.

The majority of lymphoceles collapse after one or two aspirations or the insertion of a fine tube and continuous suction drainage. When aspiration fails, the only effective treatment is surgical ligation of the leaking lymphatic.[47] In an easily accessible area, such as the groin, the leaking lymphatic can usually be found by gently opening the wound, injecting 2 mL Patent Blue Violet into the subcutaneous tissues of the upper thigh and gently massaging the thigh until the dye appears out of the leaking lymphatic in the wound. The leaking lymphatic can then be ligated or oversewn and the wound closed with suction drainage. If a leaking point cannot be found, the subcutaneous tissues of both sides of the wound must be firmly oversewn with a continuous stitch in the expectation that the stitch will occlude the leaking vessel.

A similar surgical approach can be applied to a lymph fistula from a groin wound, but if the leak is not too copious, it is simpler to wait for up to 3 weeks (keeping leg exercise to a minimum) for spontaneous closure. We have found that the mild tissue inflammation produced by a small dose of therapeutic irradiation will often cause closure.

An iliac lymphocele that re-collects after repeated aspiration can also be cured by ligating the leaking lymphatic, but in this case the leak may be from a vessel on the distal, proximal or lateral side of the lymphocele and thus not always demonstrable with the Patent Blue Violet subcutaneous injection method. It is therefore advisable to define the precise site of the leak by performing a preoperative lymphogram, taking frequent films when the Lipiodol reaches the level of the lymphocele, in order to determine the exact site where fluid leaks from the lymphatics and enters the cyst (Fig. 19.4).

Iatrogenic postoperative chylous ascites that does not respond to repeated paracentesis plus a low-fat diet with medium chain triglycerides or even a period of total parenteral nutrition (*see* Chapter 16)[48] should also be treated by oversewing the leaking area after determining its position with a preoperative lymphogram.

LYMPHANGIOMA CIRCUMSCRIPTUM

Lymphangioma circumscriptum is a mainly subcutaneous cavernous lymphangioma that extends into and through the skin. First described by Fox and Fox in 1879[49] and in more detail in 1893 by Francis,[50] it has been the subject of great interest to dermatologists and the cause of many case reports over the years.

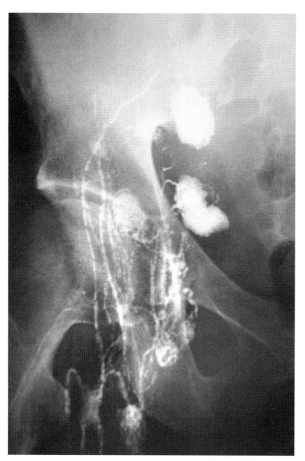

Figure 19.4 *A lymphocele on the side wall of the pelvis, which developed following a kidney transplant. Pedal lymphography showed normal lymphatics up to the right groin and then Lipiodol filling a large, bilobed lymph cyst immediately above the inguinal ligament. A direct injection of contrast medium into the cyst, which was palpable, would not have revealed whether the leaking lymphatics were proximal or distal to the cyst.*

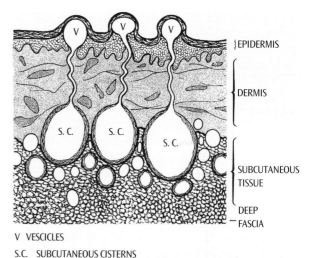

V VESCICLES
S.C. SUBCUTANEOUS CISTERNS

Figure 19.5 *A diagramatic representation of the relationship between the muscular deep subcutaneous cysts of a lymphangioma circumscriptum (s.c.) and the small vesicles (v) on the skin surface. The latter are blow-outs from the former produced by the regular contractions and resulting high pressure that occurs in the subcutaneous cysts. Reproduced from reference 51.*

Pathology

Although the prominent clinical feature of the lesion is translucent vesicles on the skin, it has long been recognized that there are also cysts beneath the skin. The relationship between the two was a subject of much debate, until Whimster,[51] in 1976, described the pathophysiology of the lesion. The subcutaneous cysts have a thick muscular wall (the feature that makes this a cavernous lymphangioma).

The skin vesicles are thin-walled saccular dilatations from the cysts of the subcutaneous lymphangioma that penetrate through the dermis to appear on the skin surface as vesicles (Fig. 19.5). Measurement of the pressure within the subcutaneous cysts[51] revealed that the walls contract rhythmically and contract in response to percussion (Fig. 19.6). The skin vesicles often appear long after the subcutaneous cysts have first been noticed.

These observations, and the fact that skin excision and grafting with a split-skin or pedicle graft, without excision of the deep cysts, is associated with the reappearance of the skin vesicles on the graft, has led to the conclusion that the prime pathological abnormality is the muscular-walled subcutaneous cavernous lymph cysts and that the skin vesicles are simply 'blow-outs' from the deep cysts produced by their repeated contraction.

The deep cysts are closed spaces, connecting neither with each other nor with the normal lymphatics that run around them.[52] They must therefore be small blind segments of primitive lymphatics that have failed to connect into the developing lymphatic system in utero. An appreciation of the underlying physiology that produces the skin vesicles is essential when planning effective treatment.

Clinical features[53]

The skin lesion consists of scattered translucent vesicles, up to 5 mm in diameter, in otherwise normal skin. These lesions are filled with clear yellow lymph and sometimes a little blood. Small quantities of blood make the vesicles pink or red, but if there is clotting, the vesicles turn a dark purple/black and eventually peel off like scabs (Fig. 19.7). The vesicles may break open and leak lymph for a few days. After drying up, they gradually refill. Patches of vesicles in an area rubbed by clothing may leak and become infected, which often causes the skin to become hyperkeratotic. As the years pass, the patch of vesicles gradually increases in size.

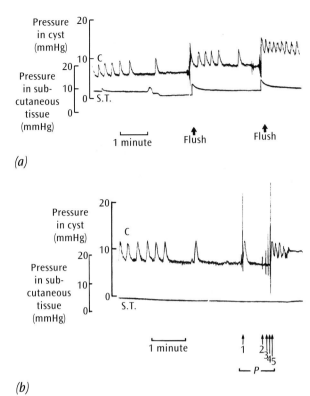

(a)

(b)

Figure 19.6 *The pressures in one of the subcutaneous cysts of a lymphangioma circumscriptum (C) and in the adjacent subcutaneous tissues (S.T.). (a) At rest, there were regular contractions every 5–10 seconds, which increased in frequency when the catheter was momentarily flushed. (b) The response to external percussion: five taps (P) on the cysts doubled the frequency of contraction. It is interesting that the frequency of contraction of these cysts is similar to that found in normal conducting lymphatics (see Chapter 3). Reproduced from reference 51.*

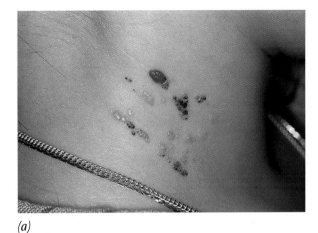

(a)

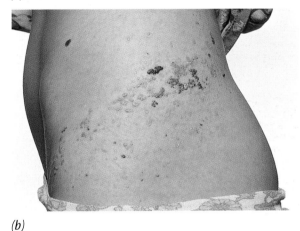

(b)

Figure 19.7 *Two examples of lymphangioma circumscriptum. (a) A small lesion less than 10 cm in diameter. (b) A large lesion covering the whole of the flank. The size of the lesion has a significant effect on the surgeon's ability to excise all of the subcutaneous cysts and thus effect a cure.*

Beneath every patch of vesicles, except for those with an area of less than 10 cm², is a subcutaneous collection of cysts that makes the subcutaneous layer thicker and the skin lesions more prominent. It is not always possible to find subcutaneous cysts large enough to palpate individually or to test for fluctuation. The thickened, swollen area beneath the skin vesicles fades away well beyond the limits of the skin vesicles.

The majority of skin lesions present at birth or within the first few years of life, but they occasionally appear after the age of 45 years. Females appear to be slightly more affected than males, but this may be a false impression related to a female concern about appearance. The skin vesicles may appear years after noticing the diffuse subcutaneous swelling.

Lymphangioma circumscriptum may appear anywhere on the skin but is most common on the limb–trunk junctional areas such as the upper chest wall, the neck and axilla, and the buttock and inguinal regions (Fig. 19.8). The condition can also occur deep to the mucous membranes and produce vesicles on the mucosal surface of the cheek, lip and tongue (Fig. 19.9).

Investigation

The diagnosis is made on the clinical appearance. The best description we have heard is that of a 6-year-old boy who said, 'My friends keep telling me that I've got "Rice Krispies" stuck to my skin.' The assessment of the extent of a lesion with a large amount of subcutaneous swelling may be helped by an ultrasound scan. Lymphographs are of no value except when lymph or chylous reflux is a possible differential diagnosis, at which point a lymphogram made via a vesicle may be helpful.

Treatment

Any treatment intended to produce a permanent cure must include the removal of all the subcutaneous cysts.

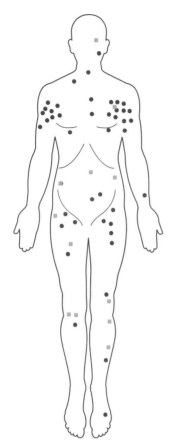

Figure 19.8 *The distribution of lymphangioma circumscriptum based upon Peachey et al.'s 65 cases.*[53] • *Larger than 1 cm² with palpable subcutaneous swelling (43).* ■ *Smaller than 1 cm² with no palpable subcutaneous swelling (12).*

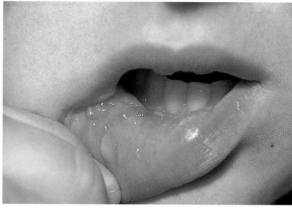

(a)

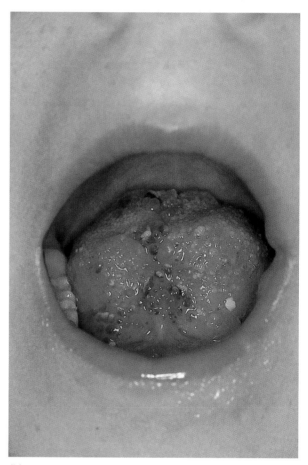

(b)

Figure 19.9 *Lymphangioma circumsciptum in and beneath the oral mucous membrane. (a) Typical golden-coloured lymph-filled vesicles beneath the buccal mucous membrane. (b) Lymphangioma circumscriptum affecting the superior and inferior surfaces of the tongue. The tip of the tongue had been excised 5 years earlier to remove large vesicles that were interfering with eating and speaking.*

Many superficial forms of treatment can remove the superficial vesicles, but if this is all that is achieved, recurrence is inevitable.

The superficial treatments that have been tried include carbon dioxide laser vaporization,[54,55] tuneable dye laser,[56] superficial radiotherapy[57,58] and simple electrocautery or diathermy. All may abolish the vesicles, but the effect is only temporary. Such treatments may be used as an adjunct to excision when the skin lesions are too extensive to excise in one sitting, even when all the subcutaneous cysts have been removed, or when the patient prefers temporary relief and repeated, non-invasive treatments to a more major surgical procedure.

Surgical excision should be designed to remove as many of the skin vesicles as possible consistent with a primary suture, plus the far wider excision of all the subcutaneous cysts (Fig. 19.10).[59] The necessary wide subcutaneous excision presents, however, two difficulties. First, the subcutaneous abnormality may be so large that its total removal would leave two thin potentially ischaemic skin flaps. In these circumstances, staged excisions should be planned 6–9 months apart, removing the central part of the skin lesion and as much subcutaneous tissue as possible at the first operation, and the original scar, more subcutaneous tissue and the remaining vesicles at the second.

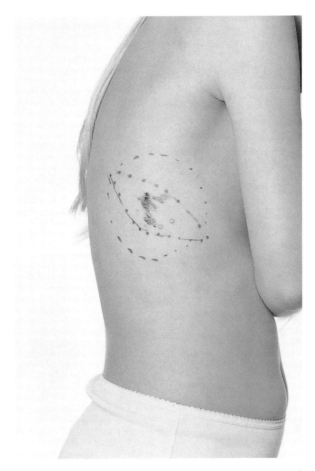

Figure 19.10 *The outline of the area of skin to be removed to eradicate the surface vesicles of a lymphangioma circumscriptum and the outline of the extent of the palpable subcutaneous cysts that must be removed to prevent recurrence. Although palpation can give a guide to the extent of the subcutaneous excision (useful information for preoperative counselling), the full extent of the excision can only be determined by the surgeon at operation. The excision must be continued until dry tissue with no minute fluid-filled cysts is reached. In this case, the subcutaneous cysts extended 3–5 cm beyond the outlined palpable thickening.*

Second, the excision of all the subcutaneous tissues over a much larger area than the region of excised skin leaves a significant depression, which around the buttock or outer thigh can be quite disfiguring. It is important to warn patients of this effect, especially if they are undergoing the procedure solely for cosmetic reasons. The extent of the skin excision is thus determined by the ability to obtain primary closure, and the extent of the subcutaneous excision by the viability of the skin flaps.

The limits of the subcutaneous excision can only be determined by the surgeon during the operation. As the flaps are raised, it is possible to see the cysts in the subcutaneous tissue. As the distance from the centre of the lesion increases, the cysts become smaller and the subcutaneous tissues less wet. Dissection should continue until cyst-free, normal, 'dry' fatty tissue is reached (Fig. 19.10). The whole subcutaneous mass down to the deep fascia should then be excised. After careful skin closure, suction drainage and local pressure are essential until the skin flaps are firmly fixed.

A review of 29 patients treated in this way, six of whom had staged operations, that was undertaken 2–8 years after their operations[59] showed all but three of the lesions to be controlled and the patients to be satisfied with the treatment. None of the small lesions (less than 10 cm maximum diameter) recurred. In those with large (over 10 cm maximum diameter) lesions, one lesion was too extensive to excise even with two operations, and the other two individuals had troublesome residual vesicles. No patient had developed new vesicles, and the vesicles that had to be left in the skin overlying the area of excised subcutaneous tissue regressed – an indication that the subcutaneous excision was the critical part of the operation.

In some places, such as the face, subcutaneous excision is not possible. On two occasions, we have partially removed the abnormal tissue of the cheek and chin by vigorous liposuction. This procedure, combined with needle-point diathermy destruction of vesicles on the buccal mucous membrane and/or partial excision of vesicles on the tongue, has provided worthwhile relief.[60]

SUBCUTANEOUS SPONGIFORM LYMPHANGIOMATOSIS

This condition is described separately because it does not fit into any of the three categories of lymphangioma described at the beginning of this chapter: it does not have well-defined boundaries, the cystic spaces communicate with each other and sometimes with the normal lymphatics, and it may be associated with multiple bone cysts (see below). For these reasons, the term 'lymphangiomatosis' – which implies a diffuse unrestricted form of lymphangiomatous malformation rather than a circumscribed lymphangioma – seems to be the most suitable name. The few clinical descriptions that exist all mention it in passing as an abnormality associated with skeletal lymphangiomatosis[61–63] rather than a condition in its own right.

Pathology

The multiple, subcutaneous interconnecting spaces have an extremely thin lining of flattened epithelium (Fig. 19.11).[64] The spaces contain a clear yellow fluid, sometimes stained pink with blood, or a coagulated, jelly-like lymph that may be reddish-purple in colour (Fig. 19.12). The spaces are not closed so cannot be called cysts; they are merely spaces lined with lymphatic endothelium.

Microscopically, these spaces infiltrate between collagen bundles and around the structures of the dermis and

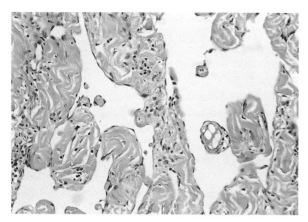

Figure 19.11 *A haematoxylin and eosin-stained cross-section through the tissues of spongiform lymphangiomatosis, showing them to be full of interconnecting lymph spaces lined with smooth, shiny epithelium. The tissues are disrupted (see Chapter 4).*

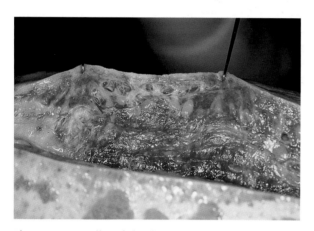

Figure 19.12 *A slice of the tissue removed from the patient illustrated in Fig. 19.13. The subcutaneous tissues can be seen to contain multiple cystic spaces and the tissues between them much haemosiderin.*

subcutaneous tissues, leaving islands of normal tissue. We have described this appearance as the 'hair-dryer' effect – the normal tissues looking as if they have been blown apart but otherwise preserved.[64] There are often lymphoid aggregates around the spaces and extensive deposits of haemosiderin in the surrounding stroma.

Clinical features

Subcutaneous lymphangiomatosis[64] causes swelling of the subcutaneous tissues, usually of the lower limb but sometimes of the arm. The swelling generally appears at birth or during early childhood.

Unlike normal lymphoedema, the swelling is soft, malleable and moveable. When the leg of the patient shown in Fig. 19.13 was elevated, all the fluid immediately ran up into the thigh, and the distension of the lower leg

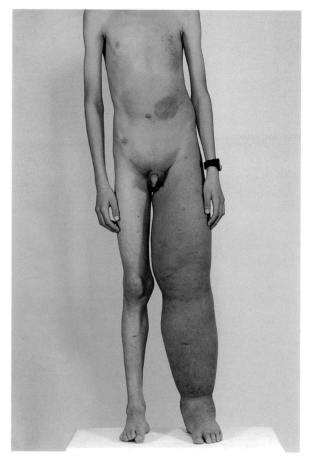

Figure 19.13 *Spongiform lymphangiomatosis. The swelling in this leg ran down to the ankle when the patient stood up but ran up to the thigh and groin within 30 seconds of the patient lying down and elevating the leg. The skin is hyperkeratotic and pigmented with haemosiderin. The swelling did not pit: it simply moved away when pressed.*

and foot collapsed, a clinical sign noted by Harris and Prandoni in 1950 in their report on a case of skeletal lymphangiomatosis.[61] The texture of the subcutaneous tissue, and the way in which the fluid within it moves around, is identical to that of water moving about in a large sponge, hence our use of the descriptive adjective 'spongiform'. *Normal interstitial lymphoedema cannot be moved about in this way.*

The skin overlying the swelling becomes hyperkeratotic and pigmented, the result of minor degrees of bleeding into the subcutaneous, cyst-like cavities. There are no vesicles on the skin. Infection is uncommon, and the only physical disabilities are those caused by the size and weight of the limb and the cosmetic disfigurement. Patients may have had a number of long bone fractures during the first few years of their life.

Investigation

Because this abnormality may be associated with skeletal and visceral lymphangiomatosis,[65] it is important to

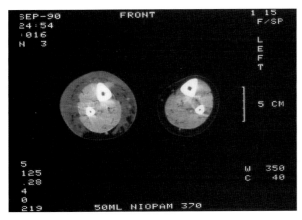

Figure 19.14 *Transverse computed tomography scan of the lower limb of a patient with spongiform lymphangiomatosis, showing multiple cystic spaces in the subcutaneous tissues of the right leg.*

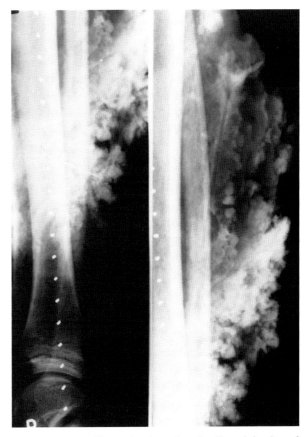

Figure 19.16 *Radiograph taken after the direct injection of a non-ionic contrast medium into a cystic space in the lower leg of a patient with spongiform lymphangiomatosis, showing interconnecting lymph-filled spaces throughout the subcutaneous tissues.*

perform a full skeletal *X-ray* survey to exclude bone involvement, and *CT* or *NMR* scans to exclude other asymptomatic lymphangiomata in the mediastinum or abdomen. A CT scan of the limb will define the extent of the subcutaneous changes (Fig. 19.14).

Lymphangiograms usually show a mixture of a few normal lymphatics and many dilated lymphatics joining the interconnecting cyst-like subcutaneous spaces (Fig. 19.15). Delayed films taken 2 or 3 days later may show Lipiodol in bone cysts. A direct injection of contrast medium into one of the fluid-filled spaces will spread throughout the lesion (Fig. 19.16) and give a good indication of its size and shape. The lymphangiogram should be continued until the lymphatics of the abdomen and chest are displayed if lesions in these sites are suspected.

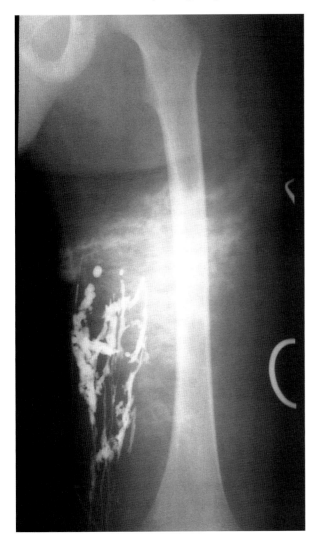

Figure 19.15 *Pedal lymphangiogram of a patient with spongiform lymphangiomatosis, showing normal lymphatics joining dilated irregular lymphatics and the Lipiodol beginning to fill lymph spaces around the whole thigh. One normal lymphatic continues up the thigh, bypassing the lymphangiomatosis.*

Treatment

Compression stockings have little or no effect, and repeated aspiration gives only temporary relief. In two patients, we have flushed the spaces through with a weak sclerosing agent (diluted ethanolamine) and then kept the spaces closed with suction drainage and external compression until their walls appeared to be sealed together. This produced two 6 month periods of relief in patients with swelling confined to the lower leg. Larger lesions would, however, require a dangerously large injection of sclerosant.

Simple surgical reduction – the staged Homans' operation (*see* Chapter 10) – is easy and effective. The spaces assist the dissection of the skin flaps and the visualization and preservation of the skin's nutrient arteries, but some degree of recurrence from spaces left in the deep dermis must be anticipated. Alternatively, a complete excision with a skin graft from normal skin – the Charles operation (*see* Chapter 10) – completely removes the lesion and guarantees a cure of the area excised. Unfortunately, many of these lesions occupy the whole length of the limb so a mixture of total excision below the knee and subcutaneous excision above is often the best compromise.

SKELETAL LYMPHANGIOMATOSIS

Lymphangiomatous spaces in bone were first described by Bickel and Broders in 1947.[66] Since then, many more cases have been reported, often associated with other lymphatic abnormalities.[67,68] Subcutaneous spongiform lymphangiomatosis, as described in the previous section, is probably part of a spectrum of disease that at one extreme affects only the subcutaneous tissues and at the other affects only the bones, with mixed varieties in between.

We know very little about the lymphatics of bone. None of the standard textbooks on lymphatic anatomy mentions their existence, yet the periosteum is richly endowed with lymphatics,[66] and lymphatics can also be seen accompanying the blood vessels in the haversian canals.[66,61] Whether the large cyst-like spaces lined with lymphatic endothelium that develop in bone are derived from these lymphatics or are part of a generalized abnormality of all the lymphatics is not known. The finding of lymphatic abnormalities in all the bones, including those which were radiologically normal, during the post mortem of a 1-year-old infant with skeletal lymphangiomatosis, together with other soft tissue lymphatic abnormalities,[69] supports the latter hypothesis. Lymphangiomatosis is probably a widespread genetic abnormality of lymphatics that affects all tissues to varying degrees and thus causes many varied forms of clinical presentation.

Clinical features

Skeletal lymphangiomatosis commonly presents in the first 20 years of life as an underlying cause of repeated fractures or is discovered on routine X-rays obtained when investigating other complaints, such as swelling of a limb, back pain, chest pain or dyspnoea.[67] All the bones can be affected, but the long bones of children and young adults are the ones that are most often broken. Compression fractures of the vertebrae can cause back and nerve root pains.[68]

Cysts that gradually increase in size may become visible or palpable masses, be locally painful and tender and affect the movement, use and growth of a limb. Cysts close to joints may restrict movement and cause effusions. Lesions in the ribs may cause pleuritic pain, and pleural effusions may cause dyspnoea.[70] Hepatic and splenic involvement may cause abdominal pain and distension.[71] There may also be symptoms and signs related to other lymphangiomatous lesions in the soft tissues and viscera.[63,72]

Investigations

The whole skeleton should undergo *X-ray* examination. Typical lesions (Fig. 19.17) are demineralized areas, usually spherical, with a sclerotic border, and often expanding the bone. Previous fractures may have caused bone distortion and thickening. *CT* and *NMR* scans may be required to assess the adjacent soft tissue involvement, particularly when the spinal cord or nerves are becoming compressed.[68]

As the radiological changes are non-specific, it is important to exclude, by suitable haematological and metabolic tests, other conditions that cause areas of bone demineralization, for example hyperthyroidism, von Recklinghausen's disease, polyostotic fibrous dysplasia

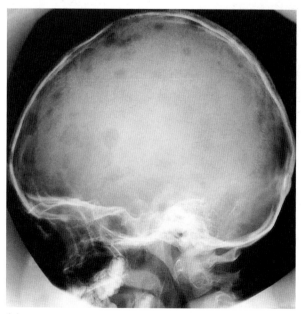

(a)

Figure 19.17 *Four examples of lymphangiomatous cysts in bones. (a) In the skull of an 8-year-old boy.*

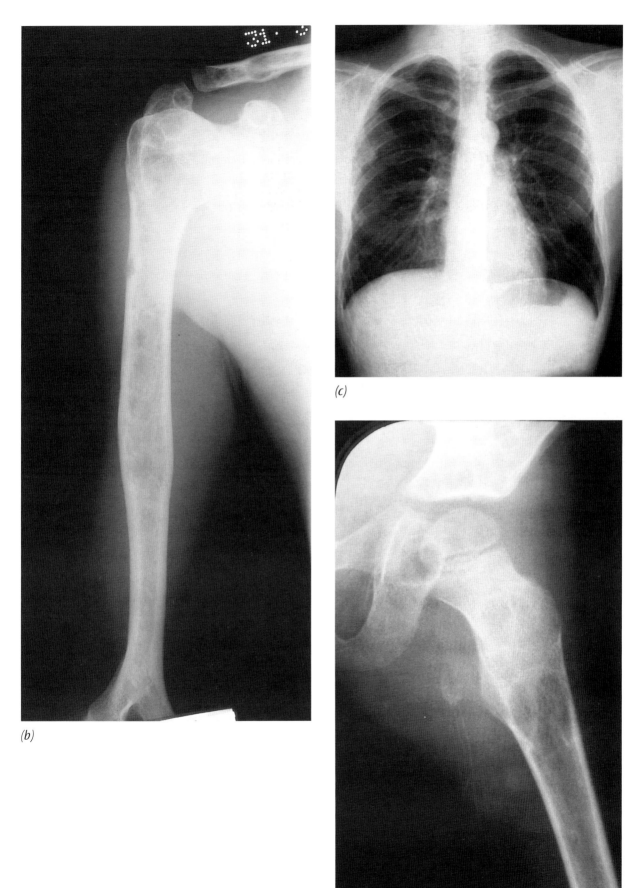

Figure 19.17b–d (b) In the humerus of a 30-year-old man. (c) In the ribs of a 30-year-old man. (d) In the femur and pelvis of a 10-year-old boy.

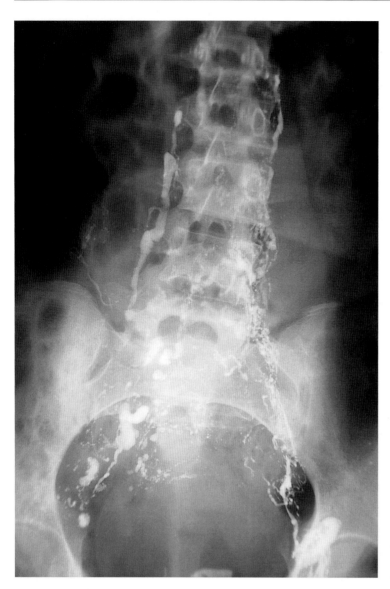

Figure 19.18 *The lymphangiograph of an 18-year-old woman with cysts in all her bones (clearly visible in the bones of her pelvis), which revealed retroperitoneal megalymphatics with reflux down to the floor of the pelvis.*

(Albright's syndrome),[73] multiple haemangiomata, multiple myeloma, secondary neoplastic deposits and diseases of lipid metabolism. Lymphangiography is not helpful with regard to the bone cysts, although some Lipiodol may enter them, but may show other concomitant lymphatic abnormalities such as megalymphatics and reflux (Fig. 19.18).

Extensive lesions can almost completely destroy the bone and suggest a diagnosis of vanishing bone disease (Gorham's syndrome)[65] so *biopsy* of one of the lesions may be necessary to establish the diagnosis, especially if only one bone is involved and there are no other lymphatic abnormalities.[74] The cysts contain a clear or slightly milky fluid with no diagnostic features.

Treatment

There is no specific treatment for the bone cysts, but fortunately they tend to stop enlarging after the age of 20–30 years and thereafter cause no further symptoms.

The non-involved bone is normal so fractures respond to standard treatment and heal well. Symptoms caused by compression fractures of the spine should be treated by nerve decompression and if necessary by fixation and fusion of the relevant vertebrae. The treatment of any non-skeletal lymphatic abnormalities that may be found is as described elsewhere.

LYMPHANGIOSARCOMA

Lymphangiosarcoma is the only malignant disease of the lymphatics. Although often known by the eponym Stewart–Treves sarcoma,[75] Stewart and Treves were not the first to describe it – this should be credited to Lowenstein, who, in 1906,[76] described a case in the arm and then Kettle, who described a case in the leg in 1918.[77] Because it is a rare and fatal condition, many individual case reports have been published, these being well summarized in 1967 by Danese *et al.*[78] and in 1995 by Gebhart *et al.*[79]

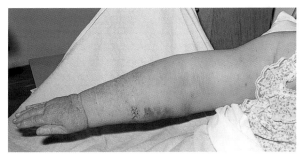

Figure 19.19 *The purple nodules of a lymphangiosarcoma on the medial side of the forearm of a woman with severe lymphoedema of the arm that had been present for 15 years and began following a radical mastectomy. The patient thought that these patches were simple bruises.*

The true prevalence of the condition is not known. Over the past 30 years, during which we have seen more than 5000 patients with lymphoedema (mostly primary), we have encountered only six cases.[80]

Clinical features

Lymphangiosarcomata arise in chronically lymphoedematous tissues. The majority of reported cases have arisen in oedematous upper limbs 10–20 years after a radical mastectomy (Fig. 19.19), but the disease can occur in any long-standing lymphoedema, including cases of primary (Fig. 19.20) and filarial lymphoedema of the lower limb.[81,82] It has also been reported to have developed in lymphangioma circumscriptum.[83]

The patient complains of the appearance of painless, reddish-purple nodules in and deep to the skin of the swollen limb, these increasing in size and number over a period of months. As the nodules grow, they may ulcerate, bleed and become infected. The oedema usually increases as the nodules spread. As time passes, nodules appear beyond the oedematous tissues – on the chest wall and abdomen. At this stage, the patient feels ill, loses appetite and begins to lose weight. The cause of the long-standing oedema is usually apparent from the history.

Investigation

The only diagnostic investigation is a tissue *biopsy*. It is better to excise a complete nodule as incisional biopsies do not heal well and ulcerate.

As the cause of the oedema is usually known there is nothing to gain from investigating the lymphatics of the limb with a lymphogram. The nodules do not appear to have a lymph circulation that connects with the few remaining lymphatics of the limb and are therefore not filled by the Lipiodol.[84]

This sarcoma spreads rapidly to all the viscera and bones so both should be investigated in order to detect

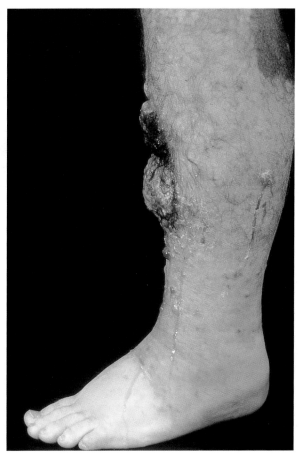

Figure 19.20 *A protuberant, rapidly growing lymphangiosarcoma in a 50-year-old man who had suffered from primary lymphoedema of the leg since adolescence.*

and quantify the extent of any metastatic spread. Most patients have widespread metastasis by the time of presentation.

Treatment

Few patients live for more than 6–12 months after diagnosis. The clinician must make a careful assessment of the balance between the risks and complications of any treatment and the near certainty that it will fail.

Surgery, usually amputation at the shoulder, is usually contraindicated by the presence of widespread metastases. Patients with multiple, ulcerating, painful and smelly lesions occasionally request an amputation for symptomatic relief knowing it will not be curative.

Some temporary remission of the growth of the metastases and an occasional 'cure' has been reported with radiotherapy, intravenous chemotherapeutic agents such as cyclophosphamide, intra-arterial infusions and combinations of all three.[85–91] It is to be hoped that cytotoxic agents will eventually be developed that will control this distressing, fatal complication of long-standing lymphoedema.[92]

REFERENCES

1. Landing BH, Farber S. Tumours of the cardiovascular system. In: *Atlas of tumour pathology*, Section III, Fasicle 7. Washington, DC: Armed Forces Institute of Pathology, 1956.

2. Bill AH, Sumner DS. A unified concept of lymphangioma and cystic hygroma. *Surgery, Gynecology and Obstetrics* 1965; **120:** 79–86.

3. Kittredge RD, Finby N. The many facets of lymphangioma. *American Journal of Roentgenology* 1965; **95:** 56–66.

4. Redenbacher EAH. *De ranula sublingua speciali cum casu congenita.* Monachii: Lindauer, 1828.

5. Broomhead IW. Cystic hygroma of the neck. *British Journal of Surgery* 1964; **17:** 225–44.

6. Morley SE, Ramesar KC, Macleod DA. Cystic hygroma in an adult: a case report. *Journal of the Royal College of Surgeons of Edinburgh* 1999; **44:** 57–8.

7. Pui MH, Li ZP, Chen W, Chen JH. Lymphangioma: imaging and diagnosis. *Australasian Radiology* 1997, **41:** 324–8.

8. Koeller KK, Alamo L, Adair CF, Smirniotopoulos JG. Congenital cystic masses of the neck: radiologic–pathologic correlation. *Radiographics* 1999; **19:** 121–46.

9. Sermon A, Gruwez JA, Lateur L, De Wever I. The importance of magnetic resonance imaging in the diagnosis and treatment of diffuse lymphangioma. *Acta Chirurgica Belgica* 1999; **99:** 230–51.

10. Fung K, Poenaru D, Soboleski DA, Kamal IM. Impact of magnetic resonance imaging on the surgical management of cystic hygromas. *Journal of Pediatric Surgery* 1998; **33:** 839–41.

11. Chevernak FA, Isaacson G, Blakemore KJ, Bregg WR. Foetal cystic hygroma, cause and natural history. *New England Journal of Medicine* 1983; **309:** 822–25.

12. Sun CC, Grumbach K, DeCosta DT, Meyers CM, Dungan JS. Correlation of prenatal ultrasound diagnosis and pathologic findings in fetal anomalies. *Pediatric Developmental Pathology* 1999; **2:** 131–42.

13. Nakajo T, Saeki M, Ogata T, *et al*. Cystic lymphangioma – treatment based on analysis of 273 cases. *Japanese Journal of Pediatric Surgery* 1984; **16:** 931–8.

14. Ikeda K, Suita S, Hayashid Y, *et al*. Massive infiltrating cystic hygroma of the neck in infancy with special reference to bleomycin therapy. *Zeitschrift für Kinderchirurgie* 1977; **20:** 227–36.

15. Yara J, Hashimoto T, Tsuruga N, *et al*. Bleomycin treatment for cystic hygroma in children. *Archives of Japanese Surgery* 1977; **46:** 607–14.

16. Orford J, Barker A, Thonell S, King P, Murphy J. Bleomycin therapy for cystic hygroma. *Journal of Pediatric Surgery* 1995; **30:** 1282–7.

17. Ogita S, Tsuto T, Tokiwa K, Takahashi T. Intra cystic injection of OK-432, a new sclerosing therapy for cystic hygroma in children. *British Journal of Surgery* 1987; **74:** 690–1.

18. Ishida N, Hoshino T. *A streptococcal preparation as a potent biological response modifier, OK-432*, 2nd edn. Amsterdam: Exerpta Medica, 1985.

19. Nagoo K. Studies on treatment of pleural carcinomatosis with special reference to effect of OK-432. *Chiba Medical Journal* 1982; **58:** 345–53.

20. Ravitch MM, Rush BF Jr. Cystic hygroma. In: Welch KJ, Randolph JG, Ravitch MM, *et al*. eds. *Paediatric surgery*. Chicago: Year Book Medical Publications, 1986: 533–9.

21. Takiff H, Calabria R, Yin L, Stabile BE. Mesenteric cysts and intra-abdominal cystic lymphangiomas. *Archives of Surgery* 1985; **120:** 1266–9.

22. Roisman I, Manny J, Fields S, Shiloin E. Intra-abdominal lymphangioma. *British Journal of Surgery* 1989; **76:** 485–9.

23. Harrow BR. Retroperitoneal lymphatic cyst (cystic lymphangioma). *Journal of Urology* 1957; **77:** 82–9.

24. Gray SW, Skandalakis JE. *Embryology for surgeons*. Philadelphia: WB Saunders, 1972.

25. Walker AE, Putnam TC. Omental, mesenteric and retroperitoneal cysts: a clinical study of 33 cases. *Annals of Surgery* 1973; **178:** 13–19.

26. Baker AH. Developmental mesenteric cysts. *British Journal of Surgery* 1961; **48:** 534–40.

27. Rekhi BM, Esselstyn CB, Levi I, *et al*. Retroperitoneal cystic lymphangioma: a report of two cases and a review of the literature. *Cleveland Clinical Quarterly* 1972; **39:** 125–8.

28. Fouty WJ, Sacher EC, Cronemiller PD, Valaske MJ. Rare retroperitoneal tumours presenting as abdominal conditions requiring operation. *Journal of the International College of Surgeons* 1964; **42:** 233–9.

29. Galifer RB, Pons JG, Juskiewenski S, Pasguie M, Gaubert J. Intra-abdominal cystic lymphangiomas in childhood. In: Rikham PP, Hecker W, Prevot J eds. *Progress in pediatric surgery*, Vol. II. Baltimore: Urban & Schwarzenberg, 1978: 173–238.

30. Dietz WH, Stuart MJ. Splenic consumptive coagulopathy in a patient with disseminated lymphangiomatosis. *Journal of Pediatrics* 1977; **90:** 421–3.

31. Henzel JH, Porier WJ, Burget DE, Smith JL. Intra-abdominal lymphangioma. *Archives of Surgery* 1966; **93:** 304–8.

32. Norfleet CM, Fitzsimmons LE, Smith LC, Carlson KP. Ureteral obstruction due to retroperitoneal lymphatic cyst (cystic lymphangioma). *Journal of Urology* 1959; **81:** 737–9.

33. Thomas AMK, Leung A, Lynn J. Abdominal cystic lymphangiomatosis: report of a case and review of the literature. *British Journal of Radiology* 1985; **58:** 467–9.

34. Negus D, Whimster I, Wiernik G. Peritoneal lymphangiectasis. *British Journal of Surgery* 1966; **53**: 740–2.

35. Barnett LA, Branch LNJ. Retroperitoneal cystic lymphangioma. *Journal of the American Medical Association* 1960; **173**: 1111–16.

36. Kalish M, Dorr R, Hoskins P. Retroperitoneal cystic lymphangioma. *Urology* 1975; **6**: 503–6.

37. Raskowski HJ, Rehbock DJ, Cooper FG. Mesenteric and retroperitoneal lymphangioma. *American Journal of Surgery* 1959; **97**: 363–7.

38. Brown L, Reimann HM, Rosenow EC, Gloviczki P, Divertie MB. Intrathoracic lymphangioma. *Mayo Clinic Proceedings* 1986; **61**: 882–91.

39. Halliday DR, Dahlin DC, Pugh DG, Young HH. Massive osteolysis and angiomatosis. *Radiology* 1964; **82**: 637–44.

40. Pedicelli G, Mattia P, Zorzoli AA, Sorrone A, DeMattino F, Sciotto V. Gorham syndrome. *Journal of the American Medical Association* 1984; **252**: 1149–51.

41. Pilla TJ, Wolverson MK, Sundaram M, Heiberg E, Shields JB. CT evaluation of cystic lymphangiomata of the mediastinum. *Radiology* 1982; **144**: 841–2.

42. Edieken J. Roentgen diagnosis of diseases of bone. In: Harris JH ed. *Golden's diagnostic radiology*, Section 6, Vol. 1. Baltimore: Williams & Wilkins, 1981: 138–49.

43. Brewster DC. Early complications of vascular repair below the inguinal ligament. In: Brehard VH, Towne JB eds. *Complications of vascular surgery*. Orlando: Grune & Stratton, 1985: 37–53.

44. Williams RA, Vetto J, Quinones-Baldrich W, Bougard FS, Wilson SE. Chylous ascites following aortic surgery. *Annals of Vascular Surgery* 1991; **5**: 247–52.

45. Jansen TT, Debruyne FM, Dalaere KP, deVries JD. Chylous ascites after retroperitoneal lymph node dissection. *Urology* 1984; **23**: 565–7.

46. Calkins CM, Moore EE, Huerd S, Patten R. Isolated rupture of the cisterna chyli after blunt trauma. *Journal of Pediatric Surgery* 2000; **35**: 638–40.

47. Kwann JHM, Bernstein JM, Connolly JE. Management of lymph fistula in the groin after arterial reconstruction. *Archives of Surgery* 1979; **114**: 1416–18.

48. Busch T, Lofti S, Sirbu H, Dalichan H. Chyloperitoneum, a rare complication after abdominal aortic aneurysm repair. *Annals of Vascular Surgery* 2000; **14**: 174–5.

49. Fox T, Fox TC. On a case of lymphangiectodes with an account of the histology of the growth. *Transactions of the Pathology Society of London* 1879; **30**: 470–6.

50. Francis AG. Lymphagioma circumscriptum cutis. *British Journal of Dermatology* 1893; **5**: 33, 65.

51. Whimster IW. The pathology of lymphangioma circumscriptum. *British Journal of Dermatology* 1976; **94**: 473–86.

52. Edwards JM, Peachey RDG, Kinmonth JB. Lymphangiography and surgery in lymphangioma circumscriptum. *British Journal of Surgery* 1972; **59**: 36–41.

53. Peachey RDG, Lim CC, Whimster IW. Lymphangioma of the skin. A review of 65 cases. *British Journal of Dermatology* 1970; **83**: 519–27.

54. Eliezri YD, Sklar JA. Lymphangioma circumscriptum: review and evaluation of carbon dioxide laser vaporization. *Journal of Dermatology and Surgical Oncology* 1988; **14**: 357–64.

55. Bailin PL, Kantor GR, Wheeland RG. Carbon dioxide laser vaporization of lymphangioma circumscriptum. *Journal of the American Academy of Dermatology* 1986; **14(Pt 1)**: 257–6.

56. Weingold DH, White PF, Burton CS. Treatment of lymphangioma circumscriptum with tunable dye laser. *Cutis* 1990; **45**: 365–6.

57. Denton AS, Baker-Hines R, Spittle MF. Radiotherapy is a useful treatment for lymphangioma circumscriptum: a report of two patients. *Clinical Oncology (Royal College of Radiology)* 1996; **8**: 400–1.

58. O'Cathail S, Rostom AY, Johnson ML. Successful control of lymphangioma circumscriptum by superficial X-rays. *British Journal of Dermatology* 1985; **113**: 611–15.

59. Browse NL, Whimster I, Stewart G, Helm CW, Wood JJ. Surgical management of lymphangioma circumscriptum. *British Journal of Surgery* 1986; **73**: 585–8.

60. Manders EK, Egan N, Davis TS. Elimination of lymphangioma circumscriptum by suction-assisted lipectomy. *Annals of Plastic Surgery* 1986; **16**: 532–4.

61. Harris R, Prandoni AS. Generalised primary lymphangiomas of bone: report of a case associated with congenital lymphoedema of the forearm. *Annals of Internal Medicine* 1950; **33**: 1302–5.

62. Hayes JT, Brody GL. Cystic lymphangiectasis of bone. *Journal of Bone and Joint Surgery* 1961; **43A**: 107–17.

63. Tsyb AF, Mukhamedzhanov IK, Guseva LI. Lymphangiomatosis of bone and soft tissue. *Lymphology* 1983; **16**: 181–4.

64. Gomez CS, Calonje E, Ferrar DW, Browse NL, Fletcher DM. Lymphangiomatosis of the limbs. *American Journal of Surgical Pathology* 1995; **19**: 125–33.

65. Gorham LW, Stout AP. Massive osteolysis (acute spontaneous absorption of bone, phantom bone, disappearing bone): its relation to haemangiomatosis. *Journal of Bone and Joint Surgery* 1955; **37A**: 985–1004.

66. Bickel WH, Broders AC. Primary lymphangioma of the ilium: report of a case. *Journal of International Surgery* 1947; **29**: 517–22.

67. Gutierrez RM, Spjut HJ. Skeletal angiomatosis. *Clinical Orthopedics and Related Research* 1972; **85**: 82–95.

68. Edwards WH, Thompson RC, Varsa EW. Lymphangiomatosis and massive osteolysis of the cervical spine. *Clinical Orthopedics and Related Research* 1983; **177:** 222–9.

69. Morphis LG, Arcinue EL, Krause JR. Generalized lymphangioma in infancy with chylothorax. *Pediatrics* 1970; **46:** 566–75.

70. Berberich FR, Bernstein ID, Ochs HD, Schaller RT. Lymphangiomatosis with chylothorax. *Journal of Pediatrics* 1975; **87:** 941–2.

71. Asch MJ, Cohen AH, Moore TC. Hepatic and splenic lymphangiomatosis with skeletal involvement. Report of a case and review of literature. *Surgery* 1974; **76:** 334–9.

72. Najman E, Fabecic-Sabadi V, Temmer B. Lymphangioma in the inguinal region with cystic lymphangiomatosis of bone. *Journal of Pediatrics* 1967; **71:** 561–6.

73. Albright F, Butler AM, Hampton AO, Smith P. Syndrome characterized by osteitis fibrosa disseminata and endocrine dysfunction with precocious puberty in females. *New England Journal of Medicine* 1937; **216:** 727–46.

74. Jumbelic M, Fenerstein IM, Dorfman HD. Solitary intraosseous lymphangioma. *Journal of Bone and Joint Surgery* 1984; **66A:** 1479–81.

75. Stewart FW, Treves N. Lymphangiosarcoma in post-mastectomy lymphoedema. *Cancer* 1948; **1:** 64–81.

76. Lowenstein, 1906. Cited in Danese CA, Grishman E, Oh C, Dreiling DA. Malignant vascular tumours of the lymphoedematous extremity. *Annals of Surgery* 1967; **166:** 245–53.

77. Kettle, 1918. Cited in Danese CA, Grishman E, Oh C, Dreiling DA. Malignant vascular tumours of the lymphoedematous extremity. *Annals of Surgery* 1967; **166:** 245–53.

78. Danese CA, Grishman E, Oh C, Dreiling DA. Malignant vascular tumours of the lymphoedematous extremity. *Annals of Surgery* 1967; **166:** 245–53.

79. Gebhart M, Chasse E, Petein M. Lymphangiosarcoma. Reports of 3 cases and review of the literature. *European Journal of Surgical Oncology* 1995; **21:** 211–14.

80. Mulvenna PM, Gillham L, Regnard CF. Lymphangio-sarcomata – experience in a lymphoedema clinic. *Palliative Medicine* 1995; **9:** 55–9.

81. Gajraj H, Barker SG, Burnand KG, Browse NL. Lymphangiosarcoma complicating chronic primary lymphoedema. *British Journal of Surgery* 1987; **74:** 1180.

82. Muller R, Hadju SI, Brennan MF. Lymphangiosarcoma associated with chronic filarial lymphoedema. *Cancer* 1987; **59:** 179–83.

83. King DT, Duffy DM, Hirose FM, Gurevitch AW. Lymphangiosarcoma arising from lymphangioma circumscriptum. *Archives of Dermatology* 1979; **115:** 969–72.

84. Kinmonth JB. *The lymphatics,* 2nd edn. London: Arnold, 1982.

85. Rawson AJ, Frang JK. Treatment by irradiation of lymphangiosarcoma in post-mastectomy lymphoedema. *Cancer* 1953; **6:** 269–72.

86. Southwick HW, Slaughter DF. Lymphangiosarcoma in post-mastectomy lymphoedema: five year survival with irradiation treatment. *Cancer* 1955; **8:** 158–60.

87. Greenspan FM. Angiosarcoma responsive to cyclophosphamide after failure of the combination of thiotepa and methotrexate. *Cancer Chemotherapy Reports* 1961; **11:** 147–55.

88. Herman JB, Ariel IM. Therapy of lymphangiosarcoma of the chronically oedematous limb: a five year cure of a patient treated with intra-arterial radioactive yttrium. *American Journal of Roentgenology* 1967; **99:** 393–9.

89. Tragus ET, Wagner DE. Current therapy for post-mastectomy lymphangiosarcoma. *Archives of Surgery* 1968; **97:** 839–42.

90. Tong D, Winter J. Post-mastectomy lymphangiosarcoma. *British Journal of Surgery* 1974; **61:** 76–8.

91. Malhaire JP, Labat JP, Simon H, *et al.* One case of Stewart–Treves syndrome successfully treated at two years by chemotherapy and radiation therapy in a 73-year-old woman. *Acta Oncologica* 1997; **36:** 442–3.

92. Breidenbach M, Rein D, Schmidt T, *et al.* Intra-arterial mitoxantrone and paclitaxel in a patient with Stewart–Treves syndrome: selection of chemotherapy by an ex vivo ATP-based chemosensitivity assay. *Anticancer Drugs* 2000; **11:** 269–73.

Index

Indexer: Dr Laurence Errington

Note: The text makes comprehensive reference to the figure numbers and to the relevant material in those figures. Therefore, figures appearing on a different page to the related text have not been given an additional page reference. Only important items mentioned exclusively in figure legends have been given page references.